Molecular
Biology
Intelligence
Unit

The Molecular Mechanisms of Cancer Predisposition

Neil F. Sullivan, M.B.A., Ph.D.

Newcastle University Ventures Ltd.
Newcastle Upon Tyne, U.K.

Anne E. Willis, Ph. D.

Department of Biochemistry
University of Leicester
Leicester, U.K.

R.G. Landes Company
Austin

Molecular Biology Intelligence Unit
THE MOLECULAR MECHANISMS OF CANCER PREDISPOSITION
R.G. LANDES COMPANY
Austin

CRC Press is the exclusive worldwide distributor of publications
of the Molecular Biology Intelligence Unit.
CRC Press, 2000 Corporate Blvd., NW, Boca Raton, FL 33431. Phone: 407/994-0555.

Submitted: September 1994
Published: December 1994

Please address all inquiries to the Publisher:
R.G. Landes Company, 909 Pine Street, Georgetown, TX 78626
or
P.O. Box 4858, Austin, TX 78765

Phone: 512/ 863 7762; FAX: 512/ 863 0081

ISBN 1-57059-193-8
CATALOG # LN9193

Library of Congress Cataloging-in-Publication Data

Sullivan, Neil F., 1959-
The molecular mechanisms of cancer predisposition / Neil F. Sullivan, Anne E. Willis.
p. cm.—(Molecular biology intelligence unit)
Includes bibliographical references and index.
ISBN 1-57059-193-8
1. Carcinogenesis. 2. Cancer—Susceptibility. 3. Cancer—Molecular aspects.
4. Cancer—Etiology. I. Willis, Anne E., 1962- . II. Title. III. Series.
{DNLM: 1. Disease Susceptibility. 2. Neoplasms—etiology. ap 202 S951m 1994}
RC268.5.S827 1994
616.99'4071—dc20
DNLM/DLC 94-38487
for Library of Congress CIP

While the authors, editors and publisher believe that drug selection and dosage and the specifications and usage of equipment and devices, as set forth in this book, are in accord with current recommendations and practice at the time of publication, they make no warranty, expressed or implied, with respect to material described in this book. In view of the ongoing research, equipment development, changes in governmental regulations and the rapid accumulation of information relating to the biomedical sciences, the reader is urged to carefully review and evaluate the information provided herein.

To Our Readers

R.G. Landes Company publishes four book series: *Medical Intelligence Unit, Molecular Biology Intelligence Unit, Neuroscience Intelligence Unit,* and *Biotechnology Intelligence Unit.* Our goal is to publish the most recent information in biomedical science for sophisticated researchers and physicians.

To achieve this goal we have accelerated our publishing program to conform to the fast pace in which information grows in biomedical science. Most of our books are published within *90 to 120 days* of receipt of the manuscript.

As you might expect, this causes a few problems for us; sometimes it makes our office more like a big city newspaper than a scholarly publisher. So as you look through this book you may see something that isn't just right. Please let us know. Or if you have an idea for improving our books, we'd like very much to hear from you. If the problem you describe hasn't already been discovered or if your idea is provocative enough to promote a discussion here, we'll give you a free book of your choice. Just list three titles in order of preference and we'll send you one, based on availability—with our thanks. Our address is printed on the copyright page of each of our books.

Carol Harwell
Publications Director
R.G. Landes Company

CONTENTS

PROLOGUE

In this book we are attempting to raise issues germane to the study of mechanisms for predisposition to cancer. We will illustrate the value of the human cancer prone inherited diseases as models for the cancer process, in the context of broader arguments which relate to the etiology and molecular biology of cancer. In doing so, we hope to show how the myriad of changes which lead to neoplasia are beginning to be identified. Since the researcher usually has access only to either normal or end point tissue, it is rare that intermediate stages can be defined and studied. Improvements in therapy could be envisaged if intermediate stages could be identified and as such, we hope this text will serve to generate debate in this direction.

We have assumed a basic knowledge of cell and molecular biology regarding intracellular structure and function, including DNA structure, transcription, translation etc.. Thus we have built upon these principles to describe the development of the tumor cell and the molecular changes which may contribute to the transformation of a normal cell. The field is full of interesting and informative research papers, most of which deserve mention. This is of course impossible to do in such a short text, and thus we have attempted to select papers which offer either a good introduction to a subject or particularly profound research information.

We hope that you enjoy reading this book as much as we have enjoyed writing it and that it stimulates thought and discussion in your laboratories and classrooms.

Dedication

This book is dedicated to May and Jim Sullivan

and to Edward Willis.

CHAPTER 1

Introduction: Cancer in Context

Cancer is a disorder which affects almost all multicellular organisms and which usually appears as a mass of cells, known as a tumor. The disease was first identified as having a cellular composition by Müller in 1830 and since then it has been convincingly demonstrated that cancer is the result of a series of genetic changes which develop towards an often lethal endpoint. The definition of a tumor cell is necessarily heuristic as our current operational definitions are continuously influenced by a wealth of new information. However, the advent of both molecular biology and new techniques in cell biology now affords possibilities for unraveling these processes.

In man, all of the four main tissue types have been associated with cancer. The bone marrow normally gives rise to cells of the reticuloendothelial system (white and red blood cells) which are either in circulation or are present as fixed populations within given tissues such as the liver and lymph nodes. Disruption of the cellular status quo in these tissues can result in the diseases commonly known as leukemia and lymphoma. The nervous tissues consist of the brain, the central and peripheral nervous system and the supporting cells. Here disorders such as neuroblastoma, meningioma and neurofibrosarcoma occur. The mesenchymal tissues consist of connective tissue, bone, muscle and blood vessels which are associated with the cancers known as fibrosarcoma, osteosarcoma, rhabdomyosarcoma and hemangiosarcoma, respectively. Finally, there are cancers derived from the epithelium of organs such as skin and liver, exemplified by melanoma and carcinoma.

These tissues are usually arranged in an interdependent way. For example, skin epithelium is supported by a layer of muscle and connective tissue (mesenchyme) which is both innervated and supplied with blood. Other tissues retain a similar pattern but vary in terms of the arrangement of the mesenchyme and the specific nature of the cells involved. The size attained by a given organ is precisely controlled throughout life with tissue replacement occurring via proliferation of a pool of stem cells which are capable of differentiation into the required cell types. Organ size is presumably regulated by positive and negative influences which control the extent of hypertrophy (increase in cell size), selective cell death (apoptosis) and hyperplasia (increase in cell number).

It has been suggested that only a minority of cancer patients have genetic predisposition as a primary determinant of their disease, and indeed, epidemiological studies do indicate that the children of parents with a particular form of cancer have only a small (two- to three-fold) increased risk of contracting a similar cancer. However, we will argue that this could reflect the operation of more profound mechanisms which involves cancer predisposing genes of low penetrance and the reduced probability of acquisition of consequential genetic changes. Using modern molecular biology techniques, genes for some of these familial cancers have been identified and localized to particular chromosomes. We will discuss the evidence which relates to particular examples, those of predisposition to lung, stomach and breast cancer. However, in a small proportion of patients, mutations are inherited and often appear to involve the same mixture of genes as the sporadic cancer. To date, only a few inherited mutations have been identified (Table 1.1), and the evidence which suggests predisposition to cancer is often correlative and rarely indicates causal relationships. However, the elucidation of the underlying genetic mechanisms of predisposition to cancer is of the highest importance and will doubtless provide insights into the pathology of both the inherited and sporadic forms of a given cancer. Indeed, the extent to which inherited mutation augments the action of environmental agents is one of the key questions in cancer biology today.

There have been several models proposed to explain the progression towards carcinogenesis, none of which are completely satisfactory. The promoter/initiator hypothesis, whereby the sequential action of particular classes of environmental carcinogens (taken to mean chemical or radiation) results in cancer, will be used as a benchmark since this is the most widely accepted hypothesis. A fuller discussion of both this and the initiation, promotion, malignant conversion and progression model for the accumulation of complementing "all or nothing" changes[1] will follow in later chapters, but for now the basic premises will suffice. An initial lesion in DNA (there are other possible targets), which could be due to the action of a carcinogenic chemical, viral infection, radiation or a DNA replication error may persist for the lifetime of the individual. The affected cells are said to be initiated. The action of a tumor promoting agent, which in itself cannot produce tumors, then follows, perhaps by further carcinogenic action, the action of hormones, normal growth promoters or an inflammatory response. Initiated cells have at least one

Table 1.1. Dominantly acting genetic tumor predisposition

Syndrome	Chromosome (Gene)	Tumor
Familial adenomatous polyposis	5q (APC)	Colorectal adenoma
Familial breast cancer	17q	Breast carcinoma
Familial melanoma	9p	Malignant melanoma
Gorlin Syndrome	9q	Naevoid basal cell carcinoma
Hereditary non-polyposis colorectal cancer	2p	Colon carcinoma (and several others)
Li-Fraumeni	17p (p53)	Many tumor types
Multiple Endocrine Neoplasia type 1	11q	Parathyroid glands, pancreatic islet cells
Multiple Endocrine Neoplasia type 2	10	Pheochromocytoma
Neurofibromatosis type 1	17q (NF1)	Neurofibrosarcoma, leukemia
Neurofibromatosis type 2	22q (NF2)	CNS tumors
Retinoblastoma	13q (Rb)	Retinoblastoma
von Hippel-Lindau	3p	Many tumor types
Wilms' tumor	11p (WT1)	Kidney lesions

transformation predisposing step although they may not necessarily grow abnormally. Using our simple definition, this must follow from the action of the promoting agent when the cells enter a growth and division cycle. However, it is important to note that some agents can induce cell division without predisposing to tumor development. Tumor promoting agents may interfere with the differentiation process as stem cells enter the differentiated population, whilst still leaving these cells sensitive to the normal action of growth inhibitory factors. Thus a spectrum of preneoplastic and fully transformed cells could be found, which may not necessarily grow or die at the requisite time. Workers exposed to the action of particular industrial carcinogens may not develop cancer for over 20 years and probably contain many initiated cells. By the same arguments therefore, only a tiny proportion of those cells previously initiated will eventually produce tumors. Carcinogenic agents surround us throughout our lifetimes, whether these be X rays due to sunlight, medicine or dentistry, ultra violet irradiation (sunlight), exposure to viruses, cigarette smoke or the constituents of our diet (e.g. well cooked meat). There are examples of tumors which are both age and organ specific, e.g., in the embryo, Wilms' kidney tumor, neuroblastoma; in the young (leukemia, bone, testis); and in the old (prostate, colon, bladder, skin). In the latter case we might rationalize by suggesting an age dependent: (a) increase in susceptibility to carcinogens, (b) cumulative effect of continuous exposure to low doses of carcinogens throughout life or (c) humoral change to the hormonal system or decreased efficiency of the immune system. For the embryonic and juvenile cancers it is less clear still; we may consider, for example, over-activity of growth factors involved in cell proliferation. There are as yet no clear answers but for the undoubted association with genetic change, whether this be by chromosomal aberration, gene mutation or gene loss.

1. CANCER INCIDENCE AND EPIDEMIOLOGY

Over their lifetime, one in three people will develop cancer and in over 70% of cases it will be in those over 60 years of age. Cancers of the lung account for approximately 15% of all new cancers diagnosed with two-thirds of these being in males. This figure in part represents the post 1940 male tradition of smoking and to it should be added a percentage of other cancers thought to be related to exposure to cigarette smoke, e.g., esophageal and stomach. For women, the most common cancer is that of the breast (approximately 18% of all new cancer diagnoses) followed by those of the reproductive system (ovary, cervix and uterus together account for 10% of all new diagnoses). In males, prostate cancer contributes 10% to all new cases diagnosed.

In both sexes there are high frequencies of skin cancers and tumors of the gastrointestinal system (19% and 13% in males and females; figures include colon, stomach, rectum and esophagus) although with the exception of malignant melanoma nearly all new cases of skin cancer are curable and 5-year survival rates are high (97%). What is notable, however, is that despite intensive research, the 5-year survival rate for many types of tumors, e.g., lung cancer, is still very low (7%), with the exception of malignant melanoma. Lung cancer in women is currently showing an alarming rate of increase.

One of the most important ways in which to study cancer is that of epidemiology, the identification of suspected cancer risk factors.[2] These include smoking, diet, exposure to sunlight, reproductive habits, industrial and environmental pollution and genetic makeup. All vary from country to country as do the rates of particular forms of cancer. For example, there appears to be a general increase in cancer as one moves from southern to northern Europe, particularly in common cancers such as lung, breast and colon. The rarer cancers such as those of the larynx, esophagus and liver tend to be more frequent in southern Europe. The incidence of malignant melanoma is increasing at 3% per annum in northern Europe—a figure considered epidemic in proportion. This is most likely linked to the recent preoccupation of northern Europeans with one or two week high dose UV irradiation holidays in southern Europe. Other social factors have impact upon cancer incidence; for example, the overall incidence of breast cancer in Spain is two-fold lower than in the UK, probably due in part to the tendency for earlier child birth. We may expect other significant correlations to appear as the effects of 'Iron Curtain' pollution are revealed and the long term effects of nuclear weapons testing and/or nuclear power plant mishaps become apparent. There is weak evidence for leukemia clusters in children around particular UK nuclear power plants, although we must consider if other leukemia clusters situated around the country are of similar epidemiology. The latter clusters have been correlated with living in regions of radon gas and high social class!

2. MOLECULAR CLUES TO THE CANCER PROCESS

In humans, cancer is a result of multiple steps which arise from alteration of the genome in a manner that is inconsistent with the cellular status quo.[3] We must identify exactly which genetic changes are necessary and decide whether it is the accumulation of transformation associated changes or the order of acquisition which is important. Furthermore, many of these genes are expressed in a variety of tissues whilst others show a more restricted distribution. What determines this and is it relevant to the development of a tumor in that tissue? In addition, only a tiny population of affected cells will eventually form a tumor yet all contain the inherited mutation. What are the parameters of the clonal selection which must occur?

The epidemiological evidence suggests that there will be on average four to six rate limiting and independent steps necessary for a diagnosable cancer to develop.[4] This follows from the observation that in age dependent cancers the rate of tumor development is proportional to the fourth to sixth power of elapsed time. There are of course exceptions to this rule but it does provide an idea of the magnitude of the problem. In certain cases, the epidemiology suggests that a minimum of two changes may be sufficient (e.g. elimination of both alleles of a tumor suppressor gene) but for the majority, several changes are likely to be required. To date the evidence does not suggest that there are a fixed number of genetic events associated with any particular tumor type.

Usually, genetic abnormalities are both acquired and accumulated during the lifetime of the individual but in some cases these genetic changes are inherited. This may be either inheritance of a genetic change which directly affects the transformation state of particular cells within a tissue or one which increases susceptibility to, for example, environmental carcinogens. As some of the genetic abnormalities which are associated with cancer are identified, so they begin to appear in patients with familial cancer predisposition and vice versa. It would come as no surprise if each sporadic human cancer was found to have an inherited partner. However, due to variability in penetrance of cancer predisposing inherited genetic changes, it is difficult to distinguish between the rare cancer prone syndromes of high gene penetrance and cancer predisposition in the general population due to genes of low penetrance.

The genetic changes which can occur in a cell and contribute to augmentation of transformation related pathways can be classified as either: (a) oncogenes, (b) mutator genes which act in a dominant fashion or (c) those which normally act to suppress transformation—the tumor suppressor and DNA repair associated genes. In addition, epigenetic changes such as genomic imprinting may be involved. Many such genes have now been identified and examples from several cellular pathways have been implicated in aberrant control of cell growth. Whether we find defined patterns of genetic change associated with particular tumors at particular stages remains to be seen, but the inherited cancer prone syndromes do offer us a step towards resolution of this issue. By identification of the pattern of premalignant lesions, we can both delimit the biological consequences of these changes and ask the nature of the *extra* changes which lead to particular types of tumor. As we shall see later, particular inherited syndromes can be associated with either specific tumor types or a broad range.

A model which we find useful is that of the 'vicious downward spiral' (Fig. 1.1) whereby any given change can make subtle increases in selection pressure for subsequent growth enhancing changes, with a net cumulative effect. This implies that once the cancer process has begun, i.e., has acquired a mutation which has escaped either the DNA repair or immunosurveillance mechanisms, the cell is inexorably launched on the transformation pathway and clonal selection ensues. In cellular terms, there are at least four 'fail safe' mechanisms which help protect against genetic alterations, being: (a) detection of mutations and chromosomal aberrations, followed by direct repair of the DNA (genomic surveillance). In this case, inefficiencies in the DNA repair machinery will result in the accumulation of mutations, perhaps introduced as a result of imprecision during DNA replication or direct damage of DNA due to the action of radiation or chemical carcinogens,[5-7] (b) immune surveillance, whereby the expression of abnormal proteins which are produced as a result of transcription and translation of a mutated gene and are expressed on the cell surface, can be detected and the abnormal cells destroyed (c) internal mechanisms for detection of mutant proteins, e.g., in the incorrect conformation due to point mutation and (d) programmed cell death or apoptosis.

i. Oncogenes

Oncogenes were first isolated as the genes responsible for the transforming component of the RNA tumor viruses. Onkos is derived from the Greek for mass or bulk. Viral oncogenes (v-*onc*) were shown subsequently to have homologous cellular counterparts (c-*onc*) and became known as proto-oncogenes. In all cases, these genes have a normal role in cell proliferation and differentiation, but when their expression or activities are altered, they contribute to the circumvention of normal growth control mechanisms. Oncogenes, for which examples have been found at several stages of the signal transduction pathways which lead to cell cycle progression, will be discussed in chapter 2. However, for the present, we should consider that this might involve cell surface receptors, membrane proteins (e.g. G proteins), membrane and cytoplasmic protein phosphorylation reactions, changes in nuclear transcription and probably several other intracellular events.

ii. Tumor Suppressor Genes

In a classic paper, Knudson[8] first demonstrated the concept of recessive cancer mutations by predicting mutations at both alleles of a single (then unidentified) locus for a rare juvenile tumor known as retinoblastoma. These children with multiple tumors were predicted to have inherited a mutation in one allele such that a one step mutation of the second allele was sufficient to allow tumor development. Modern molecular biology has provided additional evidence for this hypothesis with both the identification of deletions at the site of the retinoblastoma gene on chromosome 13 and a correlation with allele loss in tumor tissue. In addition, reintroduction of the normal gene suppressed tumorigenicity.

A number of more complicated examples have since been elucidated, perhaps the best known of which is the Wilms' kidney tumor, where studies involving loss of heterozygosity have revealed allele loss at either of two loci on different chromosomes. Indeed, there is a preferential loss of the Wilms' gene locus on chromosomes inherited from maternal sources, implicating a role for genomic imprinting in tumor development. Tumor suppressor genes

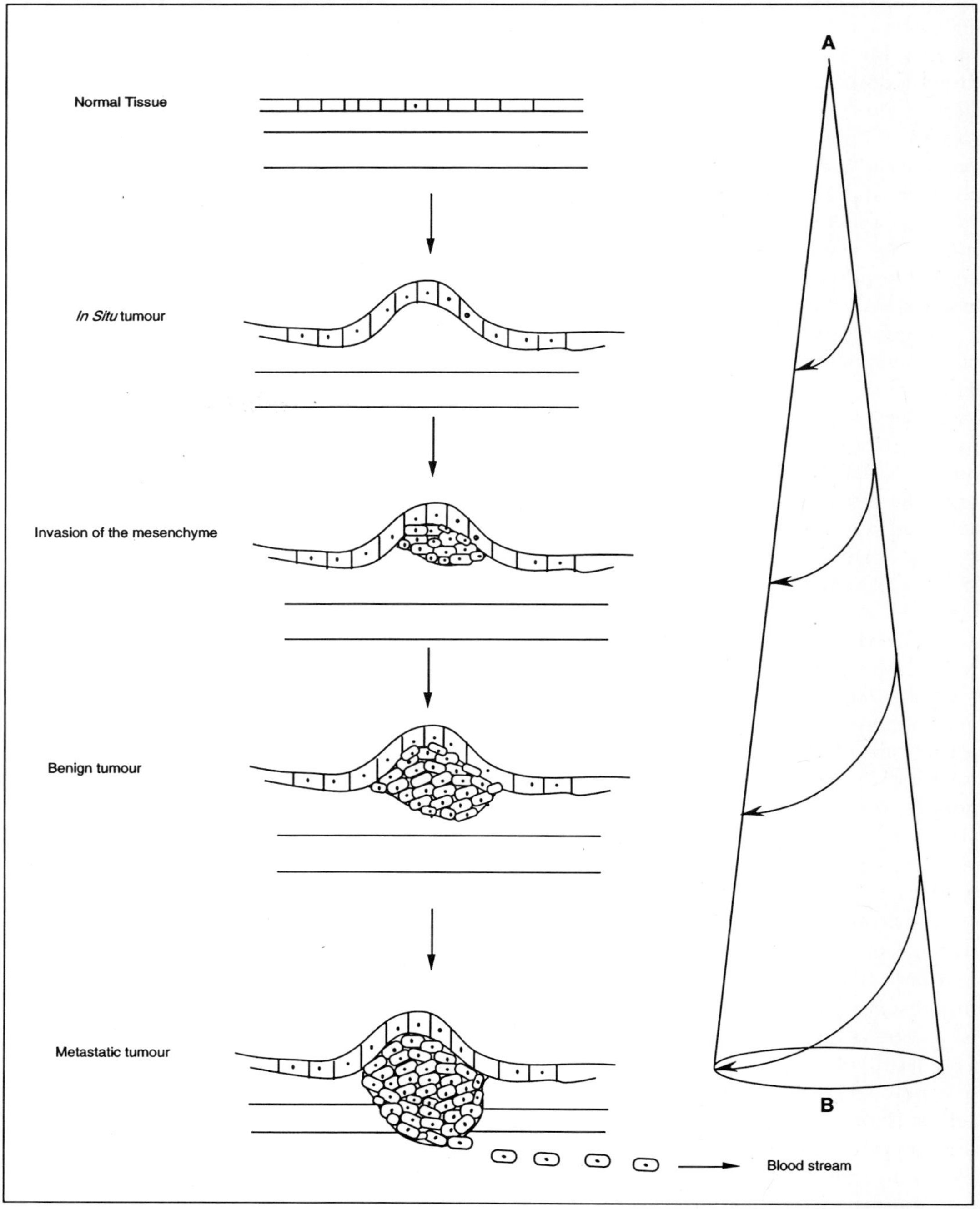

Fig. 1.1. The downward spiral towards cancer. As the initial step (A), a cell acquires one or more mutations which lead to the first histological signs of an abnormality, the in situ tumor. By this time, several consequential cellular changes may have occurred as has a degree of clonal selection. Further rounds of mutation lead to the ability to invade the mesenchyme and to the eventual formation of a benign tumor. Subsequently, the tumor may acquire metastatic capability and cells may enter the blood and lymphatic systems (B).

probably act as negative controls upon the cell cycle, perhaps being associated with differentiative rather than proliferative molecular processes, or being responsible for control of the rate of cell cycle progression. Mutations in the tumor suppressor gene p53 are the most common aberrations found to date in human cancers. Whilst in excess of 98% of these mutations can be acquired by the individual during the course of their lifetime, germline p53 mutations do have an inherited basis, as is demonstrated by the familial Li-Fraumeni syndrome.

3. CANCER SUSCEPTIBILITY

A genetic association with cancer may be indicated by early age of onset, the occurrence of multiple tumors and a Mendelian pattern of familial tissue inheritance. In considering the latter, environmental clues must also be considered since a 'cancer cluster' could reflect a higher background level of an environmental carcinogen, for example, radon in the cellar of the family home. The molecular basis of the association can be considered in three categories and will form the basis for the discussion in the rest of this book. Firstly, cancer predisposition could result from inheritance of any of the known oncogenes, although this has not yet been observed. There are, however, examples of dominantly acting cancer predisposing somatic mutations (Table 1.1). Secondly, cancer may result from inheritance of a tumor suppressor gene mutation such as the p53 or retinoblastoma gene product. The importance of tumor suppressor genes is now beginning to be realized, especially as the number of associations between both the inherited cancer syndromes and nonfamilial cancers is shown to increase. Other more complex patterns of inheritance (non-Mendelian) will also be discussed. Thirdly, and an area to which we will devote considerable attention, is cancer predisposition due to secondary effects such as mutations in genes associated with the repair of DNA. Cancer prone syndromes associated with the latter are generally recessive traits which are depicted by a recessive mutation of relatively low penetrance, although there may be some exceptions. Thus there is an opportunity for a homozygous mutant cell to clonally develop within a tissue (perhaps in conjunction with subsequent somatic mutational events), preceded by somatic mutation of the inherited allele in the heterozygote. Penetrance can be considered low since the majority of susceptible individuals (heterozygotes), together with the majority of susceptible cells within a tissue, do not progress to cancer. However, the situation increases in complexity when we consider, for example, the autosomal recessive inherited cancer prone chromosome breakage syndromes (Table 1.2). For example, in ataxia telangiectasia recessive mutations affect the cell cycle in a secondary and apparently stochastic way via the inactivation of the tumor suppressor gene p53. These syndromes must be distinguished from cancer predisposition associated with given structural or quantitative chromosomal abnormalities. The former are characterized by general genomic instability in in vitro cell culture but are cytogenetically distinct, whilst the latter involve particular chromosomal additions or deletions. Indeed, so precise is the correlation between cytogenetic alterations and particular familial syndromes that these chromosomal abnormalities have been used to map and clone the genes associated with several cancer prone disorders such as Wilms' tumor, retinoblastoma and neurofibromatosis type-1. If specific types of tumor are associated with activation of a particular set of oncogenes and/or inactivation of particular tumor suppressor genes, then we may expect the same set of oncogenes and tumor suppressor genes to be activated and inactivated in the DNA repair deficiency diseases which manifest the same specific types of tumor. By implication, therefore, deficiencies in particular DNA repair pathways (as a result of inability to repair lesions resulting from defined subsets of carcinogens) must result in activation of a particular set of oncogenes. We will discuss the possible effects of preferential

Table 1.2. Autosomal recessive inherited chromosome breakage syndromes

Chromosome breakage syndromes	Chromosomal abnormality
Ataxiatelangiectasia	Increase in chromosomal rearrangements often involving chromosome 14
Bloom's syndrome	Increased sister chromatid exchange
Fanconi's anemia	Increased chromatid breaks and exchanges
Nijmegen breakage syndrome (and Semanova syndrome)	Rearrangements involving chromosome 7 and 14. Very similar to ataxia telangiectasia
Werner's syndrome	Clonal expansion of particular rearrangements
Xeroderma pigmentosum	Chromosomal abnormalities elevated after ultraviolet irradiation

repair of actively transcribed regions and the role of chromatin structure in later sections, but meanwhile, it is important to consider the potential role of both the DNA repair and DNA replicative mechanisms in control of gene expression.

4. HOW ARE CANCER PREDISPOSING GENE DEFECTS INHERITED?

There are two clear ways in which genetic disorders may be inherited: firstly by acquiring a mutation in a single gene and secondly by inheritance of a chromosomal abnormality. Either of these may interact with environmental elements to elicit the final tumor, but without an obvious Mendelian pattern of inheritance. Mechanisms of predisposition to cancer may require, for example, the definition of subtle changes in expression of genes which mediate chemical detoxification and/or DNA repair or the effects of enzyme polymorphisms.

There are a number of clinically relevant cytogenetic changes which are of both diagnostic and prognostic significance, predominantly arising out of research into the hematological malignancies.[9] For solid tumors, there is less data available due to the difficulties encountered in cytogenetic analyses of these tissues. Cancer related chromosomal abnormalities are nonrandomly distributed in the genome[10] and may be of two forms, either directly related to the cancer in question, i.e., the sole genetic abnormality and tightly correlated with the tumor type, or of a secondary nature whereby they may be one of a number of different cytogenetic abnormalities which contribute to the growth of the cancer in different ways. The nature of the cytogenetic change may be either: (a) chromosomal translocation whereby a portion of one chromosome fuses with another, perhaps to activate an oncogene or inactivate a tumor suppressor gene, (b) amplification of particular regions to reprogram cell development by titration of tumor suppressor genes or amplification of oncogenes or (c) chromosomal deletion which might either remove tumor suppressor genes or juxtapose oncogenes. Point mutations and small insertions/deletions will also occur, but these are likely to be outside the range of detection by cytogenetic techniques. There are at least three oncogenes (c-*myc*, c-*abl* and c-*rel*) that have been shown to be rearranged by chromosomal translocation.

One of the key characteristics of leukemia/lymphoma is the presence of specific reciprocal translocations. The consistent association of such translocations with disease types has not only provided useful diagnostic criteria, but has helped identify steps in the transformation process. The first clear example was that of the Philadelphia chromosome in chronic myelogenous leukemia (CML), whereby a t(9,22)(q34;q11) occurred. Subsequently, translocations were identified in Burkitts' lymphoma t(8,14) and several other tumor types. Indeed, up to 3% of all tumors are thought to have consistent chromosomal translocations. Gene disregulation may result from juxtaposition of cellular proto-oncogenes with enhancer or promoter sequences that are active in the cell type in question. In Burkitts lymphoma, the transcription factor c-*myc* becomes under expression of the immunoglobulin heavy chain or λ or κ light chain enhancers. Similar examples occur with the T-cell receptor enhancer. Chimeric oncogene proteins may also arise via translocation, which allows expression of the transformation ability of both participants. For example, in the aforementioned CML, a *bcr-abl* fusion reveals a tyrosine kinase activity of *abl;* such activities have often been associated with transformation. The *bcr* gene product encodes a guanosine triphosphatase (GTPase) activating protein (GAP) for p21-*rac*, a c-*ras* related protein which is presumably involved in signal transduction. The GAP proteins are crucial to the modulation of c-*ras* activity and the effects of related genes such as the tumor suppressor NF1 will be discussed. Similarly, a t(5,14)(q31:q32) breakpoint has been cloned from pre-B cell acute lymphocytic leukemia and results in the positioning of a strong immunoglobulin H enhancer (chromosome 14) next to the interleukin-3 gene. Over expression of this cytokine then contributes towards leukemogenic processes. A number of other transformation associated proteins are activated by chromosomal translocation, including the retinoic acid receptor (α) protein, transcription factors (*lyl*-1, *tcl*-5), a homeobox protein (*tcl*-3), a protein involved in mediation of protein dimerization (*rbn* T1), putative cell cycle proteins (*bcl*-1, *bcl*-3 and mediators of apoptosis (*bcl*-2). In addition to the aforementioned translocations, solid tumors show a greater degree of gene amplification (via trisomy, isochromosomes, homogeneously staining regions [HSR's] and double minute chromosomes [DM's]) although identification of the culprit gene vis-á-vis phenotypic change is difficult, mainly because large regions are often amplified. Trisomy of chromosome 7 is common in epithelial tumors, whilst trisomy of chromosomes 8 and 21 are common in myelodysplastic syndrome (chapter 8). Isochromosome formation is relatively variable although i(12p) is a consistent feature of germ cell malignancies. DM's and HSR's are responsible for the 10- to 100-fold amplification of a small number of genes and is a common form of activation of the c-*myc* proto-oncogene in colon adenocarcinoma and the N-*myc* proto-oncongene in late stage (III and IV) neuroblastomas. Similarly, the epidermal growth factor gene is amplified in glial brain tumors as is *erb*b2 (*neu*) in advanced breast and ovarian adenocarcinomas. Amplifications of 11p occur in up to 20% of melanoma, squamous cell tumors and breast carcinomas.

The existence of these chromosomal rearrangements and abnormalities and the association with transformation is clear. However, the most crucial questions concerning the source of clonal advantage remains to be answered. Does the cell already have a selective growth advantage which can be augmented by selection of a chromosomal rearrangement involving proliferation pertinent genes, or does the genome undergo continual cycles of breakage repair and checking such that eventually, a growth selective rearrangement escapes surveillance and stimulates clonal selection? In some diseases, the presence of general chromosome breakage and rejoining is insufficient to be the sole cause of transformation but can predispose to cancer (section 3). In ataxia telangiectasia for example, clonal expansion of translocation positive T lymphocytes occurs in a pre-leukemic phase, but it is not known whether this directly contributes to clonal selection. However, the random nature of the breaks and rearrangements suggests that there could be a defect in a process which mediates genomic surveillance, bringing forth the implication that these rearrangements are continual and random, with the majority either having no selective advantage and/or being detected. The cell could deal with such lesions by utilizing DNA repair or apoptosis mechanisms, the failure of which could leave a cell capable of clonal selection within its population. In the former case, whereby the cell already has a selective advantage, the quest for further growth advantage will exert pressure to select for translocations which augment the growth of that particular cell type. Hence we may rationalize the expansion of, for example, the clonal expansion of pre-B cells, in acute lymphocytic leukemia within a population of B cells at different stages of differentiation.

i. Acquisition of Mutation

There are four modes in which single gene defects may be inherited and transmitted to future generations: autosomal recessive, autosomal dominant, linkage of either the X or Y chromosomes or mitochondrial. Of these, the autosomal recessive mode is probably the most common. There are both exceptions and grey areas where these definitions begin to break down, but for now, we will consider each in turn.

a. Autosomal recessive

Here the phenotype is only expressed in those homozygous for the mutation, i.e., both alleles carry an abnormality in the gene. Since heterozygotes have one normal allele, they are phenotypically, but not necessarily biochemically, normal. The frequency of occurrence invariably increases with the extent of population inbreeding and estimates of gene frequency across the population as a whole will obviously be inaccurate. In addition, the frequency varies according to ethnic group and indeed, this can be highly relevant to the decisions which relate to prenatal screening.

b. Autosomal dominant

Here the heterozygotes exhibit the disease phenotype although there may be different degrees of severity. This is due to a variation in the extent of gene expression and gene penetrance, i.e., the extent to which the gene can affect the final phenotypic characteristics. From a molecular point of view, it is interesting to note that the penetrance of dominant cancer syndromes is dependent upon the age of the individual concerned.

c. X linked recessive inherited syndromes

In general, only males can be affected by such syndromes since females will obviously have two X chromosomes and be heterozygous. Some of the latter may however, express certain disease characteristics. This contrasts to the X linked dominant inherited syndromes in which the disease phenotype is expressed in both females and males. Females may exhibit the full phenotype if, in the rarest of cases, both X chromosomes acquire a similar mutation, if there is a chromosomal translocation between an autosome and an X chromosome or if the individual is affected by Turner's syndrome.

d. Mitochondrial

Mitochondria are inherited from the egg, rarely, if at all, from the sperm. This means that a certain proportion of the DNA from maternal sources can transfer inherited mutations to offspring, whether these are male or female.

ii. Genomic Imprinting

Depending on parentage, certain genes are expressed differently in embryonic development and manifest as phenotypic variation in autosomal dominant disorders. For example, neonatal myotonic dystrophy occurs only if the gene is maternally inherited. These effects may be due to gene inactivation by DNA methylation, but the molecular basis is, at the moment, largely unclear. Genomic imprinting may be apparent as retention of paternal alleles in particular tumor types (embryonal rhabdomyosarcoma, Wilms) where it is known that a paternal tumor suppressor gene is inherited.[11] This has a number of important implications regarding the tumor suppressor genes and inherited predisposition to cancer since the two hit model proposed for retinoblastoma[8] did not predict such a bias, and in other examples, the marked sex bias of autosomally inherited tumors implies that other genetic mechanisms are activated. One suggestion is that this occurs via a genomic imprinting mechanism whereby a male derived tumor suppressor gene is inactivated, perhaps by hypomethylation leading to a loss of imprinting (LOI) and hence either gene activation or inactivation.[12] Alternatively, hypermethylation may contribute to differential locus mutability. Such mechanisms are often referred to in the literature as epigenetic. Two hypotheses for the involvement of genomic imprinting in tumor formation are illustrated (Fig. 1.2).

iii. Limitation by Sex

Certain autosomal disorders, e.g., ovarian cancer can obviously only be expressed in females.

5. WHAT MAKES A 'TRANSFORMED' CELL?

Before we discuss the particular molecules and genes thought to be involved in disrupting cellular growth control, we will first review the properties of the transformed cell. It would not be unreasonable to suppose that cellular abnormalities have a molecular basis and that the selective pressures which contribute to the accumulation of mutation in these genes must confer advantage in one or more of these characteristics, in addition to effects upon the cell cycle. For these discussions a transformed cell will be defined as one which has any deviation from the growth associated behavior pattern that it would normally be expected to have.

i. Characteristics of the Transformed Cell

a. Transformed cells are often aneuploid, i.e., their chromosomal complement may be abnormal or unstable.
b. In addition, transformed cells are often heteroploid, and even within an individual tumor there can be a range of cells with different numbers of chromosomes.
c. There can be a loss of contact inhibition, the normal process whereby cells stop growing upon meeting their compatriots in any given tissue. The consequences of loss of contact inhibition could be multiple layering of, for example, epithelial cells.
d. Transformed cells often have a higher saturation density in in vitro culture, perhaps again a reflection of factors which control cell-cell proximity. This is particularly relevant to the cells of the reticuloendothelial system whereby production and response to circulatory growth factors may help limit uncontrolled expansion of circulating B and T cells.
e. Transformed cells often exhibit anchorage independence and in vitro will form colonies in soft agar with a higher efficiency than normal cells. In vivo this may be equivalent to a reduced requirement for attachment to the extracellular matrix.
f. Transformed cells often exhibit higher secreted protease activity, e.g., urokinase or plasminogen activator. This may help in invasion of surrounding tissues or release of the growth constraints furnished by the extracellular matrix or intracellular adhesion.
g. As tumors grow beyond 1 mm in size, they must have access to a source of dissolved oxygen and nutrient. Many transformed cells secrete factors which aid angiogenesis and hence vascularization of the developing tumor.
h. Tumor cells often exhibit the property of invasiveness, whereby they acquire the capability to infiltrate neighboring tissues, or indeed, in the case of metastasis, distant tissues. This is a step beyond loss of normal intracellular contact signals since these cells may now develop affinities for other types of cell, perhaps by expressing different cell adhesion or extracellular matrix molecules.
i. Tumor cells must, in the final instance, have the ability to form tumors when xenografted into nude mice.

Thus the cellular decline towards the transformed state is probably initiated by chromosomal rearrangement and/or acquisition of mutations that alters the expression

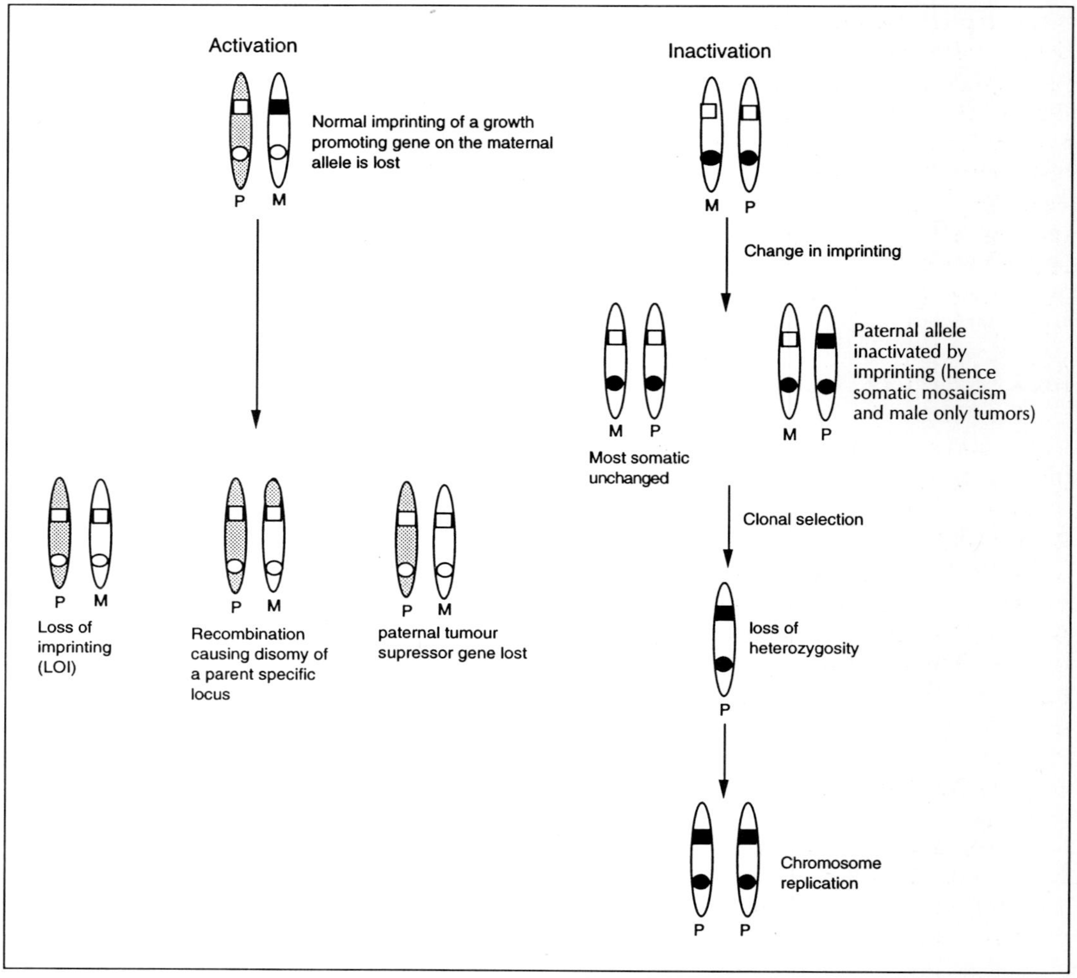

Fig. 1.2. Loss of heterozygosity and imprinting: two hypotheses for the involvement of genomic imprinting in cancer development.

of genes involved in growth regulation, thus affording the opportunity for clonal expansion. This is likely to be paralleled by changes which allow growth outside of the normal cellular environment, perhaps by loss of molecules which regulate either normal cell-cell contact and/or interactions with the extracellular matrix. In some cases, cells may attain the ability to lodge and invade completely different tissues and finally, tumor cells may ensure their own nutrient supply by secretion of factors which aid in their own vascularization.

ii. On the Nature of Cell Immortalization

The phenomenon of immortalization, i.e., the ability of a cell to proliferate indefinitely in in vitro culture has probably not received the attention due to it over the past few years. Immortalization or 'establishment' is a prerequisite for many cell culture systems and cell transformation models. It can be induced by over expression of particular cellular transcription factors such as c-*myc* and also be viral oncogenes such as the adenovirus E1a gene product or the SV40 large T antigen. But what constitutes immortalization at a mechanistic level? It is worth taking a sideways step to examine this property in more detail. Each somatic cell has within it a preprogrammed number of divisions within the tissue, and upon the relevant stimulus, can often be triggered to re-enter the cell cycle. For example, this is important in wound healing as fibroblasts migrate to the site of a cut or hepatocytes aid in liver regeneration. This is in general a defense mechanism for somatic cells and is not related to their normal (differentiated) cellular function. Stem cells could theoretically divide indefinitely, each time giving a replacement of itself and a derivative which will be the precursor of one or more differentiated cell types. We may envisage different degrees of proliferative capacity within each stem cell compartment, this in itself being preprogrammed. As one moves back in development, we intuitively suspect that the proliferative capacity of stem cells will increase until we reach (at least) the embryonic stem cell of the blastocyst, the last cell type after fertilization that can be said to give rise to all tissues of the resultant fetus. We must now consider several points:

1. How are the number of divisions preprogrammed?
2. How are they counted?
3. How does the cell use this number to either signal entry into a new cell cycle or trigger apoptosis, and
4. How can these controls be overcome, e.g. by excess activity of a transcription factor such as c-*myc*?

There is very little experimental evidence which relates to any of these points, although it is fairly easy to come up with a scheme to facilitate the above criteria. The point is, however, that such pathways must exist and they remain to be identified. For now, we may assume that the immortalized cell has forgotten how to count its past number of divisions.

iii. The Cell Cycle, Functionality and the Cellular Defense Mechanisms

All life is a series of choices, whether this be choice of a partner, choice of a residence, choice of food etc. In order to make these choices, we come upon decision points and, guided by the available information, we launch off in one direction or another, being unable to sit on the fence forever. So too with cells, which must address the choice between reproduction (proliferation), functionality (differentiation) and death (apoptosis).

Cancer cells proliferate when they shouldn't, avoid the jobs they should do and often do something different (and not very well) and have found ways to escape the normal death processes. Therein lies a blurring of the normal decisions which relate to proliferation, differentiation and apoptosis (Fig. 1.3), an irrepressible chaotic trend whereby normal functionality is altered in the interest of short term gain. What then are the decisions to be made?

Any population of cells in any tissue reflects a subtle balance between renewal, functionality and death. All cells are resident at some point in the cell cycle (by definition) and within this, there are decision points. These may be purely manifested in the cell cycle of the here and now, use information from past cell cycles or be in preparation for events in future cell cycles. There are three directions which the cell may take: (a) it may proliferate, (b) it may differentiate or (c) it may decide to self-destruct. The choice will depend upon several factors, which can be broadly classified into internal and external categories (Table 1.3). Let us suppose that there is a cell in a resting or quiescent state. A change in circumstance (e.g. via the growth factor milieu or exposure to DNA damaging agents) may cause the cell to reconsider its position. If the signals are consistent with growth and replication then so be it; if they are consistent with a requirement for greater functionality then we may expect a couple of cell divisions preprogrammed to lead to a more differentiated state. If only some of the necessary factors are present for proliferation (cellular confusion) or functionality is no longer required, then in the normal course of events we would expect the cell to die. Under the

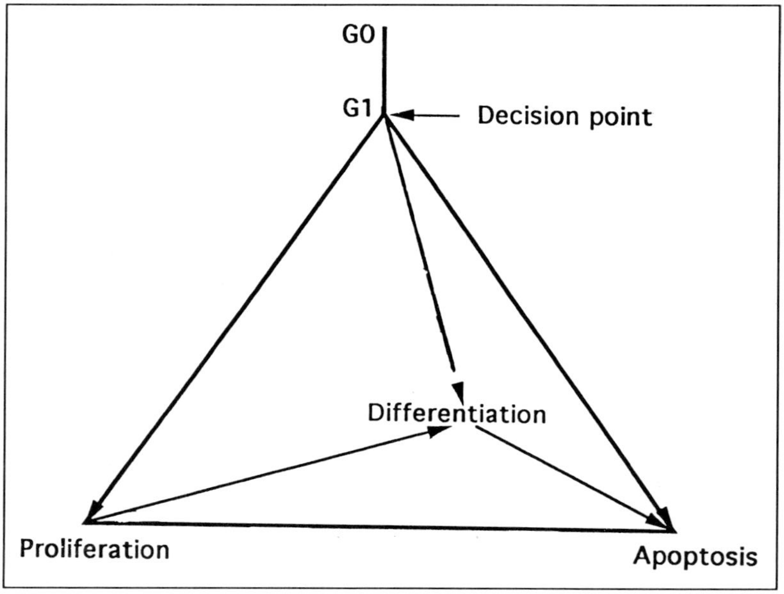

Fig. 1.3. The cellular choices.

Table 1.3. Determinants of the cellular fate

External signals	Internal facilitators	Responses
Cytokines/hormones	Genetic predisposition	Quiescence
Cell to substrate interactions	Cell type	Proliferation
Cell to cell interactions	Tissue type	Differentiation
	Metabolic state	Apoptosis
	Epigenetic position	
	State of repair	

influence of extracellular factors and internal facilitators the cell enters the cell cycle and must then make an appropriate decision. Proliferation is an orderly sequence of events (DNA replication, chromosome condensation, mitosis etc.) which is regulated by the cell itself, using a series of checkpoints which are designed to stop late events occurring before the completion of earlier events. For example, certain evidence suggests that there is a protein complex that can determine the replication state of the DNA and hence provide the necessary signals for mitosis to proceed.

The proliferative capacity of a cell is, roughly speaking, inversely proportional to the extent of differentiation. If some of the signals necessary for either of these processes are absent, then the cell is likely to detect that something is wrong upon reaching the next checkpoint and at this point it may decide to instigate a death pathway. Escape from such altruistic behavior is highly important in cancer development. Excess cell proliferation is an obvious route to tumor development, but an important point to remember is that proliferation and mutagenesis go hand in hand. If any lesions remain in place prior to DNA replication then at cell division the mutation will be transmitted to the daughter cells. An important factor in mutagenesis is the rate of cell division, the two being directly proportional. Conversely, nondividing cells would be expected to have a lower mutation frequency and a lower frequency of cancer development, which is indeed the case. Any agent which may increase cell division (cytokines, chemical, hormones, chronic infection) may thus also increase cancer risk. Many such compounds are induced as a result of normal metabolism or are taken in the diet, e.g., oxidants could increase cell division indirectly, perhaps via an inflammatory response and resultant wound healing. We might thus expect antioxidants to decrease the rate of cell division by decreasing the mutation frequency.

What are the effects of mutation in stem cells? A mutation in a stem cell will be amplified in the cycle of renewal and in the incompletely differentiated progeny that still have the capacity to proliferate. If this is a growth enhancing mutation, the effect will be to accelerate the process of clonal selection.

References

1. Harris CC. Human tissues and cells in carcinogenesis research. Cancer Research 1987; 47:1-10.
2. Henderson BE, Ross RK, Pike MC. Toward the Primary Prevention of Cancer. Science 1991; 254:1131-1137.
3. Hansen MF, Cavenee WK. Tumour suppressors: Recessive mutations that lead to cancer. Cell 1988; 53:172-173.
4. Peto R, Roe FJC, Lee PN et al. Cancer and ageing in mice and men. British Journal of Cancer 1975; 32:411-426.
5. Ames BN, Gold L. Too many rodent carcinogens: Mitogenesis increases mutagenesis. Science1990; 249:970-971.
6. Ames B, Gold L. Carcinogenesis debate (letter). Science 1990; 250:1498-1499.
7. Ames B, Gold L. Chemical carcinogenesis: Too many rodent carcinogens? Proc Natl Acad Sci 1990; 87:7772-7776.
8. Knudson AG. Mutation and cancer; A statistical study. Proc Natl Acad Sci 1971; 68: 820-823.
9. Solomon E, Borrow J, Goddard AD. Chromosome aberrations and cancer. Science 1991; 254:1153-1160.
10. Mitelman F. Clustering of chromosomal breakpoints in neoplasia. Cancer Genetics and Cytogenetics 1986; 19:67-71.
11. Scrable HJ, Sapienza C, Cavenee WK. Genetic and epigenetic losses of heterozygosity in cancer predisposition and progression. Adv Cancer Res 1990; 54:25-62.
12. Leach RJ, Magewu AN, Buckley JD et al. Preferential retention of paternal alleles in human retinoblastoma: Evidence for genomic imprinting. Cell Growth and Differentiation 1990; 1:401-406.

SECTION 1

The Biology of the Cancer Cell

In this section we will discuss some basic molecular and cell biological aspects of cancer, a means of introduction to the ways in which cell growth and development could be disregulated. This will include a discussion of oncogenes, growth factors, tumor suppressor genes, DNA repair pathways, immune surveillance mechanisms, models for chemical carcinogenesis and finally the metastatic process itself.

We will then discuss the progression towards colon cancer, where several steps in the transformation pathway have been identified, and to some extent, ordered. This example neatly illustrates the 'multiple step' nature of the cancer process.

CHAPTER 2

Genetic Influences upon Cell Growth

1. THE CELLULAR TAPESTRY

We have already seen that the number of cells in a tissue is precisely controlled by the balance between proliferation, differentiation and cell death; furthermore, that these mechanisms are by and large under genetic control. Epidemiological evidence demonstrates that multiple genetic changes are required for tumor formation and within each type of tumor, a different subset of several genetic changes could have occurred in any given group of cells. The process of clonal selection, whereby each genetic or epigenetic change enhances the growth properties of a given cell is operative. Each alteration, however slight, expands the population of modified cells giving them a growth advantage and thus creates an expanded target pool for subsequent genetic changes. What then, are the nature of these changes? Assuming no prior knowledge, we might envisage several mechanisms whereby the cellular status quo could be disrupted, leading to: (a) a growth advantage and (b) changes in the rate of progress through the cell cycle. Disregulation of genes involved in cell surface interactions and cell adhesion will be important, as will that of genes which control passage through the cell cycle, differentiation and apoptosis. We may envisage both positive and negative influences upon entry, exit and progression through the cell cycle, which will ultimately decide whether the cell divides, differentiates or dies. The interactions between the molecules involved can be thought of as a delicately balanced ecosystem, perhaps a rain forest with all of the delicate and consequential nuances therein. Small changes in one factor can have profound effects upon the whole system, which then reacts to restore the balance. These small changes are part and parcel of normal evolution, small eco-experiments to find out what will work and what will not, all the time pushing the system to find out areas of selective advantage. One might consider then, that a slight loss in the ability to react to and correct these changes may result in the development of an 'early' tumor cell, which then builds upon its advantage by failing to restore the balance resulting from subsequent exploration with different areas of possible advantage. In one particular environment, change A may be favored, in another B or C. Hence, we may consider that each cell environment has a set of "most likely" clonally selectable changes which may differ from that of a neighboring cell environment, from that of a neighboring organ or indeed, from the equivalent position in a different individual.

From this perspective, one can propose that any attempt to compartmentalize the genetic changes into 'boxes' is likely to be unsatisfactory as there will always be considerable overlap between these boxes and exceptions to the rule. The transformation related genetic changes form a continuum of cause and effect, some of which are more profound than others. This has lead to terminology such as 'oncogene', 'antioncogene', 'proto-oncogene' and 'tumor suppressor gene' for identification of the most obvious examples. However, it remains our thesis that many genes not currently identified under the above labels will also contribute to clonal selection and hence be 'transforming' changes. It is not, therefore, the case that oncogenes are equal and opposite to either antioncogenes or tumor suppressor genes, and each serves to counter the other. It is more likely that each plays an important role in the cellular tapestry, the absence or excess of which disrupts the integrity of the whole picture. Both oncogenes and tumor suppressor genes may act in either a dominant or recessive fashion, examples of which will be discussed in the next few sections. Other examples of dominant negative and gene dosage related mechanisms will be considered.

We do not propose a lengthy listing and discussion of the characteristics which pertain to each and every oncogene and tumor suppressor gene. This is material which has been adequately covered by others. However, the points germane to our discussion relate to: (a) general mechanisms of signal transduction which affect alterations in either cell cycle progression or cell biological properties and (b) how the cancer prone inherited diseases give us insight into transformation related steps which may have already occurred.

2. ONCOGENES AND ANTIONCOGENES

We will begin our discussion by identification of the four areas in which oncogenes have been discovered. None can be considered an 'oncogene' without due recourse to the cellular milieu and we must continue to give due attention to the interaction with internal cellular biochemical events such as phospholipid turnover. Oncogenes have been found in extracellular signaling molecules (v-*sis*), at the plasma membrane (*ras, src, abl*), in the cytoplasm (*raf, erb*-A) and in the nucleus (*myc, myb, ski, jun, fos*). Events at the membrane and in the nucleus dominate the literature, but it remains to be seen if they will dominate the transformation pathways. At the plasma membrane, enzymes with tyrosine kinase activity are of importance to signal transduction and probably regulate the activities of other proteins via a cascade of phosphorylation. These can be considered to be of two classes: the receptor based tyrosine kinases (e.g. the platelet derived growth factor receptor) and the nonreceptor tyrosine kinases (e.g. *c-src*, *c-abl*). These phosphorylation events then signal changes in other kinases, regulatory proteins, G proteins, phospholipid dependent enzymes and probably others, to initiate internal cellular processes such as inositol phospholipid turnover, calcium mobilization, ionic exchange and the activation of transcription factors. In general, it appears that there is a degree of cooperation between the transcription factor class of oncogenes and those of other categories, in order to elicit the transformed phenotype.

Firstly, we will discuss a key member of the signal transduction mechanism, the p21-*ras* oncogene, and secondly we will continue with a discussion of the 'oncogenic' receptor and nonreceptor based tyrosine kinases. Thirdly, the link with examples of cytoplasmic oncogenes and pathways towards activation of transcripton will follow.

i. p21-ras Mediated Signal Transduction

The p21-*ras* proteins belong to a large family of guanine nucleotide binding proteins with GTPase activity, which includes the important class of signal transducing proteins (G proteins) and factors involved in translational control. These proteins are biologically inactive when bound to guanosine diphosphate (GDP) and active when bound to guanosine triphosphate (GTP) (Fig. 2.1). There are several members of the p21-*ras* family (Ha-, Ki-[A,B alleles], N- and others) of oncogenes which all participate in transformation by accentuation of their normal function, i.e., transmission of signals from plasma membrane associated tyrosine kinases to a cytoplasmic cascade of threonine and serine kinases on the path towards the nucleus. Other members of the p21-*ras* family are also worthy of mention because of the diversity of cellular functions with which they are associated.[1] The *rab* proteins are involved in intracellular vesicle transport, *ran* proteins are nuclear GTPase's involved in mitosis, *raf* proteins are necessary for G protein ADP-ribosylation by cholera toxin and the *rho/rac* proteins are involved in cytoskeletal organization. Upon growth factor binding, actin reorganization occurs at the plasma membrane and requires *rac*, whilst *rho* is necessary for the formation of actin stress fibers. In particular, *rac* proteins may be important in mutagenesis, since they act in the NADPH dependent generation of superoxide radicals in phagocytes.

The *ras* proteins have often been compared to an important class of cellular signal transducing molecules called the G proteins. These consist of three subunits: α, β and γ of which the α subunit binds to either GTP or GDP.[2] One function of the G proteins is to activate the enzyme adenylate cyclase and hence synthesize cAMP. The latter activates a cAMP dependent protein kinase, protein kinase A, which is active in signal transduction. A number of other G proteins have been discovered (Table 2.1) and have been characterized by their sensitivity to various toxins. The p21-*ras* protein is considered to be a Gα protein by virtue of its ability to bind guanine nucleotides and its having an intrinsic GTPase activity. However, it is less than half the size of other Gα proteins (21 kDa versus 45 kDa), has little or no sequence homology and does not activate adenylate cyclase. The p21-*ras* gene family must therefore be considered to be a separate type of G protein. However, in some tissues there are G protein activating mutations which may contribute to the transformation process; 43% of pituitary adenomas exhibit mutations in the domain of Gαs which inhibits the GTPase activity. This is likely to inhibit cAMP production thus leading to a reduction in the protein kinase A cascade, which intuitively speaking would constitute a nontransforming change. Clearly, more experiments must be performed in order to understand the significance of such mutations in this tumor type.

The GTP bound form of p21-*ras* has an intrinsic GTPase activity with a relatively low rate of GTP hydrolysis; this can be stimulated up to 100-fold by p120 GAP, the GTPase activating protein. The action of neurofibromin (NF-1), one of the GAP family of proteins, will be discussed in the context of a tumor suppressor gene. These GAP proteins negatively regulate p21-*ras* but may also have other effector functions. The p21-*ras* protein is normally present on the inner surface of the plasma membrane whilst GAP is cytosolic. Thus in order for GAP to negatively regulate p21-*ras*, the latter protein is sequestered to the membrane.[3] Without this, it would indeed be difficult to rationalize both the transforming action of p21-*ras* and the inhibition of the transforming effects of v-*src* in the presence of excess GAP. In the latter case, there is also a decrease in the concentration of $[\text{p21-}ras]_{\text{GTP bound}}$. The *ras* GAP protein is phosphorylated on tyrosine in response to stimulation of cells with PDGF, EGF or CSF-1. This appears to induce interaction with at least two other tyrosine phosphorylated proteins, p62 and p190 in a mechanism which probably involves one

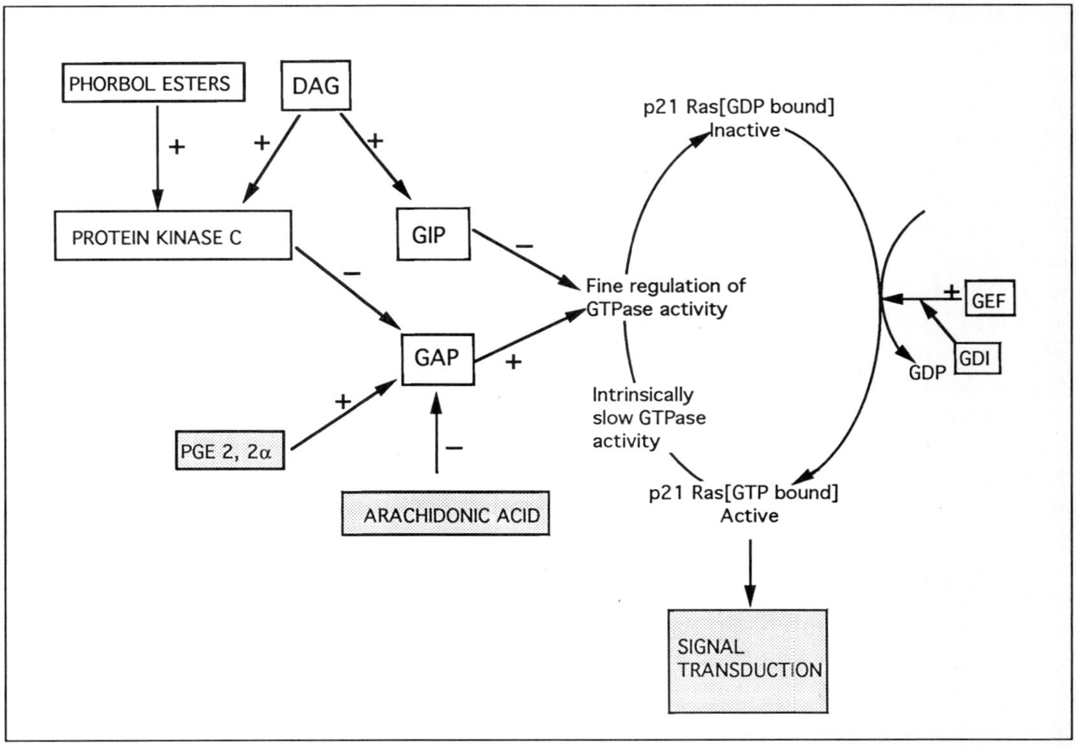

Fig. 2.1. Signal transduction via ras. *DAG, Diacyl Glycerol; PGE, Prostaglandin E; GAP, GTPase Activating Protein; GIP, GTPase Inhibitory Protein; GEF, Guanine Nucleotide Exchange Factors; GDI, Guanine Nucleotide Dissociation Inhibitors.*

or both of the two SH2 domains (see below) on *ras* GAP.[4] However, whether p120-GAP is a biologically relevant p21-*ras* effector molecule has not yet been determined and evidence is now suggesting that there is an interaction between p21-*ras* and a serine/threonine kinase known as c-*raf*-1.[5] Precedents for Gα protein GAP activities exist and phospholipase Cβ and the γ subunit of phosphodiesterase perform this function for Gq and transducin. A second hypothesis, whereby p21-*ras* is also the effector for p120-GAP, must also be considered. In this case the oncogenic form of the p21-*ras* protein would lead to persistent p120-GAP activation and thus transcriptional activation downstream of p21-*ras* via the p120-GAP *src* homology (SH-3 domains). The p21-*ras* protein is activatable by a protein which catalyzes the exchange of GDP for GTP, the guanine nucleotide exchange factor (GEF). GTP is the predominant guanine nucleotide in human cells and as such, the equilibrium heavily favors exchange of GDP. However, it should be noted that the exchange reaction will occur at a low basal rate in the absence of GEF. GEF's recognize both the GDP and GTP bound form of p21-*ras* in vitro, but the action in vivo is probably mediated by other factors.

Many extracellular factors may result in activation of p21-*ras* genes which is suggestive of both different pathways for p21-*ras* regulation and cell type dependent differences in these pathways. For example, an increase in guanine nucleotide exchange activity correlates with p21-*ras* activation on nerve growth factor treated pheochromocytoma cells (PC12) and epidermal growth factor treatment of fibroblasts, whilst similar activation of p21-*ras* results in a decrease in GAP activity as measured in vitro in phorbol ester treated T cells.

Table 2.1. G proteins

G protein	Alpha subunit	Function	Sensitivities
Gs	s	activates adenylate cyclase	cholera toxin
Gi	i	inactivates adenylate cyclase	pertussis toxin
Gp	?	activates phosphoinositide dependent phospholipase C	pertussis toxin
Go	o	ion channels in the brain	pertussis toxin
Transducin	T	activates cGMP dependent phosphodiesterase	pertussis and cholera toxin
p21 *ras*		cell proliferation	none

What then, is the mechanism by which p21-*ras* participates in signal transduction? The clues to this puzzle have in part come from studies of *Caenorhabdans elegans* whereby mutations in the *sem*-5 gene can be rescued by p21-*ras* (*let*-60) activation. The *sem*-5 gene product is an adaptor protein which appears to help proteins assemble into multiprotein complexes and a mammalian homologue, *grb*2 and other such molecules (*shc*, *crk*, and *nck*) have been identified. The *grb*2 protein associates with *sos*-1 (a guanine nucleotide exchange protein) via its SH-3 domain; current models suggest that this complex is involved in recruitment of p21-*ras* (Fig. 2.2). This process is independent of receptor activation since: (a) it is observed in vitro with recombinant proteins and (b) *grb*2-*sos* complexes occur in inactivated cells. The most likely explanation, therefore, is that ligand binding to a receptor causes it to dimerize and autophosphorylate. This then facilitates binding to molecules involved in signal generation, such as the phospholipases, phosphatidylinositol 3-OH kinase and *grb*2, via a special region known as the SH2 (or *src* homology) domain. This induces a conformational change in *grb*2 such that its interaction with *sos* is strengthened via binding to a second SH3 domain which in turn facilitates recruitment of p21-*ras* to the local area, followed by nucleotide exchange. The latter generates the active $[\text{p21-}ras]_{\text{GTP bound}}$ moiety, which then triggers the p21-*ras* dependent kinase cascade.[6-8] Why then do several receptor and nonreceptor tyrosine kinases appear to deliver their message through a conserved molecule such as p21-*ras*? How does the cell achieve specificity or diversity in the signals it receives? First of all, the adaptor proteins (which may be legion) have a semi-permissive interaction with other proteins via the SH2 domains. Whether this applies to the SH3 domain is not yet clear. Secondly, the SH2 and SH3 domains occur in a large number of the proteins which participate in the signal transduction pathways and a single domain within a protein, e.g., an SH2 domain within phospholipase C could allow interaction with a restricted set of tyrosine kinase receptors. Together, it becomes apparent that the scope for variety in protein-protein interactions in response to a given signal is enormous. We must not forget the possible subtle regulation involved with the other proteins with which p21-*ras* interacts. For example, the *grb*2 and/or *sos* proteins may be modified by other signals from the receptor tyrosine kinase which then modulates their ability to participate in coupling. Alternatively, the accumulation of $[\text{p21-}ras]_{\text{GTP bound}}$ may be irrelevant if GAP activity is high; the latter may require inhibition for signal transduction to proceed. Another mammalian p21-*ras* activating protein *ras* GRF does not require receptor tyrosine kinase activity and has a relatively restricted tissue distribution when compared to the *sos* proteins. The *ras* GRF protein does not contain the proline rich SH3 domains and is probably subject to membrane

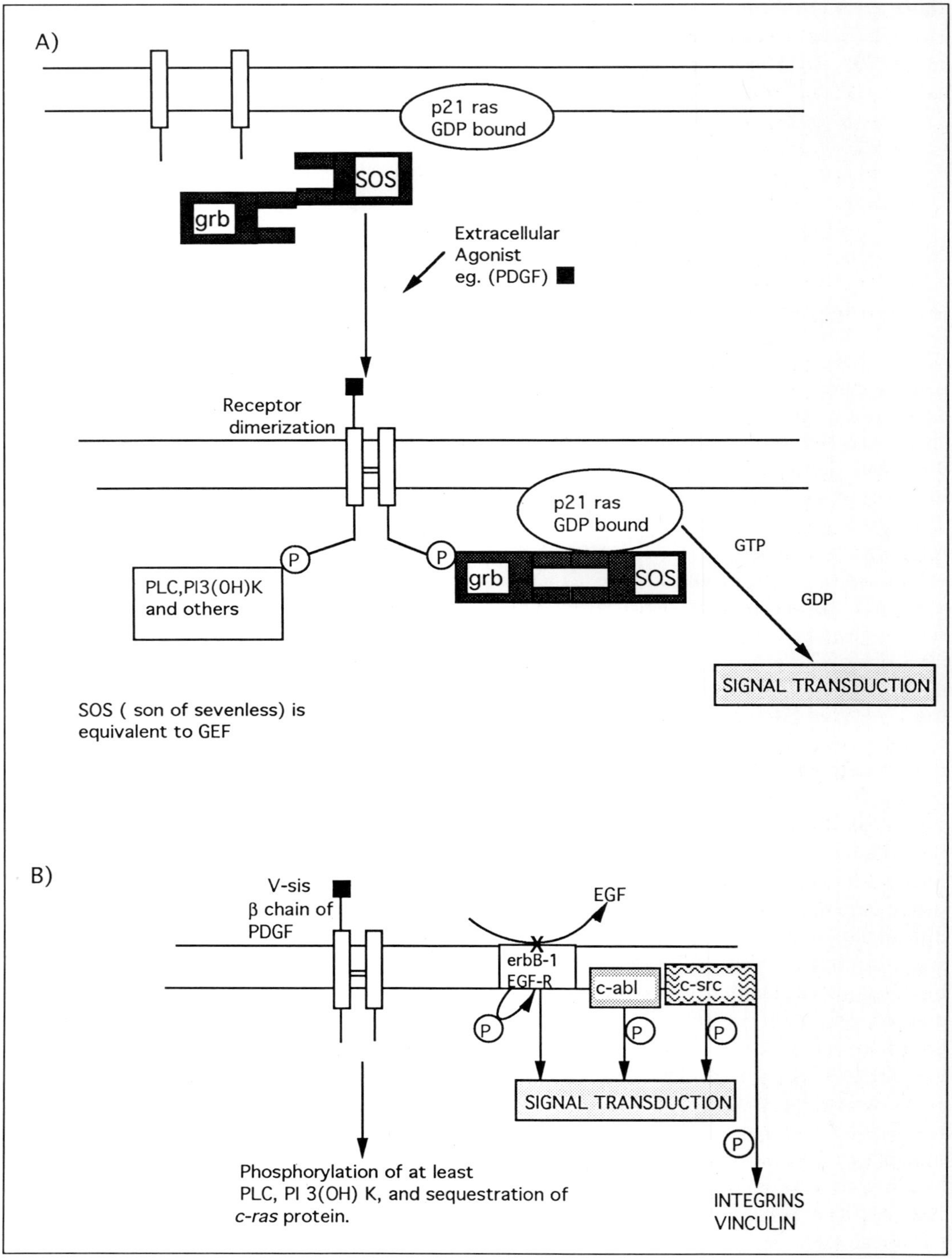

Fig. 2.2. Oncogene activation at the membrane.

recruitment via a different mechanism. Finally, we must not forget direct posttranslational modification of the p21-*ras* protein itself. Such mechanisms involve both farnesylation and palmitoylation. The C-terminus of p21-*ras* (amino acids: – CAAX, where C = cysteine, A = any aliphatic amino acid, X = a terminal methionine or serine) can undergo proteolysis of the terminal three (– AAX) amino acids, farnesylation on the C residue and carboxymethylation of the farnesylated C. In conjunction with palmitoylation of neighboring C residues, these modifications enable the targeting of p21-*ras* to the plasma membrane. The farnesyl group from farnesyl diphosphate, an intermediate in cholesterol biosynthesis is transferred to the p21-*ras* protein by farnesyl protein transferase (FTPase) and has provided an interesting candidate for the prevention of p21-*ras* associated transformation. In this case, inhibitors of FTPase are being designed which prevent the farnesylation and hence membrane localization of p21-*ras*.[9,10]

ii. The p21-*ras* Oncogene in Cancer Biology

We will now consider the types of tumors with which p21-*ras* has been associated and in the light of the above biochemical discussion, address the question as to why p21-*ras* is such a potent oncogene. Mutations in the p21-*ras* gene have been associated with up to 20% of all human cancers, in particular mutations in codons 12, 13 and 59-61. The incidence of mutated p21-*ras* genes shows a strong variation with different tumor types (Table 2.2) which ranges from 80% in pancreatic carcinomas to some tumor types where mutated p21-*ras* genes have not been observed. Presumably, other genetic and/or biochemical events have the same ultimate effect as p21-*ras* mutation. Alternatively, in some cell types p21-*ras* mutations may trigger a differentiation pathway. The type of p21-*ras* mutation may also correlate with tumor type, for example, Ki-*ras* mutations are predominant in lung, pancreatic and colon adenocarcinomas. Ha-*ras* mutations are common in squamous cell carcinomas and N-*ras* mutations have been observed in multiple myeloma.[11] The latter is of interest since in other lymphoid malignancies p21-*ras* mutations of any type are relatively rare. Within this classification there is a distinct difference in the spectra of mutations observed in lung and colon cancer, where in lung adenocarcinoma, 53% of the mutations identified are G to T mutations in the first base of codon 12 (GGT), thus changing a glycine to serine. In colon cancer, the equivalent mutation occurs in only 10% of cases whilst G to A mutations in the 12th and 13th codon (GGC) account for 38% and 22% of the observed Ki-*ras* mutations. In lung cancer, the equivalent frequency is 15% and 3%. These differences may be attributable to the carcinogenic influences of cigarette smoking on the lung and pancreas, but probably not in the colon. The precise genotoxic agents present in tobacco smoke have not yet been identified, so the mechanism of mutation is unclear. The association between chemical carcinogenesis and p21-*ras* mutation has been clearly demonstrated in rodent model systems where the observed mutational spectra may be correlated with particular DNA adducts (Table 2.3).[12]

Table 2.2. Incidence of* ras *gene mutations

Tumor type	**% with *ras* mutation**
Colon carcinoma	47
Pancreatic carcinoma	81
Lung adenocarcinoma	32
Thyroid tumors	56
Endometrial adenocarcinomas	47
Ovarian adenocarcinoma	75
Squamous cell carcinomas (UV nduced)	47
Oral squamous cell carcinomas (tobacco)	35
Mammary adenocarcinoma	2
Hepatocellular carcinoma	4
Cervical carcinoma	4

Table 2.3. Carcinogen action on the Ha-ras gene: mutational preferences

Tumor	Codon	Position	Change	Carcinogen
Rat mammary	12 (CGA)	2	G to A	M N U
Mouse hepatic	61 (CGA)	2	A to T or G	VC, HO-DHE
		1	C to A	HO-AFF
Mouse skin	61 (CAA)	2	A to T	DMBA

MNU, N-methyl-N-nitrosourea; VC, vinyl carbamate; HO-DHE, 1'-hydroxy-21, 31 dehydroestradial; HO-AFF, N-hydroxy-2 acetylaminofluorene; DMBA, 7, 12-dimethylbenz[a]anthracene

iii. Why is p21-*ras* an Oncogene?

It is most likely that the point mutations in p21-*ras* at codons 12, 13 and 59-61 lead to conformational changes in three dimensional structure of the p21-*ras* protein which results in the equilibrium between p21-$ras_{[\text{GTP bound}]}$ and p21-$ras_{[\text{GDP bound}]}$ being heavily in favor of the former. Even though only one allele may be mutated, there may be enough mutant p21-*ras* in the membrane to elicit a signal transduction event in the absence of an effector, i.e., the mutation is dominant and constitutive. It is likely, therefore, that these mutations are either in or close to the GTP binding domain and somehow prevent the intrinsic and/or *ras* GAP enhanced GTPase activity.[1]

iv. Nonreceptor Tyrosine Kinases

This group of tyrosine kinases are so designated because of a lack of extracellular sequences, although many can associate with proteins that do have extracellular domains. There are at least eight different classes of such kinases, most of which seem to have several members.[13] Both 'oncogenic' and 'antioncogenic' potential have been identified within these classes of genes and we will now describe the associated biochemistry. Historically speaking, the archetypal nonreceptor tyrosine kinase is the p60 c-*src* protein, other members being p59 c-*fyn* and p60 c-*yes* for example. In structure all tyrosine kinases have a 300 amino acid region of homology, defined as the kinase domain and designated SH1, for *src* homology. Additional homologous regions which are not found in the receptor tyrosine kinases include SH2, SH3 and an amino terminal sequence that is associated with myristoylation and attachment to the membrane, via a recently identified protein. Many proteins use myristoylation as a means to attach to the membrane and this is not specific to this class of enzymes. SH2 and SH3 domains are found in other proteins such as phospholipase Cα, phosphatidylinositol 3-OH kinase (PI_3-OH kinase), *ras* GAP, the p74 c-*ras* serine/threonine kinase, *grb*2, *sos* and *crk*. Such domains may be integral to the mechanism by which the latter two proteins function as adaptor proteins.

The intrinsic tyrosine kinase activity of c-*src* and its family members is low, perhaps suggesting either that cellular targets may be involved in signal amplification or repression of c-*src* activity. With regard to the latter, the *csk* protein may be responsible for C terminal c-*src* tyrosine phosphorylation, which inhibits its activity. They may be activated by cytokine binding, thus implicating other membrane associated proteins. For example, binding of PDGF to its receptor in fibroblasts leads to p60 c-*src* dependent tyrosine kinase activity. This may in part be regulated by tyrosine phosphorylation such that if a particular carboxy terminal residue which is outside the kinase domain is not phosphorylated (e.g. by replacement of the tyrosine residue with phenylalanine), then the transforming abilities of p60 c-*src* increase. Enzymes which dephosphorylate tyrosine residues, e.g., the lymphocyte CD45 antigen, may have important roles in such pathways. Another important interaction of c-*src* is likely to be with PI_3-OH kinase, although this enzyme appears to be associated with a number of tyrosine kinases, whether these be of the receptor or nonreceptor type. A link between serine kinases and tyrosine kinases has been demonstrated and members of the c-*src* family may activate p74 c-*raf*. This is unlikely to be the direct SH2 domain dependent mechanism which pertains to PI_3-OH kinase and *ras* GAP, since p74 c-*raf* does not contain an SH2 domain and is only weakly phosphorylated on tyrosine. Several other proteins are likely to be phosphorylated by the c-*src* family, some of which include the lipocortin/calpactin family, which undergo calcium dependent membrane association.

One possible function of the p60 c-*src* complex may be in enzyme recruitment whereby the p60 c-*src* protein in a complex with another protein (X), brings X to the membrane where it can more efficiently interact with its own substrate. This is supported by experiments in which removal of the myristolation domain from both c-*src* and c-*abl* prevents fibroblast transformation, but still permits tyrosine phosphorylation on cytosolic proteins.

Despite these possibilities, the exact function of the c-*src* protein remains unclear. However, several lines of evidence now point towards a role for it in the cell cycle, since: (a) in fibroblasts c-*src* is partially dephosphorylated during mitosis, resulting in a two- to four-fold increase in tyrosine kinase activity, (b) *cdc*2 dependent phosphorylation events occur on c-*src* serine and threonine residues during mitosis and (c) PDGF treatment of fibroblasts stimulates c-*src* kinase activity with accompanying PDGF receptor association. The latter may be important in cell type specific amplification of the signal from the activated receptor. Evidence suggests that c-*src* acts upstream of p21-*ras* in signal transduction and although the precise in vivo substrates have not been identified, there are some interesting candidates: Gα subunits, protein phosphatase 2A, actin binding proteins (cytoskeletal rearrangement during G2-M?) and the focal adhesion kinase (FAK). The latter possesses its own tyrosine kinase activity and colocalizes with proteins in the focal adhesion plaques, such as tensin, vinculin and talin. Similarly, FAK can be activated by the action if the integrins and a number of extracellular effectors, such as bombesin, vasopressin and endothelin. These data point to FAK as a convergence point for signals which regulate cell motility, shape and adhesion.[14] This provides a molecular mechanism by which an altered extracellular cytokine environment could modulate the way in which the cell interacts with the extracellular matrix and neighboring cells. As we shall see in our discussion of colon cancer, modification of such interactions can be a source of growth advantage and hence clonal selection.

It is also worth noting that c-*src* activation may be one of the first cellular responses to ultraviolet (UV) irradiation. As a result of UV treatment, the transcriptional activation of several genes occurs, including that of c-*jun*. The latter can be blocked by dominant negative mutants of v-*src*, Ha-*ras* and c-*raf*-1, thus not only implicating all of these proteins but suggesting that the initial 'knee jerk' response to UV irradiation is initiated at the plasma membrane. Obviously this will be in addition to, or part of, the normal DNA repair processes which will occur at a later stage as the 6-4 pyrimidine-pyrimidone photoproducts and cyclobutane pyrimidine dimers are detected. Additional effects of UV irradiation are: (a) generation of free radicals via lipid peroxidation and (b) oxidative 'stress' via a reduction in the intracellular poll of reduced glutathione. By using N-acetyl cysteine, a precursor of glutathione, the UV dependent activation of c-*src* and the transcriptional induction of c-*jun* can be inhibited.[15] Furthermore, tyrosine kinase inhibitors enhance the cytotoxic effect of certain wavelengths of UV, suggesting that this response may have a role in cell protection and that certain oncogenes may increase radioresistance, perhaps via the transcriptional induction of genes involved in protection against oxidative stress, e.g., quinone reductase and glutathione-S-transferase. Taken together, these data illustrate a subtle mechanism whereby oncogene activation may interfere with cancer treatments which involve the generation of free radicals, i.e., by increasing the effective threshold level for cytotoxicity

A second important class of nonreceptor tyrosine kinases includes the c-*abl* gene, unique because of several distinct subcellular localizations of the protein and different functional options in cell cycle regulation and signal transduction.[16] Constitutive activation of the c-*abl* tyrosine kinase, e.g. by fusion to *bcr* in some human leukemias (the Philadelphia translocation) leads to a protein which is capable of participating in transformation. This may in part be by regulation of events which occur upon actin filaments and/or by binding to DNA, since the c-*abl* protein can sometimes be translocated to the nucleus. During mitosis, the c-*abl* protein is hyperphosphorylated, which also prevents its binding to DNA.[17] Whether this modulates cytoskeleton dependent gene expression is not yet clear, but such a mechanism would be indeed be necessary upon entry into the cell cycle.

v. Receptor Tyrosine Kinases

These kinases bind cytokines and hormones via extracellular sequences and in doing so are induced to dimerize, autophosphorylate on tyrosine residues and phosphorylate internal cellular proteins on tyrosine residues. In general, these proteins have an SH1 domain, but lack the SH2 and SH3 domains (Fig. 2.3). The oncogene forms of these receptors generally allow tyrosine kinase activity in the absence of ligand binding and there are examples of mutations within the cytosolic domain, amino acid substitutions in the transmembrane domain and deletions in the extracellular domain which lead to enhanced tyrosine kinase activity, presumably by

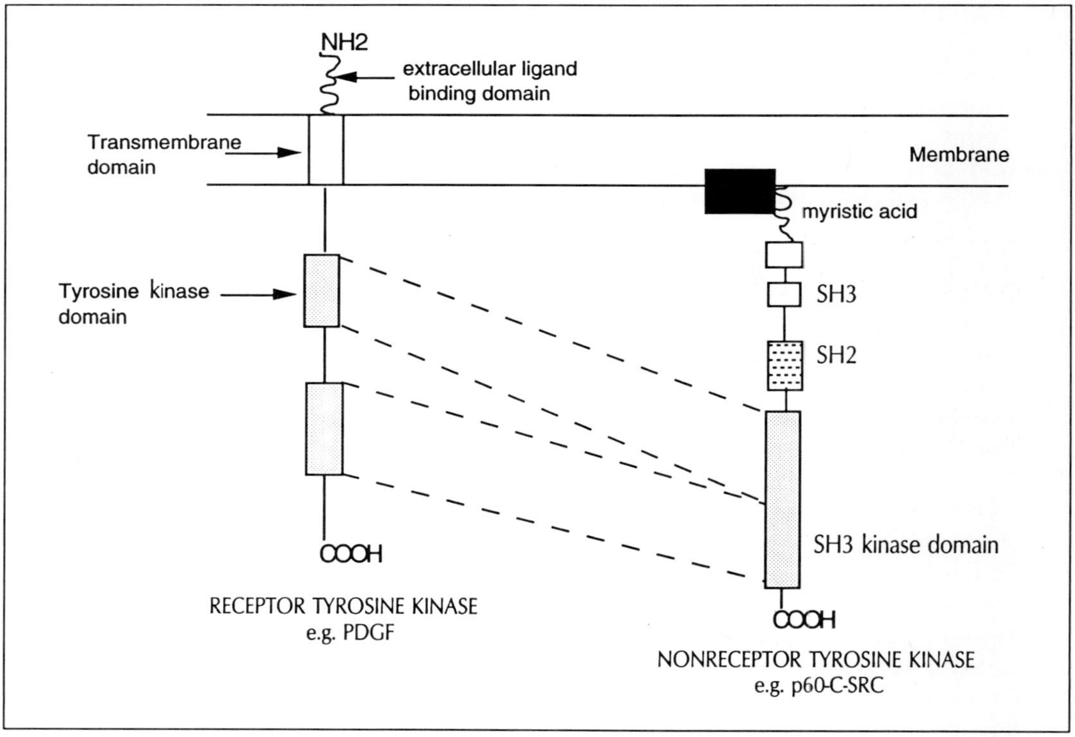

Fig. 2.3. Comparison of archetypal receptor and nonreceptor tyrosine kinases.

enhancing the dimerization and autophosphorylation activities. The latter creates binding sites for specific enzymes to bind via their SH2 domains, akin to the mechanism proposed for c-*src* and that already described for *grb*2-*sos*. Using the PDGF receptor as an example, there are at least four key proteins that are tyrosine phosphorylated in response to ligand binding; PI_3-OH kinase, *ras* GAP, phospholipase Cγ1 and p74 c-*raf* (Fig. 2.4). However, the c-*raf* protein is mostly phosphorylated on serine, a phenomenon which can be mimicked by other agents, such as insulin or the phorbol esters. Since other growth factors may augment the mitogenic effect of PDGF, there are probably other targets which the PDGF receptor does not phosphorylate. In addition, the PDGF receptor is the only receptor known to activate all four of the above proteins. The inefficiency of PDGF as a mitogen could be explained by PDGF receptor down regulation, but the occurrence of a transforming oncogene homologous to the BB form of PDGF, i.e., v-*sis* is supportive of a key role for PDGF and its receptor in signal transduction. It is unlikely that any single target is sufficient for initiation of cell cycle progression in any single cell type, a hypothesis supported by deletion analysis on the receptors. For example, removing a domain from the CSF-1 receptor which reduces association with PI_3-OH kinase leaves the mutant receptor capable of transformation in some cells but not others. This deletion does not affect the association or phosphorylation of *ras* GAP.[18] Arguments relating to the activation or nonactivation of any particular pathway may be considered somewhat naive since the additional variables of duration and magnitude of response are

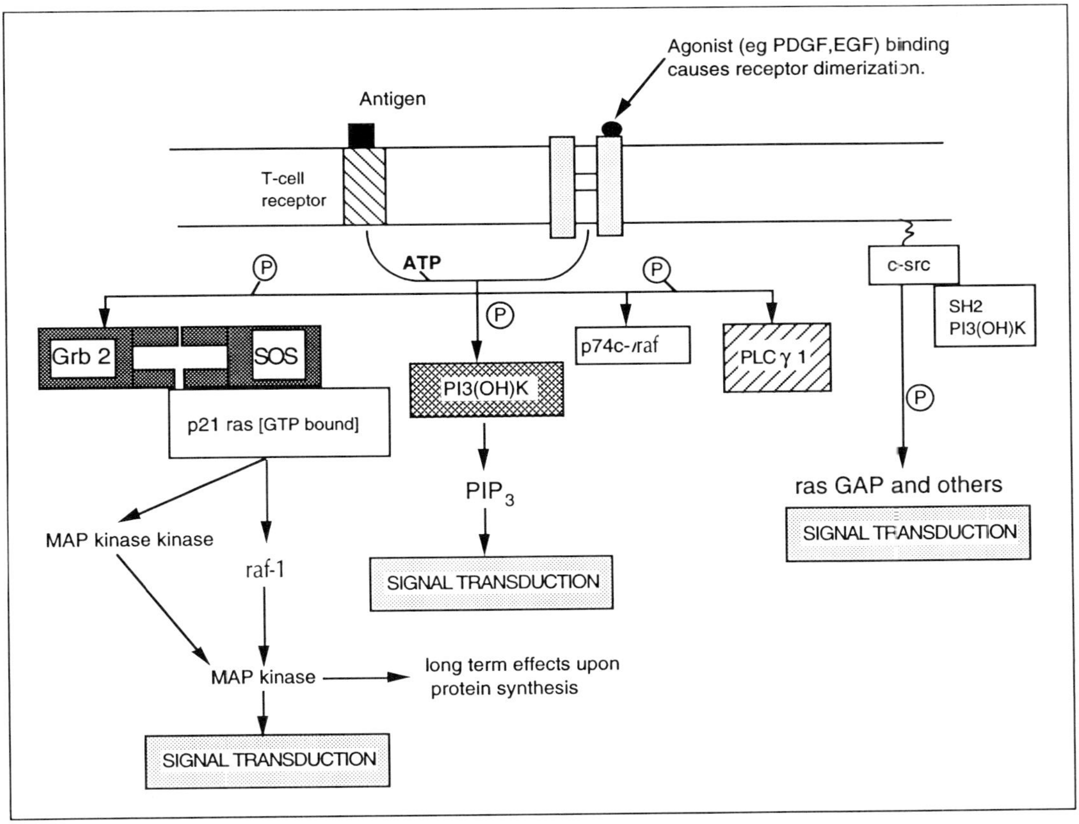

Fig. 2.4. Receptor and nonreceptor tyrosine kinases. $PI_3(OH)K$ - Phosphatidylinositol 3-hydroxy kinase.

likely to be significant factors. It is known that in order to lead to proliferation, PDGF must be continuously present for at least 1 hour and whilst some responses such as PI_3-OH kinase activation occur rapidly, others may require longer. For example, PDGF causes breakdown of phosphatidylcholine to diacylglycerol in a process which takes at least an hour.[19] In addition, multiple pathways often appear to trigger the same cellular event, e.g., activation of c-*fos* or c-*myc* transcription can be both protein kinase C dependent and independent. To some extent this may reflect activation of factors which are required for proliferation in a more general sense. It is the pathway specific activations (if they exist!) which are likely to provide the clues to the transformation triggers relevant to one cell type compared to another.

vi. Nontyrosine Kinase Receptors

External signals may react with at least three types of cellular receptors: the tyrosine kinase linked receptors, nontyrosine kinase linked receptors (e.g. G protein linked receptors) and lymphokine receptors. For the first two, inositol[1,4,5] trisphosphate (IP3) appears to be a unifying and central feature, via an ATP driven activation of phospholipase C. For the G protein linked receptors, the activated receptor utilizes a G protein system to communicate with one of the phospholipase C family (β1). Such receptors appear to have around seven domains which span the membrane and which are connected by both intracellular and extracellular peptide loops (Fig. 2.5). There are at least two classes depending upon their sensitivity to pertussis toxin and many agonists for G protein linked receptors, e.g., 5-hydroxytryptamine, vasopressin, gastrin releasing peptide (bombesin) and acetylcholine,[20] which upon binding to the receptor introduce a conformational change in two of the intracellular loops. Exchange of GDP for GTP and dissociation of the G protein complex leave the subunits (α, β and γ) free to interact and activate different isoforms of phospholipase C (β1, β2). Binding to PLC β1 enhances the GTPase activity of $G\alpha_{[GTP\ bound]}$ and as such it may be considered to act as a GAP protein.

The activated lymphokine receptors are not thought to act through G proteins or cause phospholipid turnover and very little is known about the way in which lymphokine derived signals are transduced with the cytoplasm.

vii. Through the Cytoplasm

The multitude of potential membrane signaling events, e.g., via p21-*ras*, c-*src*, phospholipid turnover, suggests that there are likely to be a multitude of routes across the cytoplasm as the signals forge their path to the nucleus. It is therefore surprising that only a few have come to light in the literature. However, one such pathway involves p21-*ras*$_{[GTP\ bound]}$, which activates at least two serine/threonine kinases in the cytoplasm, c-*raf*-1 and a series of mitogen activated protein kinases (MAPs) (Fig. 2.6).[21] MAP kinase may also be activated independent of either p21-*ras* or c-*raf*-1 suggesting that it may be coupled to at least one other pathway. That p74 c-*raf*-1 is downstream of p21-*ras* is suggested by two lines of evidence: (a) transformation due to the viral *raf* gene does not require p21-*ras* action and (b) a kinase defective mutant of c-*raf*-1 can suppress the effects of activated p21-*ras*. However, ligand dependent stimulation of both p74 c-*raf*-1 and the MAP kinases seems to require p21-*ras* and indeed it has been shown that they lie on the same pathway with c-*raf*-1 upstream of the MAP kinase system.[21,22] It has subsequently been shown that activated p21-*ras* can form a direct complex with the serine/threonine MAP kinase (MAP-KK[23]) which then directly activates MAP kinase. Whether this association activates MAP-KK or sequesters already active MAP-KK remains to be demonstrated. This reaction is independent of binding to c-*raf*-1 and the two may both associate with p21-*ras* in order to elicit a signal. However, these data are consistent with p21-*ras* being a switch point between the tyrosine kinases of the plasma mem-

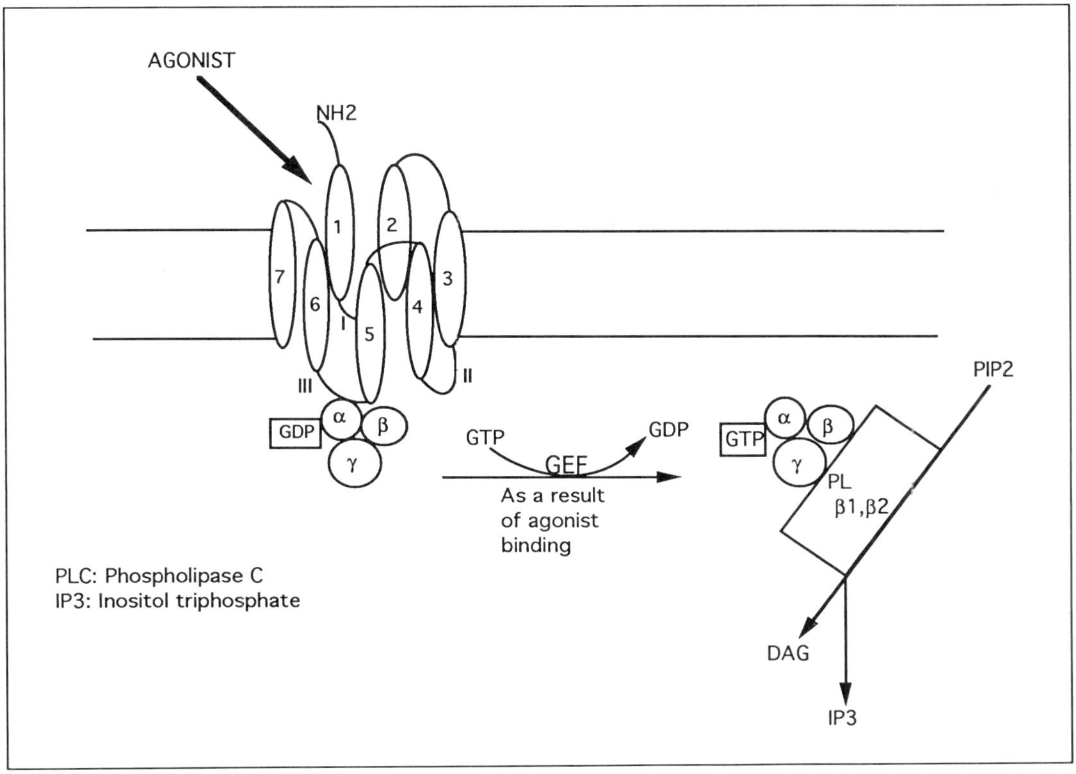

Fig. 2.5. G protein linked receptors. PLC – Phospholipase C; IP3 – Inositol trisphosphate.

brane and the cytosolic serine/threonine kinase system. Given our previous arguments it is unlikely that all of the effort in the membrane serves only to focus on one kinase (MAPK), and with the passage of time several more cytosolic events can be expected to be identified. To reiterate, it is those changes which confer cell type specific transformation that are likely to be of most interest. Furthermore, MAP kinase activation occurs within 5 minutes of mitogen stimulation and may therefore not be involved in the longer term (1 hour) potentiation of proliferation. That p74 c-*raf*-1 may not be the sole activator of MAPK in all cell types is indicated in several lines of evidence including the inability of c-*raf*-1 to activate MAPK in PC12 cells in contrast to p21-*ras* and activation of p74 c-*raf*-1 in interleukin-2 dependent T cells in the absence of MAP kinase activation.[24] There is evidence to suggest that in some cell types MAP kinase may be activated by either protein kinase C (via phorbol ester treatment) or G proteins other than p21-*ras*. The downstream substrates of the MAP kinase are at the very least likely to include transcription factors. Also involved is the p90-c-*rsk* protein, which was once thought to be responsible for phosphorylation of ribosomal protein S6 and hence activate factors which participate in translational control. These in vitro data have not been confirmed in vivo, and the more likely activator is an independent 70 kDa kinase. The MAP kinase phosphorylates a 62 kDa ternary complex factor (p62-*tcf*) which participates in stimulation of c-*fos* transcription.[25] In response to either serum or phorbol ester treatment, the transcriptional induction of c-*fos* does not require de novo protein synthesis and must therefore be brought about by the modification of pre-existing factors. Similarly, MAPK specifically phosphorylates the c-*jun* transcription factor and may in part explain

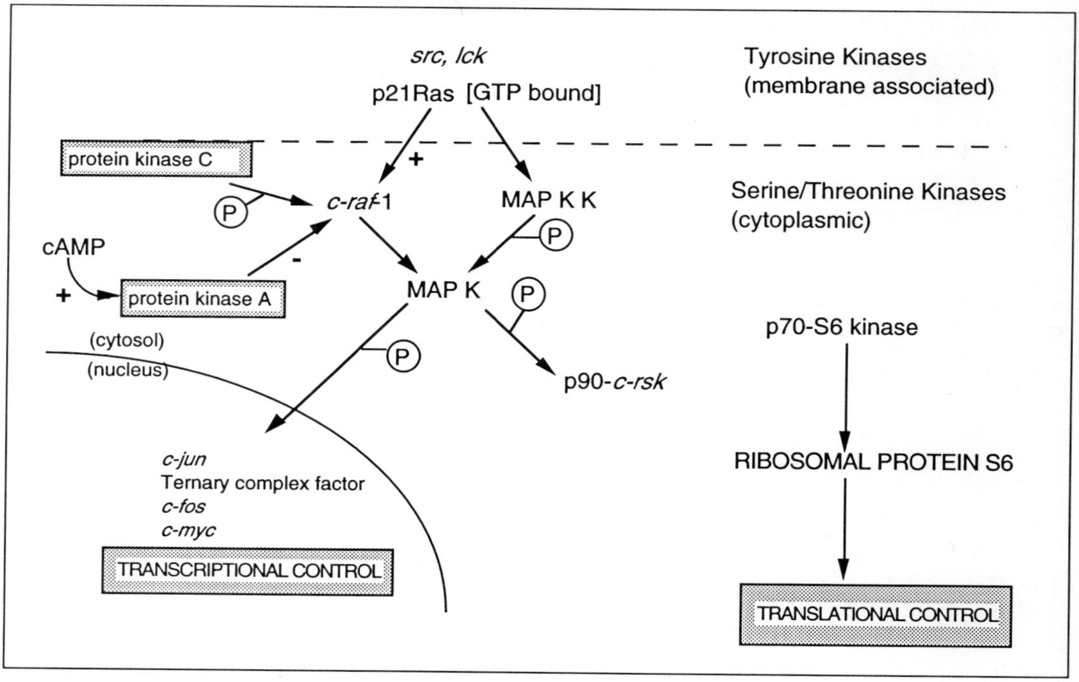

Fig. 2.6. Cytoplasmic kinases. MAP K - Mitogen Activated Protein Kinase.

the induction of this factor by various mitogenic signals.[26]

One of the key regulators of signal transduction via the p21-*ras*-*raf*-1 pathway is likely to be mediated via cAMP. The latter is increased by hormonal stimulation of Gαs to bind GTP, which then activates adenyl cyclase to produce cAMP. At least one of the effects of cAMP is to stimulate the activity of protein kinase A. In general, cAMP is inhibitory to cell proliferation across a number of cell types, both transformed by oncogenes and otherwise. This effect is likely to occur between the G0 and mid G1 phases of the cell cycle and is independent of phospholipid turnover. After cell stimulation by epidermal growth factor, activation of the c-*raf*-1 kinase is inhibited by elevation of the intracellular concentration of cAMP.[27] However, the accumulation of p21-$ras_{[GTP\ bound]}$, receptor tyrosine kinase activity and *grb*2-*sos* associations were unaffected. Since c-*raf*-1 may be phosphorylated by protein kinase A, a simple model would have inhibition of c-*raf*-1 activation by a protein kinase A dependent phosphorylation event, in such a way as to prevent interaction with p21-$ras_{[GTP\ bound]}$. This is likely to be only one of several mechanisms for modulation of transcytoplasmic signaling events; the key areas to identify will be the mechanisms for modulating apparently converging signaling pathways in different cell types.

viii. Into the Nucleus

Oncogene proteins in the nucleus by and large fall into the category of transcription factors, i.e., are involved in activation or repression of genes at the level of transcription. Many other mechanisms are of course possible and will no doubt come to light as our understanding increases. For now, we will consider the important example of c-*myb*, c-*myc*, the c-*jun*-c-*fos* interaction and the dominant negative oncogene, c-*erb*A.

a. c-*myb*

The c-*myb* gene product is an important transcriptional regulator in cells of the hematopoietic lineage and is itself generally down regulated as differentiation proceeds. The levels of c-*myb* protein vary according to the state of differentiation with low levels being detected in terminally differentiated hematopoietic cells. In human myelogenous leukemia cell lines, the down regulation of c-*myb* is an early event which generally precedes differentiation. However, c-*myb* is not strictly tissue specific and its aberrant expression has been associated with small cell lung cancer, colon adenocarcinoma and tumors of the early embryo. The c-*myb* protein is phosphorylated at several sites by MAP kinase and p34-*cdc*-2 kinase.[28] It is likely that these are important in c-*myb* attenuation, since the viral counterpart cannot be phosphorylated by MAP kinase in vitro. However, the cellular targets for c-*myb* transcriptional repression and/or activation have not yet been defined.

b. The c-*myc* enigma

There are three members of the *myc* gene family that have been associated with tumorigenesis: c-*myc*, N-*myc* and L-*myc*. All enhance cell proliferation and suppress differentiation when overexpressed, utilizing a variety of mechanisms. The *myc* proteins are probably transcription factors and all bear the characteristic structural hallmarks of such: a basic region, a helix loop helix and a leucine zipper motif. This b-HLH-LZ structure expedites both interaction with other protein partners and binding to DNA. The latter is facilitated by another protein, *max*,[29] which specifically and preferentially associates with the c-*myc* protein to form heterodimers, which in turn bind to a consensus DNA sequence (CACGTG). Several forms of *max* protein have been identified across a range of cell types, but whether these play a role in cell type specific *myc-max* transcription remains to be shown. Whilst *max* may form both homodimers and heterodimers with c-*myc*, the latter has not been shown to homodimerize in vivo. *Max* protein is always in excess, is stable and does not vary in concentration with the cell cycle. In contrast, the amount of c-*myc* protein varies according to the cytokine milieu and is a relatively unstable protein. Both *max-max* homodimers and *max-myc* heterodimers bind to the same sequence and since *max-max* lacks the ability to transcriptionally transactivate, this protein complex probably blocks transcription of potentially responsive genes. Upon synthesis of c-*myc*, e.g., after mitogen stimulation, the balance now shifts towards *max-myc* complexes and transcription may ensue. Additional levels of control may operate, for example the effects of phosphorylation modulate both DNA binding activity and other partners in the complex (e.g. the *mad* protein). However, in principle, the mechanism of action is as outlined.

With so many cancers showing aberrant regulation of the c-*myc* protein, it is hard to envisage that it has anything but a fundamental role. Needless to say, there are an extraordinary number of citations concerning the c-*myc* family of oncogenes although the key questions have yet to be answered. These are: (a) when are the c-*myc* proteins required, (b) which genes do they transcriptionally activate and (c) what is the position of c-*myc* relative to other pathways, i.e., what are the factors which govern gene cooperativity?

c. More and more c-*myc* protein; where there is a will there is a way.

Unlike with other oncogenes and tumor suppressor genes, the cell will go to extraordinary lengths to increase the amount of the c-*myc* protein. Depending upon the cell type, nearly every possible mechanism has been used to give more c-*myc* protein, in a wide variety of tissues. Furthermore, mutant c-*myc* protein is just not good enough; the evidence suggests that it has to be an excess of the normal c-*myc* protein. The important question is not how the increases arise, but why? Unfortunately there is not a satisfactory answer to the latter, save for rather nebulous arguments which are thus: that the c-*myc* protein is of such fundamental importance to the choice between proliferation, differentiation and apoptosis (Fig. 1.3, chapter 1), that any step in the direction of the transformed phenotype will lead to intense positive selection pressure for an increase in the c-*myc* protein.

d. When does c-*myc* perform its task?

There is much evidence to suggest that the *c-myc* protein plays a key role in the onset and maintenance of cellular proliferation. The rapid induction of *c-myc* after mitogenic stimulation of both fibroblasts and lymphoblasts indicates that the *c-myc* protein is involved in the G0-G1 transition.[30] Moreover, microinjection of c-*myc* protein into quiescent fibroblasts will cause these cells to enter the cell cycle even without the expression of any other immediate early gene products, thus demonstrating that *c-myc* alone is sufficient to drive the cells into a proliferative mode.[31] However, microinjection of antisense oligonucleotides directed against c-*myc* mRNA into mitogen stimulated lymphoblasts is insufficient to halt the G0-G1 transition although these cells remain blocked in G1, hence indicating that this protein is not absolutely required for the G0-G1 event to occur. In addition, this protein is expressed continuously in rapidly growing cells, independent of the cell cycle, implying that it is also required for a proliferative state.[32,33] It also appears that c-*myc* has a role in the G2-S transition as preB cells which do not express *c-myc* will enter S phase although they are not capable of proceeding into G2; the introduction of *c-myc* protein into these cells removes this block.

In contrast, it has been shown that it is necessary to downregulate *c-myc* protein levels for cellular differentiation to occur. Thus the amount of the protein is found to rapidly decrease upon induction of differentiation in a number of different systems including mouse erythroid leukemia cells (MEL), human promyelocytic HL60 cells and primary murine keratinocytes. The introduction of an antisense *c-myc* plasmid constructed into these cell types will cause them to differentiate in the absence of an inducer, whilst the overexpression of *c-myc* protein will interfere with their terminal differentiation. Hence the loss of *c-myc* expression seems to be responsible for cellular differentiation.

There is evidence which suggests that the *c-myc* protein is able to mediate apoptosis.[34] It is possible that this type of apoptosis results from a catastrophic consequence of cellular imbalance[35] although there are data which indicate that it may have a normal physiological role, for example, the receptor mediated cell death which occurs in embryonic thymocytes.[36] Thus the c-*myc* gene product also seems to be involved in programmed cell death and hence the complete removal of a cell from the cell cycle! It has been proposed that the cell death and cell proliferation pathways are either tightly coupled or are overlapping processes that are both driven by *c-myc* (Fig. 2.7). In this model, any cell which is proliferating and is a potential carcinogenic hazard can be automatically primed for death should it fail to receive the appropriate survival signal.

In this respect it has been shown that the amount of the *c-myc* protein is increased by the treatment of cells with DNA damaging agents. This response can occur very rapidly depending on the nature of the DNA damaging agent (within 20 minutes after treatment of the cell with ionizing radiation). The *c-myc* induction is caused by DNA strand breaks with the *c-myc* protein showing maximal induction when there are approximately 3000 breaks per genome.[37] Thus there appears to be another intriguing role for the c-*myc* protein. However, these results are perhaps not surprising considering a recent proposal for *c-myc* involvement in the process of apoptosis. Hence, the introduction of DNA strand breaks above a certain threshold, which are insufficient to cause death to the cell but would nevertheless probably result in the introduction of many mutations into the DNA, would result in the induction of *c-myc* protein. This protein would allow the cell to either coordinate repair process (perhaps with c-*myc* acting as a transcription factor for some of the gene products that are required) or if there was too much damage for the cell to be able to affect a repair,

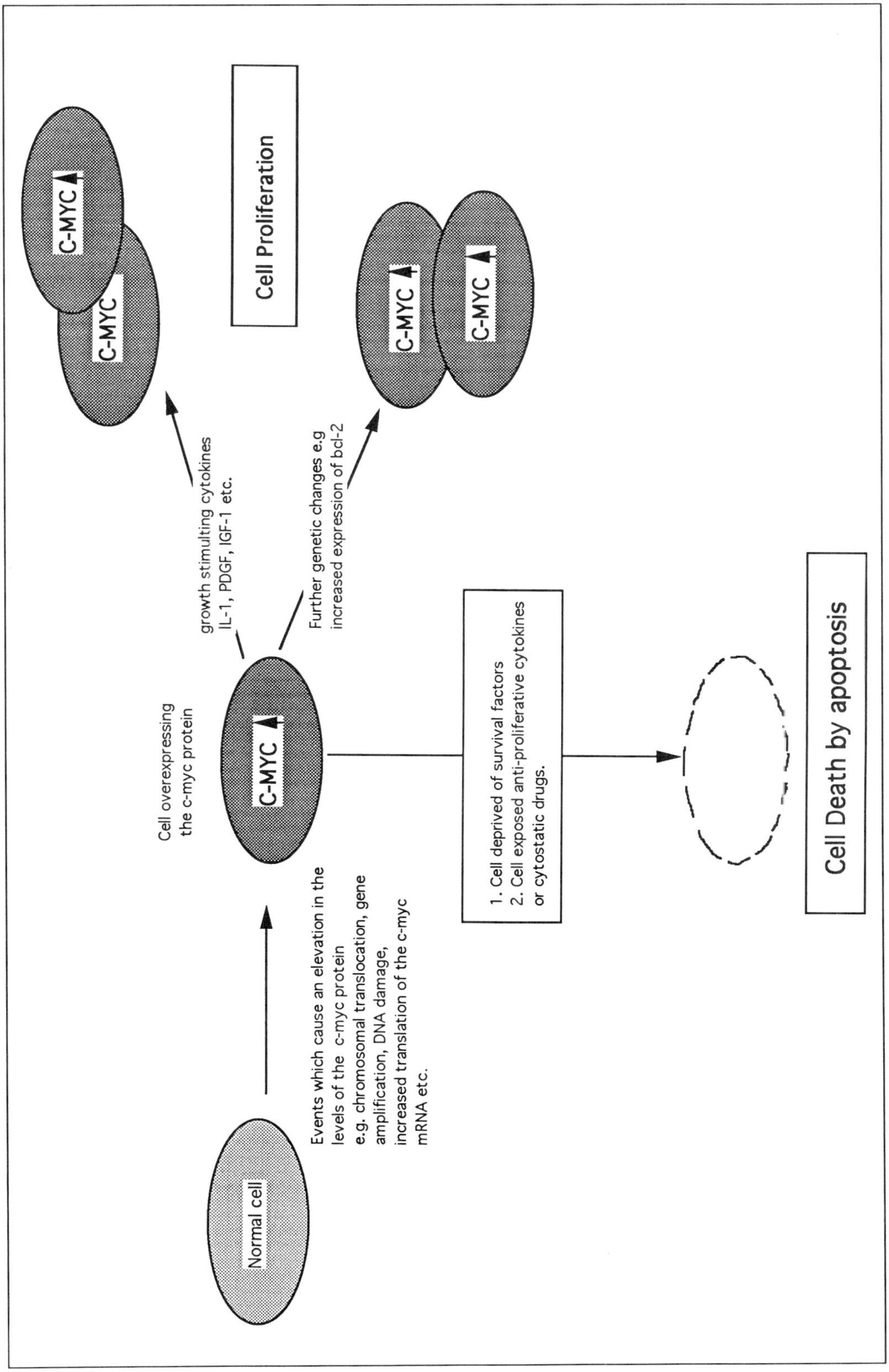

Fig. 2.7. Cellular choices influenced by c-myc.

the *c-myc* protein could be instrumental in sending the cell down the apoptotic pathway (Fig. 2.7).

e. What genes does c-*myc* activate?

Early studies have indicated that the *c-myc* protein has the ability to influence the regulation of other genes and as mentioned above the *c-myc* protein contains all the elements that are required of a transcription factor. A complete picture of the genes that are regulated by *c-myc* would allow the function of this enigmatic protein to be determined. Currently only a few genes whose transcription is influenced by the *c-myc* gene have been discovered and it is not possible to have a coherent picture of what is occurring in cellular terms. However, the identification of the DNA binding activities of *c-myc* and *max* will provide opportunities for directly testing the transcriptional activities of these proteins in mammalian cells. The *c-myc* protein is able to interact directly with the transcription initiator factor TFII-I[38] and it has been shown that the c-*myc* protein is able to regulate a variety of other promoters including the HSP70 promoter and to downregulate the expression of gene products that occur downstream of the metallothione promoter.[39,40] In addition, the expression of mr-1, which encodes plasminogen activator factor, is enhanced by c-*myc*.[41] It has recently been shown that c-*myc* is able to transcribe and hence specifically upregulate the two eukaryotic translation factors eIF4E and eIF2α.[42] This is of particular interest as both of these proteins are necessary for the proliferating cell. Indeed, over expression of eIF4E results in cells with a transformed phenotype.[43] In addition, several gene products are downregulated by the either over expression and/or deregulated c-*myc* expression. These include two variant H1 histone genes, major histocompatability complex (MHC) class 1 and *neu* 1 expression.[44]

The induction of apoptosis by c-*myc* suggests that this protein, presumably through sequence specific DNA binding, is capable of modulating apoptotic or anti-apoptotic genes. However, these genes and their corresponding protein products have yet to be identified.

f. With whom does c-*myc* cooperate?

Mechanistically one could envisage a situation whereby *c-myc* was able to interact either directly or act in concert with either the protein products of proto-oncogenes and thus enhance their reactivity or alternatively with the products of tumor suppressor genes which by binding to the *c-myc* protein would be able to neutralize its effects.

It has been shown that c-*myc* can cooperate with activated *ras* oncogene to transform primary rat fibroblasts and that *c-myc* alone in the absence of secondary mutageneic events is insufficient to cause a malignant phenotype.[45] The c-*myc* protein also cooperates with *raf* to produce lymphoid tumors in mice, and a combination of the over expression of c-*myc* and *bcl*-2 is associated with a very aggressive lymphocytic leukemia.[46,47] In addition matings between *myc* and *bcl*-2 transgenic mice result in animals with malignancies of lymphoid cell types in utero, which were not observed in mice that contained only one over expressed oncogene.[48]

In vitro, the retinoblastoma gene product pRB is able to bind to c-*myc* protein at two sites although this has not yet been conclusively shown to occur in vivo. However, TGFβ downregulates *c-myc* expression in a process which appears to be mediated by pRB.[49,50] The interaction between c-*myc* and p53 is less clear and the *c-myc* protein has not been shown to be able to bind directly to p53. The effects that p53 exert on *c-myc* probably occur at the level of transcription.

g. The c-*jun*-c-*fos* interaction

The c-*fos* and c-*jun* gene products are of the first to be induced upon mitogen stimulation of quiescent fibroblasts, and like c-*myc*, could well be near the start of a cascade of gene expression that is essential for the early part of G1.[51] Indeed, microinjection of antibodies to the c-*jun* and c-*fos* proteins inhibits entry of cells into S phase.[52] The c-*fos* protein acts as a transcription factor by associating with the c-*jun* gene product via a leucine zipper domain to form heterodimers which bind to a consensus DNA sequence for the transcription factor AP1.[53] In general, AP1 targets are associated with the activation of a large number of genes, although there are examples whereby the effect is one of gene repression, e.g., the osteocalcin gene. In addition, c-*jun* may play a role in the cellular response to ultraviolet irradiation since the c-*jun* gene itself, together with several AP1 associated genes, is rapidly activated by ultraviolet irradiation treatment.[54] The c-*jun* product can form a homodimer that is in itself able to activate transcription, but less effectively than the heterodimer with c-*fos*. In contrast, c-*fos* can only function via the heterodimer and does not form homodimers There are a number of c-*fos* related proteins (*fos* related antigens[55]), the best characterized of which is *fos*B. Similarly, there are other members of the c-*jun* family such as *jun*B and *jun*D. Each of these can form heterodimers with any other c-*jun* family member and heterodimers with c-*fos*, all of which can bind to the AP1 consensus sequence and thus give an enormous range of protein complexes with transcription regulating potential. The *jun* family of proteins has different binding affinities for the AP1 site, which in all cases is enhanced by binding to the c-*fos* protein. However, it is interesting to note that *jun*B can antagonize the transforming effects of c-*jun*, compounding the undoubted biological complexity of this system.

h. The c-*erb*A paradox

The c-*erb*A gene product is a thyroid hormone receptor (e.g. triiodothyronine T3 is bound with high affinity) forming part of a larger family of proteins which acts as a general receptor for steroid hormones, thyroid hormones, vitamin D and the retinoids. Post-ligand binding, the activated receptor binds to a specific DNA sequence element either at a promoter or enhancer and subsequently regulates transcription. Thyroid hormone receptors bind to target DNA in the nucleus in the absence of ligand binding in situ. However, the steroid hormone receptors have a different mechanism of action and in the absence of ligand binding are cytoplasmic. Ligand binding brings about nuclear translocation and confers the ability to bind to specific DNA sequences. Comparison with the transforming variant of c-*erb*A, the v-*erb*A oncogene shows that v-*erb*A acts to overcome the action of its normal cellular counterpart. Hence, c-*erb*A may normally act to suppress transformation and in this case helps differentiation. This has led to the classification of v-*erb*A as a dominant negative oncogene and hence the c-*erb*A gene must formally be classified as a tumor suppressor gene.

ix. On the Clonal Selection of Oncogenes—A Cautionary Note

Why have oncogenes been discovered? Why, amongst all of the other possible gene products have oncogenes leapt to the fore? For arguments relating to this we must again return to the concept of clonal selection. The transforming retroviruses attained growth advantage (sometimes in a species or cell specific manner) by acquiring cellular genes that helped in cell proliferation. Many genes must have been picked up, but many will have not have survived in viral form since there will have been no growth advantage. Clearly, the virus gains advantage by infecting and growing in an actively proliferating cell. We may envisage that a series of mutations of the now viral cellular transforming gene will be selected, such that more transforming potential is attained. Hence we arrive at today's mixture of mutated, truncated v-*onc* genes. Similar arguments will apply to the evolution of the DNA tumor viruses whose genes often have significant blocks of homology with cellular genes. Thus the discovery of 'oncogenes' was actually the revelation of viral selection. 'Weak' oncogenes or those gene products which gave only slight growth advantage would not have been selected via this route. Does this mean they are only less important to human cancer development? We would argue not; the mechanisms of cancer induction are quite different. Viruses have 'one shot' at cell transformation. They must accomplish their goal more or less in one cell cycle and the subtleties of multiple step carcinogenesis are lost. Human cancers clearly initiate from much humbler changes and with the acquisition of new mutations, clonal selection emerges.

Following this argument, we must ask whether 'oncogenes' are the right genes to be studying. They clearly have a role to play, mostly it seems at a late stage in the development of a cancer and their vast over expression can have profound effects. However, we must carefully consider if these data accurately reflect the genesis of human cancers or whether we should devote more attention towards the more subtle cancer predisposing changes.

3. TUMOR SUPPRESSOR GENES

The negative regulation of cell proliferation is supported by three lines of evidence: somatic cell hybrid experiments, study of familial cancers and identification of sites of loss of heterozygosity. These data have been subsequently refined to focus on a group of genes (tumor suppressors) which function to negatively regulate cell proliferation, i.e., their loss helps enable the cell to override the normal checks and balances.[56-58] As previously indicated, release of growth suppression due to the inactivation of tumor suppressor genes probably occurs via inactivation of both copies (maternal and paternal) of the gene in question.[59] In general, cancer predisposition syndromes such as retinoblastoma are considered to result from inactivation of one of the two copies of a unique tumor suppressor gene in the germ line. If truly recessive and to see a phenotypic effect, a second genetic event is expected whereby the remaining wild type allele would be selected against and inactivated. The latter could occur via a number of well documented mechanisms such as: chromosome loss, chromosome loss and reduplication, partial chromosomal deletion, mitotic recombination or a more localized event such as a specific mutation (Fig. 2.8). In the recessive model for cancer development in sporadic tumors, two sequential genetic events are required in order to inactivate both alleles. It is thus implied that the second event can only occur if there is a selective growth advantage which results from the first, i.e., there has been a degree of clonal selection, however slight. Thus a single tumor suppressor gene mutation may confer selective advantage even if the remaining wild type allele is expressed in a normal fashion. This is likely to be the case for the FAP locus in colon adenomas where allelic loss rarely occurs.[60] At the time of their original identification in the 1980s, recessive transforming changes played a secondary public role to the newly discovered dominantly acting oncogenes. The passage of time has revealed the utmost importance of the tumor suppressor genes and the nature of their interaction with other cellular gene products.

i. Somatic Cell Hybrids

In the absence of chromosome loss, hybrids between a wide variety of nontumorigenic and tumorigenic cells do not give rise to tumors in a relevant host. This was the first evidence which led to the suggestion that the suppression of tumorigenicity had a genetic basis and that this effect may in part be due to recessive changes. In particular, certain hybrid combinations of different tumor cells may also be nontumorigenic, which shows that the hypothesized recessive changes are multiple in nature. Subsequent single chromosome transfer experiments have helped identify some of the tumor suppressor loci, which may in turn be specifically associated with different types of tumors.[61,62]

Hybrid cell lines proliferate indefinitely in in vitro culture, thus expressing the characteristic of immortality. In hybrids between nonestablished diploid fibroblasts and tumor cells, the fusion cells take on the nonestablished nature of the parental cells, i.e., senesce in culture after a limited number of cell division events. Immortalized variants arise at a low frequency and

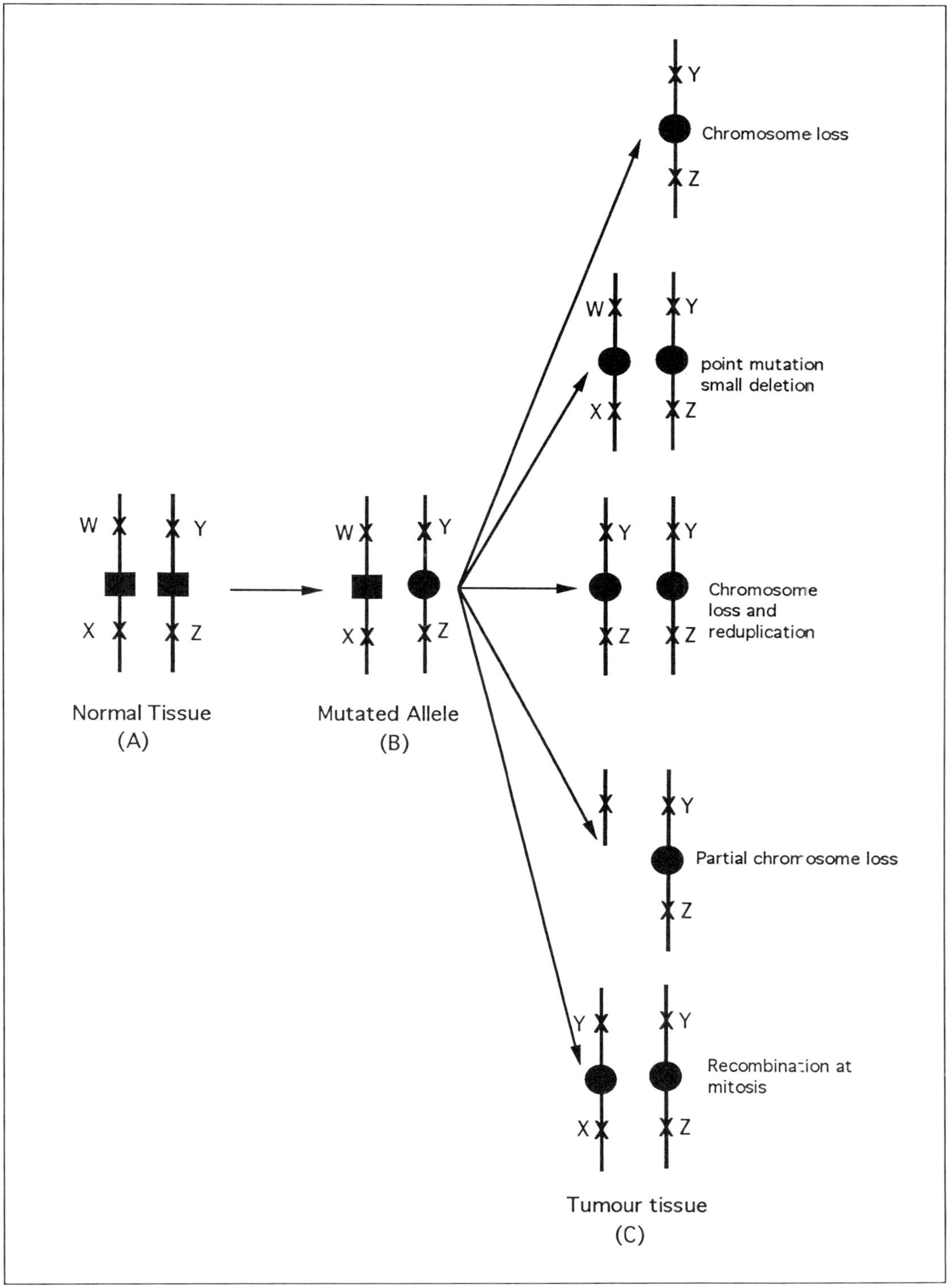

Fig. 2.8. A model for retinoblastoma tumorigenesis. In sporadic tumors, at least two mutations are required to lead to a tumor phenotype (ABC). However, retinoblastoma patients inherit one mutated allele and only one mutation is required for homozygosity at this locus (BC). As shown, this may occur via a number of different mechanisms.

do not form tumors in mice, thus showing that immortalization per se is not sufficient for tumorigenicity. As before, several different genes appear to be able to suppress the immortal phenotype.[63]

When introduced in vivo, the hybrid cells both cease to proliferate and furthermore, undergo a program of differentiation akin to that of the parent. Similar differentiation events follow the natural regression of tumor cells. Thus the suppression of tumorigenicity in somatic cell hybrids is not simply a matter of the complementation of recessive mutations within the tumor cell and more complex pathways may be triggered. For example, straightforward complementation may lead to either induction of the 'normal' differentiation program for that particular tissue or superimposition of a second pathway.

ii. Familial Cancers

Using the hybrid cell route it has not yet proved possible to identify tumor suppressor loci directly. Another approach, the study of familial cancers, has both facilitated this process and given insights into the mechanistic aspects of the cancer process. There are now several cancers for which familial cancer predisposing loci have been identified, and we will concentrate on three of them: Wilms' tumor, retinoblasma and neurofibromatosis type 1. A fourth class, that of the adenomatous polyposis coli gene in familial adenomatous polyposis, will be discussed in chapter 7.

a. Wilms' tumor

Wilms' kidney tumor is a cancer of childhood with both uni- and bi-lateral forms, the latter being associated with deletions in the chromosome 11p13 region. However, evidence is suggestive of a multilocus involvement in the etiology of Wilms' tumor, in particular 11p15. In studies of loss of heterozygosity, it is usually the maternal allele which is lost. Familial forms of Wilms' tumor do not appear to be associated with either region and as such Wilms does not show concurrence of the loci involved in both the familial and sporadic forms of the disease, as has been observed for retinoblastoma. The 11p15 region is also associated with Beckwith-Wiedemann syndrome, a deficiency in the apparatus for genomic imprinting. A putative transcription factor (so assigned because of the presence of characteristic zinc finger domains) has been identified in the 11p13 region deleted in Wilms' tumor. This gene (*WT1*) is expressed only at certain developmental stages and in a restricted range of tissues. Some Wilms' tumors exhibit a complete lack of *WT1* mRNA expression and are homozygous for deletions at 11p13. However, most Wilms' tumors show a high level expression of a mutant mRNA, and in at least one case there has been an internal deletion which has removed one of the zinc finger domains, thus perhaps preventing *WT1* acting as a transcription factor.[64] This tumor also demonstrated one normal allele so the mutant may act either in a dominant negative manner or via gene dosage. A small proportion of sporadic Wilms' tumor patients demonstrate partial loss of heterozygosity (LOH) at 11p loci in normal tissue. The tumor tissue shows the complete LOH at the same region however, implying that not only is the deletion compatible with "normality" but that the tumors arose from cells previously rendered homozygous for the LOH. This reduction to homozygosity at the 11p loci may only be relevant in the presence of other mutations.[65] Whether 11p loci participate in clonal selection events for such mutations remains to be seen.

b. Retinoblastoma

Unlike with Wilms' tumor, both sporadic and familial forms of retinoblastoma are modulated by loss of a single allele, the Rb locus. In what is probably the simplest example of a tumor suppressor gene, the mutant allele is inherited from an affected parent (creating a heterozygote) after which a somatic mutation inactivates the other allele. This inheritance is dominant with incomplete penetrance, the latter being dependent upon the somatic mutational event. Spontaneous retinoblastomas require two mutations to occur in the same cell, a relatively rare event. The genetic locus for retinoblastoma has been unequivocally identified by a deletion analysis and the demonstration of a lack of the suspect 105 kDa protein (p105-Rb) in all retinoblastoma cell lines.[66] Genetic lesions have included large deletions, small deletions in the promoter region, splicing mutations and point mutations. The p105-Rb mRNA is expressed in all tissues examined at all developmental stages and its inactivation has been shown to occur in several types of tumors besides retinoblastoma. These include small cell and non-small cell lung cancers, breast, bladder and prostate cancer, together with osteosarcoma and glioblastoma.

The p105-Rb protein probably orchestrates the cell cycle and/or the state of differentiation via an effect upon transcriptional activation. The p105-Rb protein is phosphorylated in a cell cycle dependent manner and progresses from a low degree of phosphorylation in early G1 and post mitosis to maximal during late G1 and at the G2-M transition. There are at least two proteins which can form a complex with p105-Rb both in vivo and in vitro (E2F1, *myo*D) and a further three which do so only in vitro (c-*myc*, ATF-2, PU.1).[67] All are associated with transcriptional regulation and indeed, when over expressed, E2F1 is alone sufficient to induce cells into S phase.[68] The E2F1 complex with unphosphorylated p105-Rb (which is the predominant form of Rb during G1) inhibits the transcriptional activity of the former.[69] Other Rb binding proteins have been identified by screening cDNA libraries with Rb peptides, so it is likely that other examples of regulation via Rb will be discovered. The p105-Rb protein can regulate transcription in a tissue specific manner both positively and negatively via binding to particular DNA sequences. For example, it has been suggested that the formation of the p105-Rb-E2F complex prevents the normal activity of E2F in stimulation of the transcription of gene products which are required for S phase.[70] The p105-Rb protein may also directly activate genes which are known to downregulate cell proliferation, such as TGFβ1 and β2. During growth arrest by TGFβ1, p105-Rb remains hypophosphorylated, possibly suggesting the existence of an autocrine regulatory loop. For TGFβ1, the downregulation of c-*myc* in keratinocytes may be via such a loop[71] although this mechanism is probably not general.[72] An excess of c-*myc* protein may override the p105-Rb induced growth arrest although probably via an indirect mechanism. Furthermore, p105-Rb complexes with genes involved in myogenesis (e.g. MyoD) may be responsible for the choice of pathway towards terminal differentiation in muscle cells. The p105-Rb protein can repress the expression of c-*fos* and general AP1 transcriptional activity in fibroblasts, again providing a route to control of gene expression.[73] The mechanism of action of p105-Rb in transcription is undoubtedly complex, but it is the effect upon transformation potential with which we are most concerned. How then, does p105-Rb have such a profound effect upon the cell cycle?

Only the hypophosphorylated form of p105-Rb is capable of suppressing cell proliferation, which is evidenced by: (a) the existence of point mutations which preclude phosphorylation events, (b) that differentiation of cells of the hematopoietic lineage is associated with hypophosphorylation and that (c) stimulation of quiescent T cells into a growth cycle is accompanied by phosphorylation of p105-Rb. The stepwise manner of the phosphosphorylation and dephosphorylation events pertaining to p105-Rb suggests that there may be several points at which the activity of this protein is modulated during the cell cycle. It must, therefore, be surmised that p105-Rb acts at several different stages during the cell cycle, and rather than being a crucial single point determinant, both stimulates and represses several processes at different times. However, direct microinjection of purified p105-Rb protein into cells lacking this protein can result in a reversible G1 arrest, which does not happen if the injections are performed after mid G1.[74] This may coincide with one of the cell cycle restriction points. The p105-Rb protein may be phosphorylated in vitro by *cdc*2 kinase, a universal cell cycle controlling protein, and indeed, may complex with it. The *cdc*2 kinase is a member of a family of such proteins which contains both catalytic (cyclin dependent kinases; CDKs) and regulatory (cyclins) sub-units. The cyclin family and its interactions with p105-Rb will be discussed in a later chapter. In summary then, p105-Rb can inhibit progression into S phase and mediates its effect as a tumor suppressor gene during G1. Cyclin mediated hyperphosphorylation of this protein may function to inactivate the activity as a growth suppressor.

c. Neurofibromatosis type 1

The third example which we will discuss is that of neurofibromatosis type 1 (NF1, peripheral neurofibromatosis, van Recklinghausen syndrome) which extends our discussion of Wilms and retinoblastoma to include the variable penetrance that could be associated with a mutator phenotype. In particular, there is good evidence to suggest a biochemical function for the NF1 protein acting as a tumor suppressor gene. NF1 is the most common form of neurofibromatosis with an incidence of 1 in 3000. The mode of inheritance is autosomal dominant and in 50% of cases new mutations are identified which perhaps helps explain the variable degree of disease expression. Affected individuals are at risk of optic glioma, brain glioma, leukemia, pheochromocytoma or neurofibrosarcoma, cancers predominately derived from tissues associated with the neural crest. However the clinical variability of NF1 symptoms has suggested that NF1 may be involved in the growth and development of a wider range of tissues, and indeed, it is expressed in many tissues. However, the extent of cancer predisposition compared to the general population may be distorted by the rarity of these tumors. Subsequent studies have associated loss of NF1 with malignant melanoma.[75] The latter occurs in both sporadic and familial forms by a multistep mechanism beginning with neural crest derived melanocytes.

The NF1 gene has been identified on chromosome 17q11.2 and subsequently cloned. A deletion and breakpoint analysis has unequivocally identified the gene product, called neurofibromin and shown that it has significant homology to the *ras* GTPase activating protein (p120 GAP). The notion of NF1 as a tumor suppressor gene has recently been strengthened by the identification of an example of homozygous inactivation in a malignant neurofibrosarcoma derived from an NF1 patient.[76] In this case a LOH on chromosome 17 was followed by a 200 kilobase deletion at the other locus. In a second case, a patient with malignant melanoma was shown to exhibit a monozygous deletion of the NF1 gene.[75] Other potential tumor suppressor loci are more common in melanoma as determined by LOH, notably on chromosomes 1p, 6q and 9p.

The GAP region of NF1 is capable of stimulating GTP hydrolysis of wild type *ras* protein but not that of the wild type. Thus NF1 may negatively regulate p21-*ras* mediated signal transduction pathways and this is supported by the demonstration of high levels of p21-*ras* $_{\text{[GTP bound]}}$ (i.e. active) in NF1 derived tumors. Hence, in these tumors NF1 may modulate p21-*ras* activity to a greater extent than does p120-GAP. The more general importance of NF1 to cellular metabolism is illustrated by the finding of gene aberrations in apparently unrelated tumor types, although it may be acting in a tissue specific manner or by interacting in a different pathway. For example, NF1 activity does not correlate with p21-*ras* activation in neuroblastomas or melanomas. In contrast, in a schwannoma cell line without detectable expression of NF1, over expression of p21-*ras* increased the proportion of GTP bound, consistent with a role for NF1 in negative regulation of p21-*ras*. Thus in the former case we must consider if NF1 is involved in a p21-*ras* mediated differentiation pathway and that loss of

NF1 activity may result in a lack of differentiation. Hence, NF1 may have different functions depending upon the cell type and its physiological status. It is particularly interesting that there is a high mutation frequency in NF1 resulting in the inheritance of new mutant alleles. This could be due to a variety of reasons which could include a prior defect in the DNA repair machinery thus predisposing to errors at this locus.

iii. Loss of Heterozygosity

Somatic mutations may uncover a constitutionally recessive mutation which may be manifest in various forms (chapter 1) as a loss of genetic material or a loss of heterozygosity (LOH). This can be detected by a concurrent loss of markers either side of the locus in question and may consequently reveal the presence of a tumor suppressor gene.

In combination with a pedigree analysis, LOH studies have helped identify familial and sporadic cancer predisposing loci. The tumor suppressor gene DCC (deleted in colorectal carcinoma; chapter 7) has been identified by this route, which also leads to p53 being correctly identified as a tumor suppressor gene. Disruption of the activity of the p53 gene product is particularly common in human cancers and is likely to contribute to around 50% of all cases, albeit at probably quite a late stage in the development of most cancers. The p53 gene is either lost or mutated in a number of tumor types from a wide variety of human organs, which includes: breast, lung, liver, bladder, ovary, brain, colon, esophagus, together with reticuloendothelial and hematopoietic tissues.[77-80] As such it is an extremely common genetic change in human tumors. In particular, transition mutations at CpG dinucleotide mutational 'hot spots' are common in colon, brain and the lymphoid malignancies, whilst in contrast G to T transversions are common in lung, breast and esophageal cancers, but are spread amongst a range of p53 codons. For an unknown reason, mutations at A:T base pairs are common in esophageal cancer.[81] G:C to T:A transversions are common in the smoking related non-small cell lung cancer and in each case studied the G residue is on the nontranscribed strand. Originally, the p53 oncogene was cotransfected with an activated *ras* oncogene into cells which carried two copies of a normal wild type p53 gene. Here the p53 gene was shown to cooperate with *ras* to induce fibroblast transformation.[82] This gene was subsequently shown to code for a mutant allele[83] which changed the interpretation of p53 action somewhat. Thus rather than a recessive mutation at the cellular level, p53 mutations could be considered to act as dominant negative mutations[84] perhaps via oligomerization of mutant and wild type forms in vivo.

LOH studies on chromosome 17p revealed a high frequency of these mutations in astrocytomas, colon cancer, breast cancer and small cell lung cancer which was subsequently refined to identify the p53 gene at this locus. However, gross alterations in the second p53 allele were not observed until the tumor derived p53 mRNAs were sequenced as cDNAs and shown to contain mutations.[83] Subsequently, cDNAs cloned from normal tissues were shown not to cooperate with *ras* in transformation assays and furthermore, could suppress cooperativity between *ras* and mutant p53 which led to the conclusion that the normal p53 gene product was acting as a suppressor of transformation.[85] How essential then, is the p53 gene product for normal cell growth? In order to investigate this, transgenic mice which were deficient in p53 protein were constructed by gene targeting techniques.[86] Mice homozygous for the cell allele demonstrated that p53 is dispensable for cell division, differentiation and a normal developmental program. However, it is profoundly important that these mice spontaneously developed a wide range of cancers (although biased towards malignant lymphoma and hemangiosarcoma) at an early age, with a mean time of tumor occurrence being 20 weeks after birth. These data indicate that an activated or mutant form of p53 is not obligatory for accelerated tumor development, i.e., this need not necessarily be an initiating event in tumorigenesis.[86] However, the cells of the homozygous mice are certainly likely to be predisposed on the transformation pathway, since they immediately immortalize when introduced into in vitro culture. The disposability of the p53 gene for normal development is consistent with its role as a cell cycle checkpoint protein.

The mutant protein exhibits either increased stability or changed conformation compared to the wild type. The activity of both wild type and mutant protein is controlled by either or both of the amount or the extent of phosphorylation. Levels of p53 protein increase during G1 and it is phosphorylated during S phase by both cdc2 kinase and casein kinase II. The wild type but not the mutant p53 protein is capable of binding to a consensus DNA binding site and it is likely that p53 is involved in control of transcription, either directly or via a complex with other proteins. This sequence contains two copies of a 10 base pair sequence which includes 4 copies of a half site $^{5'}$A/T-G-Py-Py-Py$^{3'}$ arranged in a symmetrical fashion. This suggests binding of p53 as a tetramer, consistent with in solution biophysical studies. The p53 protein has been shown to specifically bind to such sequences and activates genes adjacent to such sites. Many tumors contain irregularities in the p53 gene, the majority being missense mutations (Table 2.3). Some of these mutations cause conformational changes in the protein, thus disrupting its properties. In particular, these may also affect wild type molecules as complexed with mutant forms in the tetrameric complex. One would, therefore, expect that on average, one mutant and one wild type allele may lead to a mutant tetramer, and indeed, it has been demonstrated that such tetramers can no longer bind to the consensus sequence nor activate transcription. The concept of some p53 mutations as dominant negative effectors can thus be rationalized since mutant forms essentially inactivate the wild type protein. It should be noted that p53 inhibits the transcription of some genes which can be simply interpreted as the property of reducing the expression of genes which are involved in promoting cell cycle progression.

A cellular phosphoprotein, p90-*mdm* 2, has been identified and binds both mutant and wild type forms of p53 thus leading to inhibition of activity as a transcription factor.[87] The p90-*mdm* 2 sequence has been identified as an oncogene which when over expressed inhibits gene transactivation mediated by p53 and leads to an enhancement of tumorigenicity. It is particularly important that p90-*mdm* 2 has been identified as over expressed in a significant proportion of human sarcomas. Of possible relevance to cervical carcinomas, the E6 protein of the human papilloma virus inhibits transcriptional activation attributable to p53 by complexing with it and enhancing its degradation. There are now several examples of p53 complexes with proteins derived from the DNA tumor viruses, many of which have relevance to the sequestration of cellular pathways by the viruses. Inactivation of p53 by at least three of these viruses may directly lead to cancer.

Another mechanism of p53 inactivation has recently been uncovered in breast cancer whereby the p53 protein is unable to translocate into the cytoplasm and this cannot act in transcriptional activation or growth suppression.[88] Approximately one-third of breast cancer cases demonstrate cytoplasmic p53 and wild type p53 sequences, which argues for the involvement of other cellular components and not simply mutation of the nuclear transport region.

Thus overall we have at least four mechanisms by which p53 transcriptional activation can be inhibited: (1) mutation of the gene itself (missense, nonsense or splicing mutations, partial or whole gene deletions), (2) inactivation by viral proteins (Eb), (3) inactivation by amplification of other cellular genes (mdm2) and 4) relegation to the cytoplasm.

As will be expanded in later chapters the protein appears to have the characteristics of a nonessential cell-cycle checkpoint protein which functions to negatively regulate cell cycle progression. The latter may augment genetic instability and confer the mutator phenotype thus aiding in clonal selection of growth advantaged cells. A considerable amount of information has accrued concerning the function of p53 which will be discussed in later chapters as follows: the role of p53 in regulation of the normal cell cycle and after DNA damage (chapter 5), the relationship of p53 in inherited cancer predisposition (Li-Fraumeni Syndrome, chapter 16) and models for p53 induced genetic instability such as gene amplification and finally, the relationship of p53 cell cycle arrest after and γ irradiation in the cancer prone syndrome ataxia telangiectasia.

iv. A Cautionary Note on Nomenclature

It is tacitly assumed that tumor suppressor genes in some way directly affect the action of oncogenes and as such have often been referred to as antioncogenes. We believe this nomenclature has led to unnecessary confusion. Firstly, oncogenes and tumor suppressor genes both function in a dominant fashion and neither are necessarily dependent upon the other for functionality. This can be illustrated with an example of a somatic cell fusion experiment whereby a tumor cell which expresses an activated p21-*ras* oncogene is no longer capable of forming tumors when fused with a normal cell. In this case the tumor suppressor gene(s) appears to dominate the 'dominant' oncogene by pathway modulation but does not directly affect the expression or the funtionality of the activated p21-*ras* protein. Hence this behavior cannot be truly classified as 'antioncogenic'. It remains to be seen of course if the tumor suppressor genes regulate a class of oncogenes yet to be revealed, although taken to its logical conclusion one could eventually classify all genes involved in proliferation, differentiation or apoptosis in either category.

References

1. Boguski MS, McCormick F. Proteins regulating ras and its relatives. Nature 1993; 366:643-653.
2. Helper JR, Gilman AG. G proteins. TIBS 1992; 17:383-387.
3. Huang DCS, Marshall CJ, Hancock JF. Plasma membrane-targeted ras GTPase-activating protein is a potent suppressor of p21 ras function. Mol and Cell Biol 1993; 13:2420-2431.
4. Rozakis-Adcock M, Fernley R, Wade J, et al. The SH2 and SH3 domains of mammalian Grb2 couple the EGF receptor to the Ras activator mSos1. Nature 1993; 363: 83-85.
5. Zhang XF, Settleman J, Kyriakis JM et al. Normal and oncogenic p21 ras proteins bind to the amino-terminal regulatory domain of c-raf-1. Nature 1993; 364:308-313.
6. Egan SE, Giddings BW, Brooks MW et al. Association of Sos Ras exchange protein with Grb2 is implicated in tyrosine kinase signal transduction and transformation. Nature 1993; 363:45-51.
7. Buday L, Downward J. Epidermal growth factor regulates p21ras through the formation of a complex of receptor, Grb2 adapter protein, and Sos nucleotide exchange factor. Cell 1993; 73:611-620.
8. Chardin P Camonis JH Gale NW et al. Human Sos1: a guanine nucleotide exchange factor for ras that binds to GRB2. Science 1993; 260:1338-1343.
9. Kohl NE, Scott DM, deSolms J, Giuliani EA et al. Selective inhibition of ras-dependent transformation by farnesyltransferase inhibitor. Science 1993; 260:1934-1935.
10. James GL, Goldstein JL, Brown MS, Rawson TE et al. Benzodiazepine peptidomimetics: potent inhibitors of ras farnesylation in animal cells. Science 1991; 260:1937-1942.
11. Paquette RL, Berenson J, Litchtenstein A et al. Oncogenes in multiple myeloma: point mutation of N-*ras*. Oncogene 1990; 5: 1659-1633.
12. Anderson MW, Reynolds SH, Ming Y et al. Role of proto-oncogene activation in carcinogenesis. Env Health Pers 1992; 98:13-24.

13. Bolen JB. Nonreceptor tyrosine protein kinases. Oncogene 1993; 8:2052-2031.
14. Zachary I, Rozengurt E. Focal adhesion kinase: A point of convergence in the action of neuropeptides, integrins and oncogenes. Cell 1992; 71:891-894.
15. Devary Y, Gottlieb RA, Smeal T, et al. The mammalian ultraviolet response is triggered by activation of src tyrosine kinases. Cell 1992: 71:1081-1091.
16. Wang JYJ. Abl tyrosine kinase in signal transduction and cell-cycle regulation. Current Opinon Genet and Dev 1993; 3:35-43.
17. Kipreos ET, Wang JYJ. Cell cycle regulated binding of c-abl tyrosine kinase to DNA. Science 1992; 256:382-385.
18. Reedijk M, Liu X, Pawson T, et al. Interactions of phosphatidylinositol kinase, GTPase-activating protein (GAP) and GAP-associated proteins with the colony stimulating factor 1 receptor. Mol Cell Biol 1990; 10:5601-5608.
19. Larrodera P, Cornet ME, Diaz-Meco MT et al. Phospholipase C-mediated hydrolosis of phosphatidylcholine is an important step in PDGF-stimulated DNA synthesis. Cell 1990; 61:113-1120.
20. Berridge MJ. Inositol trisphosphate and calcium signalling. Nature 1993; 361: 315-325.
21. Howe LR, Leevers ST, Gomez N, et al. Activation of the MAP Kinase Pathway by the Protein Kinase raf. Cell 1992; 71: 335-342.
22. Kyriakis JM, App H, Zhang X-F et al. Raf-1 activates MAP kinase-kinase. Nature 1992; 358:417-421.
23. Moodie SA, Willumsen BM, Weber MJ, et al. Complexes of Ras-GTP with Raf-1 and Mitogen-Activation Protein Kinase Kinase. Science 1993; 260:1658-1660.
24. Turner B, Rapp U, App H, et al. Interleukin 2 induces tyrosine phosphorylation and activation of p72-74 raf 1 kinase in a T-cell line. Proc Natl Acad Sci 1991; 88: 1227-1231.
25. Gille H, Sharrocks A, Shaw PE. Phosphorylation of transcription factor p62 by MAP kinase stimulates ternary complex formation at c-fos promoter. Nature 1992; 358: 414-416.
26. Pulverer A, Kyriakis JM, Avruch J et al. Phosphorylation of c-jun mediated by MAP kinases. Nature 1991; 353:670-674.
27. Cook SJ, McCormick F. Inhibition by cAMP of *ras*-dependent activation of *raf*. Science 1993; 262:1069-1072.
28. Aziz N, Dubendorff JW, Lipsick JS et al. c-Myb and v-Myb are differentially phosphorylated by p42 in vitro. Oncogene 1993; 8:2259-2265.
29. Blackwood EM, Eisenmann RN. Max: a helix-loop helix zipper protein that form a sequence specific DNA-binding complex with c-myc. Science 1991; 251:1211-1217.
30. Kelly K, Cochran BH, Stiles D, et al. Cell specific regulation of the *c-myc* gene by lymphocyte mitogens and platelet derived growth factor. Cell 1983; 35:603-610.
31. Heikkila R, Schawb G, Wickstrome E, Loke S. Pluznik D, Watt R, Neckers L. A C-myc antisense oligonucleotide inhibits entry into S phase but not progress from G0-G1. Nature 1987; 328:445-449.
32. Hann S, Thompson CB and Eisenmann RN. C-myc oncogene protein synthesis is independent of the cell cycle in human and avian cells. Nature 1985; 314:360-369.
33. Rabbitts PH, Watson JV, Lamond A et al. Metabolism of the c-myc gene products: C-myc mRNA and protein expression in the cell cycle. EMBO 1985; 4:2009-2015.
34. Evan G, Wyllie A, Gilbert C. et al. Induction of apoptosis in fibroblasts by c-myc protein. Cell 1992; 69:119-125.
35. Harrington EA, Bennett MR, Fandi F et al. c-myc induced apoptosis in fubroblasts is inhibited by specific cytokines. EMBO 1994; 14:3286-3295.
36. Shi Y, Glynn JM, Guilbert LJ, et al. Role for c-myc in activation-induced apoptotic cell death in T-cell hybridomas. Science 1992; 257:212-214.
37. Sullivan NF, Willis AE. Elevation of c-myc protein by DNA strand breakage. Oncogene 1989; 4:1497-1502.
38. Roy A, Carruthers C, Gutjahr T. Direct role for myc in transcription mediated by interactions with TFII-I. Nature 1993; 365: 359-361.
39. Kingston RE, Baldwin AS, Sharp PA. Regulation of heat shock protein 70 gene expres-

sion by *c-myc*. 1984 Nature; 312:280-282.
40. Kaddurah-Daouk R, Green JM, Baldwin AS, et al. Genes Dev 1987; 1:347-357.
41. Prendergast GC, Diamond LE, Dahl D, et al. The c-myc regulated gene mr1 encodes plasminogen activator. Mol Cell Biol 1990; 9:1265-1269.
42. Rosenwald IG, Rhoads DB, Callanan LD. et al. Increased expression of eukaryotic initiation factors eIF-4E and eIF-2a in response to growth induction by *c-myc*. Proc Natl Acad Sci 1993; 90:6175-6179.
43. Lazaris-Karatzas A, Montine KS, Sonnenberg N. Malignant transformation by a eukaryotic initiation factor subunit that binds to the messenger RNA cap. Nature 1990; 345:544-547.
44. Lenardo M, Rustgi AK, Schieevella AR et al. Supression of MHC class-1 gene expresison by N-myc through enhancer activation. EMBO 1989; 8:3351-3355.
45. Land H, Chen AC, Morgenstern JP et al. Behaviour of myc and ras oncogenes in transformation of rat embryo fibroblasts. Mol Cell Biol 1986; 6:1917-1925.
46. Rapp UR, Cleveland JL, Fredrickson TN, et al. Rapid induction of hematopoietic neoplasms in newborn mice by a raf/myc recombinant murine retrovirus. J Virol 1985; 55:23-33.
47. Gauwerky, CE, Heubner K Isobe M, et al. Activation of myc in a masked (8;18) translocation results in a aggressive B-cell leukaemia. Pro Natl Acad Sci 1989; 86: 8867-71.
48. Strasser A, Harris AW, Bath ML, Cory S. Novel primitive lymphoid tumours induced in transgenic mice by co-operation with myc and bcl-2. Nature 1990; 348:331-333.
49. Kim SJ, Lee HD, Robbins PD, et al. Regulation of TGFb-1 expression by the product of the RB susceptibility gene. Proc Natl Acad Sci 1991; 88:052-056.
50. Rustgi AK, Dyson N, Bernards R. Aminoterminal domains of c-myc and N-myc proteins mediate binding to the retinoblastoma gene product. Nature 1991; 352:541-544.
51. Greenberg ME and Ziff EB. Stimulation of 3T3 cells induces transcription of the c-fos protooncogene. Nature 1984; 311: 433-438.
52. Kovary K and Bravo R. The jun and fos protein families are both required for cell cycle progression in fibroblasts. Mol Cell Biol 1991; 11:4466-4472.
53. Halazonetis TD, Georgepopoloss K, Greenberg ME. et al. c-jun dimerises with itself and c-fos formung complexes of different DNA binding affinities. Cell 1988; 55:917-924.
54. Rozek D, Pfeifer GP. In vivo protein DNA interactions at the c-jun promoter: preformed complexes mediate the UV response. Mol Cell Biol 1993; 13:5490-5499.
55. Franza B, Rauscher F, Josephs S, Curran T. The fos complex and fos related antigens recognise sequence elements that contain AP1 binding sites. Science 1988; 239: 1150-1153.
56. Marshall CJ. Tumour supressor genes. Cell 1991; 64:313-326.
57. Sager R. Tumour suppressor genes; the puzzle and the promise. Science 1989; 264: 1406-1412.
58. Ponder BAJ. Gene losses in human tumours. Nature 1988; 335:400-402
59. Knudson AG. Hereditary cancer, oncogenes and anti-oncogenes. Cancer research 1985; 45:1437-1443.
60. Volgelstein B, Fearon ER, Hamilton SR, et al. Genetic alterations in colorectal tumour development. N Eng J Med 1988; 319:525.
61. Shimuzu M, Yokota J, Mori N et al. Introduction of normal chromosome 3p modulates the tumorgenicity of a human renal cell line YCR. Oncogene 1990; 5:185-194.
62. Trent JM, Stanbridge EJ, McBride HL. et al. Tumorgenicity in human melanoma cell lines controlled by introduction of human chromosome 6. Science 1990; 247:568-571.
63. Pierrera-Smith OM, Smith JR. Genetic analysis of indefinite division in human cells: Identification of four complementation groups. Proc Natl Acad Sci 1988; 85: 6042-6046.
64. Haber D, Bucklet AJ, Glaser T et al. An internal deletion within an 11p13q zinc finger gene contributes to the development of Wilm's tumour. Cell 1990; 61: 1257-1269.
65. Chao L-Y, Huff V, Tomlinson G et al. Genetic mosaicism in normal tissues of Wilm's tumour patients. Nature Genetics

1993; 3:127-129.
66. Robbins PD, Horowitz JM, Mulligan RC. Negative regulation of human c-fos expression by the RB gene product. Nature 1990; 346:668-671.
67. Kouzarides, T. Transcriptional regulation by the retinoblastoma protein. Trends in Cell Biology 1993; 3:211-213.
68. Johnson D, Schwarz J, Cress D, Nevin J. Expression of transcription factor E2F1 induces quiescent cells to enter S phase. Nature 1993; 365:349-352.
69. Chellappan SR, Hiebert S, Mudryl M et al. The E2F transcription factor is a cellular target for the RB protein. Cell 1991; 65: 1053-1061.
70. Shirodkar S, Ewen M, DeCaprio JA, et al. The transcritpion factor E2F interacts wuth the RB product and p107-cyclin A complex in a cell cycle regulated manner. Cell 1992; 68:157-166.
71. Pietenpol JA, Stein RW, Morgan E et al. Factor binding element in the human c-myc promoter involved in transcriptonal regulation by transforming growth factor b1 and by the retinoblastoma gene product. Proc Natl Acad Sci USA 1991, 88: 10227-10231.
72. Zentella A, Weis MB, Ralph DA. et al. Early gene responses to transforming growth factor-β in cells lacking growth suppressive rb function. Mol Cell Biol 1992, 4952-4958.
73. Robbins PD, Horowitz JM, Mulligan RC. Negative regulation of human c-fos expression by the retinoblastoma gene product. Nature 1990; 346:668-669.
74. Goodrich DW, Wang NP, Qian YW et al. The RB gene product regulates progression through the G1 phase of the cell cycle. Cell 1991; 67:293-302.
75. Anderson LB, Fountain JW, Gitmann DH et al. Mutations in the neurofibromatosis 1 gene in sporadic malignant melanoma cell lines. Nature Genetics 1993; 3:118-121.
76. Legius E, Marchuk DA, Collins FS et al. Somatic deletion of the neurofibromatosis type 1 gene in a neurofibrosarcoma supports a tumour suppressor gene hypothesis. Nature Genetics 1993; 3:122-126.
77. Baker SJ, Fearon ER, Nigro JM et al. Chromosome 17 deletions and p53 gene mutations in colorectal carcinomas. Science 1989; 244:217-221.
78. Nigro JM, Baker SJ, Preisinger AC et al. Mutations in the p53 gene occur in diverse human tumour types. Nature 1989; 342: 705-707.
79. Takahasi T, Nauu MM, Chlba I. et al. A frequent target for genetic abnormalities in lung cancer. Science 1989; 246:491-494.
80. Iggo R, Gatehr K, Bartek J, Lane D, Harris AL. Increased expression mutant forms of p53 oncogene in primary lung cancer. Lancet 1990; 335:675-6798.
81. Hollstein M, Sidransky D, Volgelstein B et al. p53 mutations in human cancers. Science 1991; 253:49-53.
82. Jenkins JR, Rudge K, Currie GA. Cellular immortalisation by a cDNA clone encoding the transformation associated phosphoprotein p53. Nature 1984; 321:651-654.
83. Finlay CA, Hinds PW, Tan TH et al. Activating mutations for transformation by p53 produce a gene product that forms an hsc70-p53 complex with an altered half-life. Mol Cell Biol 1988; 8:531-539.
84. Herskowitz I. Functional inactivation of genes by dominant negative mutations. Nature 1987; 329:219-222.
85. Finlay CA, Hinds PW, Levine AJ. The p53 proto-oncogene can act as a suppressor of transformation. Cell 1989; 57:1083-1093.
86. Donehower LA, Harvey M, Slagle BL et al. Mice deficient for p53 are developmentally normal but susceptible to spontaneous tumours. Nature 1993; 356:215-221.
87. Chen J, Marecjal V, Levine AJ. Mapping the p53 and mdm-2 Interaction Domains. Molecular and Cellular Biology 1993; 13: 4107-4114.
88. Moll UM, Riou G, Levine AJ et al. Two distinct mechanisms alter p53 in breast cancer: mutation and nuclear exclusion. Proc. Natl Acad. Sci 1992; 89:7262-7266.

CHAPTER 3

Dynamic Interactions in Cellular Signaling

1. THE ROLE OF CYTOKINES IN CANCER BIOLOGY

Cytokines are cellular peptides usually produced in response to exogenous stimuli and which influence the behavior of target cells. They may be produced by more than one cell type and a variety of tissues, by which characteristic they can be distinguished from hormones. The action of a cytokine on a cell is determined by the expression of particular receptors on a target cell, which may act via either an autocrine (receptors on the same cell as produced the factor) or paracrine manner. There are several classes of cytokines (Table 3.1) which are responsible for the regulation of a variety of physiological processes and some of these are relevant to our discussion of transforming change. Their action is probably involved in all cell growth and differentiation processes, including wound repair, hematopoiesis, responses to changes in the local environment and tissue turnover. As a corollary, the abnormal regulation of cytokine activity has been associated with a number of disease states.

Cytokines may regulate cell growth and/or differentiation by several mechanisms both positively and negatively. They are also the likely causes of advanced cancer symptoms such as loss of body weight, aberrant nitrogen balance regulation (cachexia) and osteolysis. The former could be associated with the inhibitory effect of tumor necrosis factor α on lipoproteinlipase, an enzyme which is required for the maintenance of body fat. Examples of hematological malignancies where cytokines are probably involved are indicated (Table 3.2).

There is a close association between cytokines and the signal transduction pathways (Table 3.3) although the precise relationships and the molecular mechanisms by which these result in altered gene expression are not at all clear. The examples available to date represent oncogenes and there are as yet no examples of cytokines which represent tumor suppressor genes. However, one might expect that tumor suppressor genes could be involved in either: (a) cytokine receptor downregulation or other such mechanisms for dampening the effects of activating the intracellular signal transduction system or (b) induction of growth inhibitory cytokines.

Table 3.1. Major cytokines in human biology

Colony Stimulating Factors	Interferons	Transforming Growth Factors
Erythropoietin	IFNα	TGFα
GM–CSF	IFNβ	TGFβ-1
G–CSF	IFNγ	TGFβ-2
M–CSF		TGFβ-3
Growth and Differentiation Factors	**Lymphokines**	**Tumor Neurosis Factor**
EGF	IL-1α	TNFα
FGF (acidic and basic forms)	IL-1β	TNFβ
IGF I, IGF II	IL-2 to IL-11	
NGF		
PDGF		

Table 3.2. Hematological malignancy

Non-Hodgkins T-cell leukemia
Adult T-cell leukemia
Acute myeloid leukemia
Human T-cell leukemia
Multiple myeloma

The balance between proliferation and differentiation in any cell population is in part controlled by the relative levels of several cytokines, with concomitant factor independence (e.g. a reduced serum requirement) as the cells become more transformed. We will now consider the various classes of cytokines and examine their roles in transformation. The factors quoted are of particular note. There are no doubt many others of profound importance yet to be recognized.

i. Colony Stimulating Factors

This group of cytokines are involved in the proliferation and differentiation of cells of the hematopoietic lineage and as such, functionally overlap with the interleukins. Colony stimulating factors (CSFs) are involved in the maintenance of the stem cell population, for example, the paracrine regulation exhibited by granulocyte/macrophage colony stimulating factor (GM-CSF) which is produced by the stromal cells of the bone marrow.[1] Also involved is the macrophage colony stimulating factor (M-CSF), whose receptor is the product of the *fms* oncogene and has been shown to exhibit tyrosine kinase activity.[2]

ii. Growth and Differentiation Factors

Epidermal growth factor (EGF) is both produced by and stimulates the proliferation of several cell types. Its receptor, which is shared with transforming growth factor α (TGFα), is an oncogene (*erb*B) which has been associated with several cancers and in particular, the later stages of breast cancer.[3] Acidic and basic fibroblast growth factors (the FGFs) are structurally related and have similar growth stimulating effects, particularly upon neuroectodermal cells, vascular endothelial cells and fibroblasts. They have an angiogenic activity which acts in a paracrine manner to enhance the metastatic process. It is important to note that the normal function of the FGFs is in embryogenesis and the associated proto-oncogenes (*int*-2, *hst*) are usually only expressed in utero. However, *int*-2 has been shown to be aberrantly expressed in various human tumor types.[4]

The insulin-like growth factors (IGFs), I (somatomedin) and II (multiplication stimulating activity), have several similarities to insulin and with the exception of insulin on the IGF-II receptor, can otherwise share each others receptors. Both are present in the plasma bound to carrier proteins, which may render them inactive and provide either a means of control or a reservoir of

Table 3.3. Proto-oncogenes related to cytokines

	Normal Cellular Gene	Oncogene
Growth Factors	B chain of PDGF	*v-sis*
	FGFs	*int-2, hst, fgf-5*
Receptors	EGF receptor	*erb B*
	EGF receptor homologue	*erb B-2*
	M-CSF receptor	*fms*
	M-CSF receptor homologue	*kit*

factor. Certain hormones, such as estrogen, stimulate expression of the IGF-I gene which may in turn be associated with the observed growth stimulatory effects of IGF-I on the mammary gland. IGF-I has been shown to act in an autocrine manner upon breast carcinoma cells in vitro.[4]

Platelet derived growth factor (PDGF) is produced by several cell types (e.g. activated macrophages and endothelial cells) and not just platelets as is implied by its name.[5,6] PDGF has both α and β peptide chains, and both homodimers and heterodimers are found in vivo, although α-α PDGF is less active as a mitogen. PDGF acts via a receptor with tyrosine kinase activity and probably also protein kinase C, in order to stimulate the expression of 'early' genes in the G1 phase of the cell cycle (e.g. c-*fos* and c-*myc*) and is thus thought to have a role in committing the cell to cell cycle entry. This indeed may be one of the normal functions of PDGF in vivo, whereby it stimulates proliferation of fibroblasts in response to injury. An oncogene, v-*sis* has been identified as the β chain of PDGF. The signaling mechanism of PDGF to the nucleus is likely to be complex since in addition to the three types of PDGF, there are three types of dimerized receptor.[7] It is possible that each could provide a distinct signal to the cell, although it is the ββ form that is most closely associated with transformation.

iii. Interferons

Originally identified in protection against viral infection, interferons are now recognized to have several effects upon cellular proliferation, cellular differentiation and immune responsiveness.[8] It has been suggested that the interferons have, in general, a role in reducing cell proliferation. However, their most profound role could be in activation of natural killer cells, responsible for destruction of tumor cells.

Via cell surface receptors, interferons increase the expression of at least 30 genes.[9] One of these, double-stranded RNA activated protein kinase (PKR), has an apparent tumor suppressor gene activity via phosphorylation of the eukaryotic peptide chain initiation factor eIF-2 and subsequent impairment of protein synthesis. Dominant negative mutations of PKR introduced into either cells in culture or nude mice results in malignant transformation, perhaps by conferring an inability to regulate translation of growth associated genes.

A second potential interferon inducible tumor suppressor gene is encoded by interferon regulatory factor-1 (IRF-1) which exerts growth control via the balance of itself and IRF-2. Inhibition of cell growth by interferons may be in part due to IRF-1 activating growth inhibitory genes. It is of interest that this gene is localized to chromosome 5q31.1, a site commonly deleted in human leukemia. Such deletions have also been observed in up to 30% of patients with pre-leukemic myelodysplastic syndromes and 50% of the acute myleogenous leukemias that arise therefrom.

iv. Lymphokines

The term lymphokine is reserved for the group of cytokines which act on the immune system and constitute the intercellular signaling method used by lymphocytes. There are now at least 11 members of this family. Of these IL-6 is worthy of mention to the cancer biologist since it is active on a variety of cell types and its synthesis can be induced by the phorbol esters. It is a growth factor for plasma cells and its autocrine action may be in part responsible for the proliferation of plasma cells in multiple myeloma.[10]

In addition, IL-6: (i) promotes the G0 to G1 cell cycle transition in hematopoietic stem cells (in conjunction with IL-3), (ii) induces differentiation of murine myeloid leukemia cells into macrophages, (iii) induces maturation of megakaryocytes thus increasing platelet numbers, (iv) acts as a hepatocyte stimulating factor and (v) induces differentiation in certain neuronal cell types.[11] In multiple myeloma it is clear that IL-6 is an autocrine factor in those myeloma cells which have been freshly isolated from human bone marrow. Other cytokines such as IL-1 and TNF contribute to IL-6 induction in the bone marrow stroma indicating that paracrine mechanisms may also be operative.[10] High level over expression of IL-6 in B cells of transgenic mice leads to generation of plasmacytomas although this is to some extent dependent upon the genetic background.[12] IL-6 however, does not act as a proliferation factor for B cells and in human cells is a necessary and sufficient differentiation factor in the path to mature antibody secreting plasma cells. Indeed, in B cells it is probably IL-5 that is involved in the proliferative response.[13]

v. Transforming Growth Factors

Transforming growth factor α (TGFα) is structurally related to EGF and they share a common receptor. This receptor is also utilized by a growth factor encoded by the vaccinia virus genome. The major physiological role of TGFα is probably during embryogenesis, although some tumors do express TGFα and it may be important in the bone resorption seen in some cancer patients.

TGFβ (there are forms 1, 2 and 3) is unrelated to TGFα and has a growth inhibiting effect upon most target cells, with the exception of mesenchymal cells where it is stimulatory.[14] TGFβ may act in an autocrine manner to antagonize the effects of mitogenic factors (e.g. EGF or the FGFs). However, there is as yet no evidence to suggest that one of the steps in a transformation pathway is lack of a growth inhibitory cytokine. This may however, represent an important level of control. In breast carcinoma, cells may continue to express TGFβ but fail to respond to it, thus implicating a deficiency of the receptor. TGFβ may stimulate synthesis of extracellular matrix components and inhibit the induction (via EGF) of extracellular proteases, a useful defense mechanism indeed, since the latter are likely to be responsible for destruction of the extracellular matrix during tumor invasion.[15]

Some growth factors (e.g. EGF, TGFα) have two distinct forms, a matrix and secreted form. The secreted form usually derives from proteolytic cleavage of the matrix or membrane bound form and both generally retain the ability to phosphorylate the cognate receptor. The system increases in complexity since matrix TGFα and its receptor (the EGF receptor) may also mediate cell-cell adhesion. The extracellular matrix may be a depot for some growth factors (TGFβ, FGFβ) which can be released by cleavage of proteoglycans.

vi. Tumor Neurosis Factors

The tumor neurosis factors (TNFs) α and β are related and share a receptor.[16] TNFα is produced by macrophages, T cells and fibroblasts in response to endotoxin and the presence of other cell types. It may be involved in the cancer process at a late stage: the loss of body weight, tissue wasting and the negative nitrogen balance which leads to patient death. TNFβ is glycosylated and is produced by activated T cells and also by B cells. Despite the name, TNFs have a wide variety of physiological roles and are an important component of the inflammatory response. The in vivo antitumor effects of the TNFs are probably via increased cell killing due to activation of granulocytes and eosinophils, but they may have more direct effects via stimulation of arachidonic acid production. Metabolism of the latter can generate oxygen free radicals which directly damage DNA. It is thus of interest that TNFα expression is increased after exposure to ionizing radiation. TNFα in part mediates its cellular effects via an increase in the c-*jun* transcription factor and inhibition of the latter prevents a proliferative response to TNFα in fibroblasts.[17]

2. THE CYTOKINE MAZE

There is considerable redundancy and pleiotropy in cytokine action. Whilst cytokine activities are unique, the majority show either induction by common stimuli or overlapping biological actions. Many cytokines can induce the syntheses of other cytokines. Cytokine activity also depends upon the nature of the receptors expressed on the target cell and the state of functionality of the latter, helping to explain the contrasting biological effects of some cytokines, e.g., mitogenesis versus growth inhibition of TGFβ on mesenchymal cells and epithelial, endothelial and hematopoietic cells, respectively. Within the cell there is probably transmodulation of cytokine receptors, desensitization due to internalization and changes in gene expression, all of which contribute to cytokine action. At the extracellular level, local contacts may allow autocrine stimulation in response to high local cytokine concentrations, which will be titrated as a function of distance from the source. If the cells are phenotypically different, then cytokine action may be mediated in a paracrine manner. These effects are crucial to the development of the transformed cell, in that they are able to influence all stages in the process, from loss of growth control to tissue invasion, angiogenesis and metastasis.

3. CYTOKINE BINDING TO ITS RECEPTOR, INTERNALIZATION AND DOWNREGULATION

The cellular effects of cytokines are exerted upon specific receptors which extend beyond the cell surface and which are crucial to modulation of the effect of these agents. The generic receptor has an extracellular domain, a transmembrane domain and an intracellular domain with either enzymatic activity (e.g. tyrosine kinase) or the capability to bind to intracellular molecules. Specificity can be afforded to the external domain by converter molecules which change the affinity of the receptor for the cytokine. There are often high, medium and low affinity receptors for a given cytokine, with biological activity usually mediated via the high affinity form. To further complicate matters, certain cytokines can bind to more than one type of receptor (e.g. IGF-1 and insulin can share receptors).

Following binding of a ligand, there is often a reduction in the number of receptors found in the cell surface, caused by endocytosis. This may be: (a) part of the mode of action of the cytokine and/or (b) responsible for limitation of the biological effects of the cytokine. Within the endosome the ligand is released and either degraded by fusion with a lysosome or the receptor is returned to the surface for reuse. Thus the cell surface expression of a receptor is not just related to those factors which regulate gene expression, but also to the relative rates of membrane insertion and internalization.

Many cytokine receptors have now been cloned and often exhibit two peptide chains, one for ligand binding and the second as a nonligand binding signal transducer. This may help explain redundancy in cytokine biology since different ligand binding molecules may share the same signal transducer. The intracellular domains do not include sequences that are known to be important in membrane to cytoplasm signal transduction, and in the case of IL-6, can be deleted without observable consequence. This suggested that an additional molecule must be necessary and indeed one has been identified as a 130 kDa protein (gp130) that in itself cannot bind IL-6 (Fig. 3.1).[18,19] This protein mediates the high versus low affinity forms of the receptor and

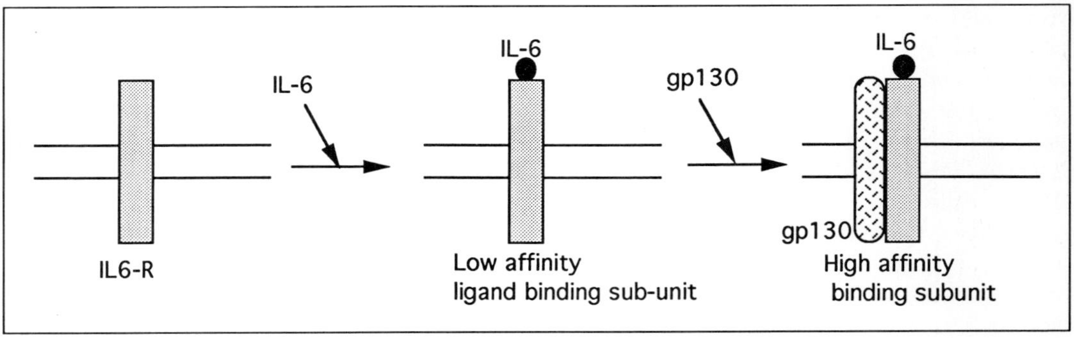

Fig. 3.1. Schematic model showing the effects of IL-6 binding to the IL-6 receptor. Within the IL-6 receptor complex, IL-6 triggers the association of a low affinity ligand binding subunit IL-6R with a non binding signal transducer. This molecule (gp130) helps to form a high affinity ligand binding complex.

is the signal transducing molecule for a number of related cytokines: leukemia inhibitory factor, oncostatin M and ciliary neurotrophic factor.[20] These factors have a wide range of activities, some of which overlap and some of which are specific.[21] The existence of a common affinity converting molecule in part helps explain the overlapping functionalities. Similarly, the human KH97 protein is the signal transducing molecule of the IL-3, IL-5 and GM-CSF receptors and increases their binding affinities to their own receptors. Stimulation of target cells by cytokines does not usually result in phospholipid turnover or an increase in the concentration of Ca^{2+} in the cytoplasm, presumably making the involvement of phospholipase C less likely. However, several cytokines activate intracellular tyrosine kinases and the binding of IL-6 to its receptor results in the homodimerization of gp130 and tyrosine specific phosphorylation events on this protein. Exactly which molecules subsequently interact with gp130 in terms of downstream signaling are not yet clear. However, candidates are beginning to emerge and the IL-2 receptor has been shown to interact with the *lck* oncogene and in IL-1 mediated transcriptional activation of IL-6 in hepatocytes, a transcription factor (NF-IL-6) has been identified and may regulate expression of a number of other genes via binding to an 'IL-6 responsive element'. This factor is activated by nuclear serine phosphorylation events although how it interacts with the IL-6 membrane signal transduction system is unclear. When cancer cells are in advanced stages of transformation, i.e., are competent to metastasize, they may acquire resistance to the effects of several cytokines at once, sometimes including those which were previously inhibitory to growth. Understanding these mechanisms are thus crucial to our attempts at clinical intervention.

Cytokine Resistance in Malignant Melanoma

We will briefly discuss the phenomenon of multiple cytokine resistances in the context of malignant melanoma, where cell lines at all stages of development are available for study. The first stage of melanoma growth (the radial growth phase) shows a plaque like lesion in the epidermis followed by a vertical growth phase in which the mesenchyme is invaded. Beyond a certain thickness the tumor may contain metastatic cells which can invade the vasculature and result in tumor spread. The critical stage, therefore, is mediated by the nature of the event(s) which leads to the ability to grow in the mesenchyme. Some of the relevant cytokines are IL-6, IL-1α, IL-1β and TNF, which inhibit proliferation in early stage melanoma cells, but not in the more advanced cells which have acquired resistance. The latter may be accompanied by the abnormal production of autocrine growth factors which confer growth autonomy and thus we must be careful to distinguish between cytokine independence in studies of advanced stage cancer cells in tissue culture and cancer cells in vivo. Indeed, βFGF is not produced by normal melanocyte cells but is of crucial importance to the growth of these cells.

4. CYTOKINE THERAPIES IN CANCER BIOLOGY

There are two areas where modulation of cytokine activity may benefit the cancer patient.[22] Firstly, by antagonizing the behavioral abnormalities of the cancer cell, and secondly, by stimulation of the immune surveillance mechanisms. This could have particular relevance to treatment of cancers associated with particular chromosome breakage syndromes, where immune dysfunction is often a symptom (e.g. Bloom's syndrome and ataxia telangiectasia).

Whilst in vitro experimental results for (e.g. interferons) have been reasonable, their use in human patients has been disappointing. There are limited applications for interferons in hematological conditions, but considerably less for the common solid tumors. IFNα therapy has been very successful for treatment of hairy cell leukemia and chronic myelogenous leukemia, whilst a number of other conditions (e.g. multiple myeloma, Kaposi's sarcoma) show partial remission. Other growth inhibitory cytokines, e.g., TNFα, are now in clinical trials, often in combination with conventional chemotherapeutics.

An alternative approach is to antagonize the receptor which stimulate the growth of tumor cells. This of course depends upon the degree of selectivity, i.e. whether the tumor shows abnormally high levels of a given receptor or if cytokine dependence is increased. Some therapies involving antibodies directed against mutant EGF receptors have been devised and can be used to target toxins to the target tumor cells.

5. SIGNALING THE NUCLEUS

i. Intercellular Signal Transduction

Once the cell has received an extracellular signal, specific internal responses are triggered, generally in order to activate nuclear processes. There are at least two types of receptors involved in these processes, the tyrosine kinase linked receptors and G protein-linked receptors. In the former case, the enzymes phosphorylate tyrosines at specific positions in the protein substrate, compared to the serine or threonine kinase activity of many other protein kinases. Many cytokine receptors have been shown to have tyrosine kinase activity (e.g. those for insulin, IGF-1, EGF, PDGF, M-CSF [*fms*], atrial natriuretic factor, *neu* [*erbB*-2] and *kit*). At least two of these, *neu* and *kit*, are proto-oncogenes. Some tyrosine kinases are associated with the plasma membrane but do not require effector binding for activity. Examples include *src* (and its family: *yes*, *lck*, *hck*, *fyn*, *lyn*), *abl*, *fgr*, *trk*, *ros*, *fps*, *sea*, *rel*, *ret* and *pim*-1. A further example is one of cross modulation whereby, for example, the IL-3 receptor does not possess intrinsic tyrosine kinase activity of its own, but may modulate this activity via other proteins.

As before, mutations, gene over expression, chromosomal translocations or deletions in these genes have been variously associated with a loss of growth control. The intracellular targets have been difficult to precisely define, but receptor dimerization and autophosphorylation is a likely key step in receptor activation.

The second class of receptor is via the GTP binding (G) proteins. Of three subunits the α subunit has an intrinsic GTPase activity which is modulated by the rate of GTP hydrolysis and the exchange of GDP for GTP. Active G proteins are those with bound GTP and are involved in activation of, at the very least, adenylate cyclase and cGMP phosphodiesterase. There are many Gα proteins broadly classified as Gsα and Giα for their respective stimulatory and inhibitory effect upon adenylate cyclase in response to cytokine or hormone action. Adenylate cyclase produces cAMP from ATP which then activates cAMP dependent protein kinase (protein kinase A), a serine/threonine kinase responsible for a number of intercellular phosphorylation events. Few cytokines seem to act directly via cAMP dependent pathways, but may do so via activation of protein kinase A (Fig. 3.2).

ii. Phospholipase C and Inositol Phospholipid Tumor

At least two forms of phospholipase C (PLC) serve to couple G protein linked receptors (PLCγ1) and tyrosine kinase linked receptors (PLCβ1) to phospholipid turnover. A typical phospholipid is based upon a modified glycol residue whereby C1 and C2 are linked to acylated fatty acids (R1, R2) and C3 has a phosphodiester linked to inositol (R3) (Fig. 3.3). The combinations of different fatty acids, inositol derivatives and enzyme specificities could potentially lead to a variety of second messenger molecules. In general, PLC hydrolyzes phosphatidylinositol 4,5 bisphosphate (PIP_2) to two second messengers, inositol 1,4,5 trisphosphate (IP_3) and diacylglycerol (DAG). The activity of PLC enzymes are linked to the action of EGF and PDGF whilst IL-1 and TNF may stimulate phospholipase A_2. The latter is on the pathway towards arachidonic acid and hence prostaglandin and thromboxane synthesis, thus implicating inflammatory processes (Fig. 3.4).

IP_3 is rapidly dephosphorylated to inositol, but its fleeting existence has a vital role in modulating calcium release from the endoplasmic reticulum, mediated via a specific receptor. Calcium binds to calmodulin which activates a variety of protein kinases in order to elicit biological effect. Other phospholipid derivatives, IP_4, IP_5 and IP_6 may have specific roles as second messengers.

iii. Protein Kinase C

Upon cellular stimulation diacylglycerol activates the calcium and phospholipid dependent class of enzymes known as protein kinase C (PKC). There are at least nine family members, all of which exhibit serine/threonine kinase activity. The tumor promoting phorbol esters also activate PKC and this is their only known cellular activity, which perhaps implicates PKC in tumor cell development. One could envisage situations whereby an aberrant form of PKC would be an oncogene and one would expect that selection for a continuously activated enzyme must be strong. In this regard it has been demonstrated that over expression of wild type nPKCε, PKCβ1 and PKCγ is sufficient to transform fibroblasts[23-25] and a mutant form of PKC has been found in a mouse sarcoma which was induced by exposure to ultraviolet light.[26] However, mutagenic activation of PKC is a relatively rare occurrence in tumors. This could indicate that PKC is of such crucial cellular importance that there are a number of fail safe mechanisms to prevent its aberrant activity. The release of calcium as a result of IP_3 production may also contribute to the activation of PKC, but it should be noted that DAG can be produced from other sources such as the hydrolysis of phosphatidylcholine by phospholipase D and its subsequent dephosphorylation. In addition, several types of DAG may be produced, depending upon the nature of the aryl residues and may therefore be responsible for differential activation of PKC isoforms. PKCα directly phosphorylates the *raf*-1 kinase and can cooperate with it in the transformation process.[27]

6. THE CELL CYCLE

i. ORGANIZATION

The cell cycle is a highly ordered process with numerous control points, which operate to organize and coordinate progression through the cycle. It consists of five main interlinked phases: (1) the G1 phase; a highly active phase in which the cell prepares for DNA synthesis, (2) S phase, in which DNA synthesis occurs, (3) the G2 phase, preparation for mitosis, (4) M phase, cell division and finally, (5) the optional Go phase which is a resting phase in which the majority of nonproliferating cells arrest (Fig. 3.5). Cell proliferation is regulated by mitogenic signals which act during the G1 phase. Late in G1, signals converge onto a cell cycle clock composed of cyclins, CDKs, phosphatases and kinases

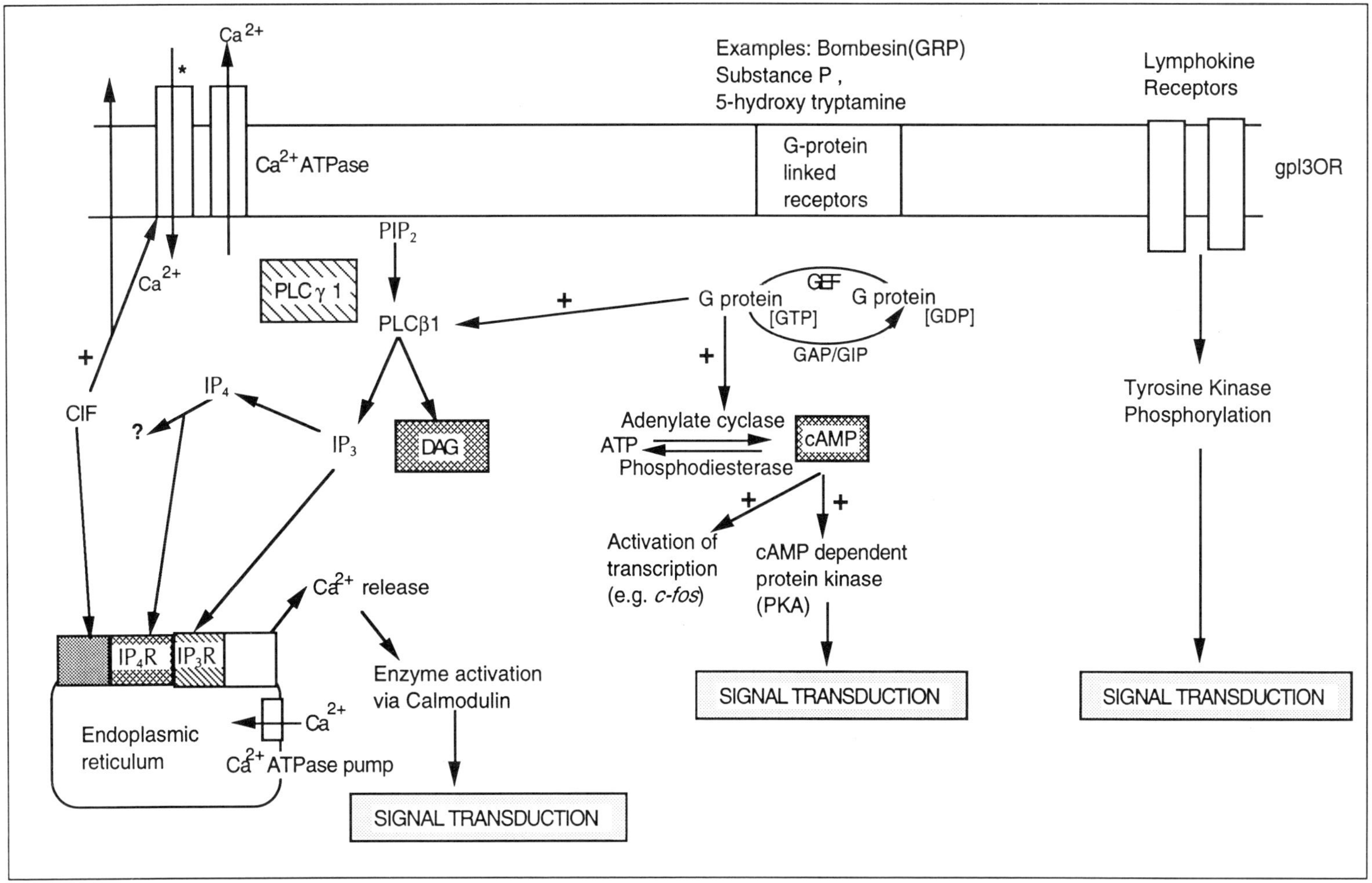

*Fig. 3.2. G Protein linked phospholipid turnover. IP_3R, Inositol trisphosphate receptor; IP_4R, Inositol 1′3′4′5-tetrakis-phosphate receptor; *, Captive entry pathway whereby the ER signals the cell membrane to allow Ca^{2+} to enter thus replenishing the depleted stores; PIP_2, Phosphatidyl-inositol biphosphate; IP_3, inositol trisphosphate; CIF, Calcium influx factor.*

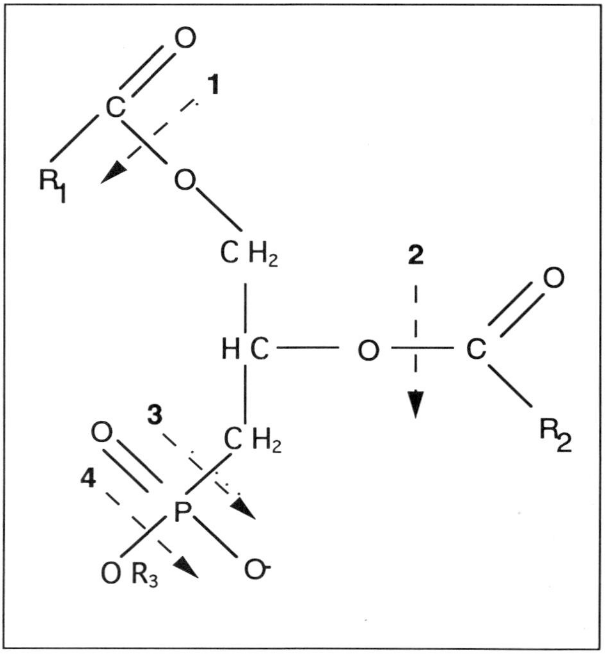

Fig. 3.3. Phospholipid structures. Numbers denote cleavage by: (1) Phospholipase A1; (2) Phospholipase A2; (3) Phospholipase C; (4) Phospholipase D.

in order to ensure commitment to S phase. Upon entry into S phase, however, progress through the cell cycle becomes independent of extracellular agents and intracellular controls are triggered. The G1 phase may be variable in duration and can begin in the preceding cell cycle. Similarly, preparation for mitosis could begin in S and continue during G2. At least four sub-phases of G1 have been identified in fibroblasts and are referred to as competence, entry, progression and assembly.[28] Little is known of the nature of biochemical events which occur during each of these subdivisions. The S phase itself has considerably more complexities than just the replication of DNA. Specific methylation and/or imprinting patterns must be copied, thus regulating gene activity or inactivity, and the nuclear structures such as nucleosomes and chromosome scaffolds must also be reproduced. Clearly, chromosome segregation at mitosis affords many possibilities for the accumulation of abnormalities. As we have already discussed, aneuploidy and rearrangement is a common feature of the genome of cancer cells and abnormal cell cycle control may play a part in this.

Genomic instability may result from aberrant cell cycle control, defects in DNA repair processes and errors in the tackle for DNA replication and chromosome segregation. The cycle is regulated at two precise points in response to DNA damage, both of which are key transitions or checkpoints: (a) the G1-S and (b) the G2-M boundaries. However, we must not close our minds to the possibilities of additional levels of cell cycle control in mammalian cells since there are at least six different points of cell cycle control in *Saccharomyces cerevisiae,* and considering other precedents, mammalian cells are inevitably more complex. From a logistic point of view, DNA damage must be repaired prior to entry into S phase, otherwise mutations could be maintained post-replication and must also be repaired prior to M phase, where DNA chain interruptions could lead to loss, rearrangement or gain of genetic material. Both checkpoints are under genetic control in yeast and mutations have been identified. It is likely that this will also be the case in human cells. The checkpoints must consist of a genomic surveillance mechanism for genetic integrity and by implication, there must also be a mechanism for transducing signals that cause the arrest of either replication or mitosis. Neither of these have yet been identified.

ii. Molecular Mechanisms of Cell Cycle Control

A series of cyclin dependent protein kinases (CDKs) regulate progression through the mammalian cell cycle. The activity of the *Cdk2* kinase appears mid-G1 phase and may be involved in phosphorylation of the retinoblastoma (Rb) protein.[29] This protein is synthesized through out the cell cycle but is phosphorylated in a phase specific manner.[30] Hence, it has

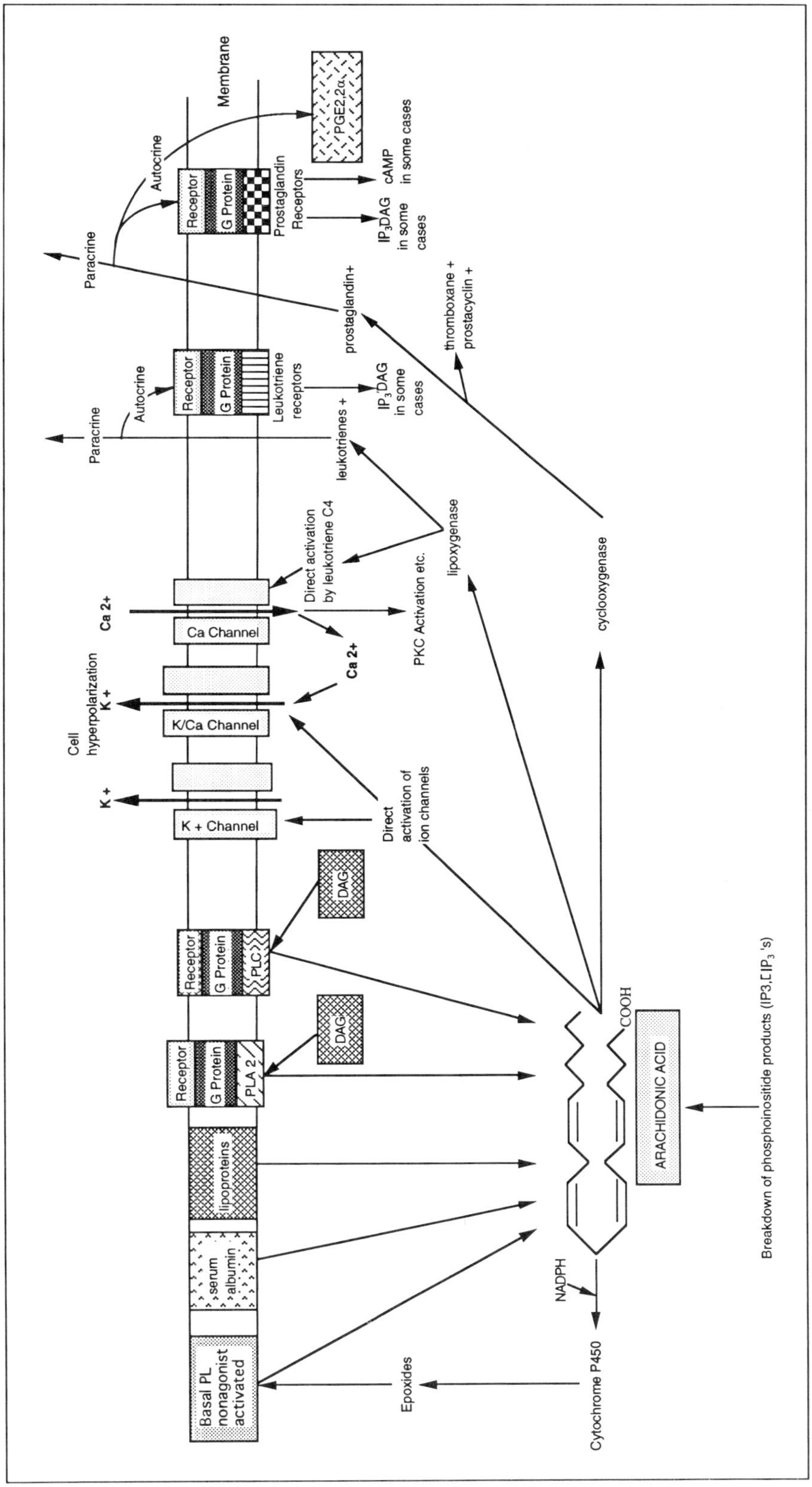

Fig. 3.4. The generalized action of arachidonic acid. Key: +, Eicosanoids; PL, Phospholipase.

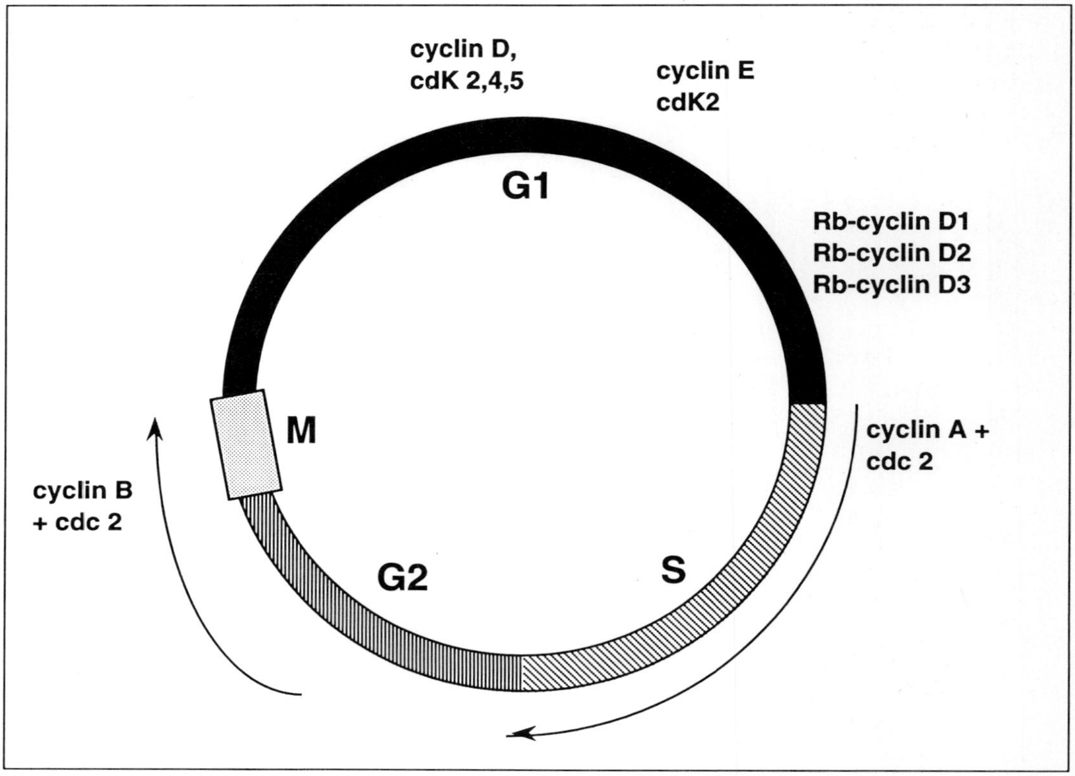

Fig. 3.5. The cell cycle.

been suggested that phosphorylation of Rb at the G1/S transition leads to its inactivation and hence allows the cell to enter into G1/S.[29] *Cdk2* is regulated by protein-protein association with cyclins and mid-G1 phase, it associates with cyclin E.[31,32] The latter complex may function in control of progression through G1[33] and it is interesting to note that its formation can be disrupted by TGFβ, a negative regulator of cell growth.[34] This effect may extend to other CDK-cyclin interactions, thus leading to a reduction in Rb phosphorylation and arrest or delay in G1 progression.[35] At least three cyclins, C, D and E are normally expressed in G1 in mammalian cells with cyclin E sharing periodic expression that peaks at the G1/S transition. In contrast, cyclin D (there are at least three family members) acts as a growth factor sensor and appears at an earlier stage of G1 compared to cyclin E. Cyclin D1 binds to the Rb protein in vitro and mutations in Rb that suppress G1 exit in vivo also prevent binding to cyclin D1. The complexes formed between cyclin D2 and D3 are more stable than those between cyclin D1 and Rb.[36] At the start of S phase *Cdk2* forms a complex with cyclin A, which may play a role in determination of the start of DNA synthesis.[37-39] Similarly, CDKs are necessary for mitosis and another kinase, p34 *cdc2*,[40] has been shown to be positively regulated by cyclin B, itself synthesized during S and G2.[41] The cyclin B-*cdc2* complex undergoes autophosphorylation which results in its activation at the G2-M transition and may help in stabilization of the complex. Other phosphorylation events maintain the kinase in an inactive form during S and G2 and their removal probably triggers mitosis. Cyclin B is degraded in a ubiquitin mediated reaction during anaphase which results in release of inactive *cdc2* and exit from mitosis.[42]

iii. The Effect of Cytokine Action upon the Cell Cycle

Extracellular growth factors may cause entry into G1 and progression through DNA synthesis. Exposure to competence cytokines is required for a considerable part of G1 with an overlap for stimulation by other factors (IGF-1, insulin) in order to circumvent a G1 restriction point and proceed.[28] Proliferation antagonistic cytokines such as TGFβ or TNF can still exert their effects at a relatively late stage in G1.[43] However, the same mixture of cytokines may result in the cell following a differentiation program or in their absence, an apoptotic pathway.[44,45] In the hematopoietic system the sequential action of cytokines controls progress along the differentiation pathway but this is reversible if the cytokine is removed. For example, hematopoietic progenitor cells will proliferate in the presence of a combination of GM-CSF and G-CSF which may be inhibited by IL-3.[46,47] The pathway followed by any given cell is determined by the nature and order of the external factors and the nature of the internal biochemical signals, i.e., whether the cell is competent to receive and disseminate the signal. The presence of multiple types of cytokine receptors is strongly suggestive of the importance of combinations of interacting stimuli. This need not imply that commitment to a particular response is a cumulative effect of cytokine complementation since exposure to one cytokine may compromise the ability to respond to a second. For example, PDGF may transmodulate EGF receptors and TGFβ may cause PDGF receptor downregulation.[48,49] The complexity of these interactions requires spatial confinement of cytokine activity and those in the circulation (PDGF, TGFβ and IGFs) are held in a latent form by either complexing with serum proteins or with platelets.[50] Others however, e.g., FGFβ are confined by the extracellular matrix which could act as a reservoir that can be sequestered by local proteolysis.[51] Thus the ultimate response to a cytokine is not just the nature of the package of cytokines to which the cell is exposed, but also the cellular context, so much so that many cytokines are observed to elicit quantitatively different effects on different cell types and may also do so in a concentration dependent manner.

iv. Control at the G1-S Checkpoint

There is evidence for a role for the p53 tumor suppressor gene in cell cycle control, particularly at the G1-S checkpoint (Fig. 3.6).[52] High levels of p53 inhibit the G1-S transition and in tumor cells which lack p53 or have a dominant mutant form, the normal delay in the G1-S transition which would be present after ionizing irradiation is no longer present.[53] Indeed, this delay can be both restored by the reintroduction of wild type p53 to tumor cells and prevented by the addition of dominant mutant p53 to wild type cells.[54] The levels of the p53 gene product are increased 3- to 5-fold after exposure of cells to γ-irradiation, UV irradiation and DNA cross-linking agents at a point in the cell cycle which coincides with the G1-S transition.[53,55,56] It is also of interest to note that the human inherited Li-Fraumeni syndrome shows heterozygosity for p53 and that cells which are homozygous for mutant p53 are genetically unstable,[57,58] which provides for a method for cancer predisposition in this syndrome. The p53 protein is a transcription factor and probably controls the expression of several genes.[58,59] It is not clear, therefore, whether the loss of genomic stability is a result of loss of the G1-S checkpoint or another function controlled by p53. An additional (and exciting) complication is provided by the example of the inherited syndrome ataxia telangiectasia whereby the G1-S checkpoint is abolished.[60] In the presence of significant numbers of DNA chain interruptions, wild type cells would normally block the initiation of new DNA replication sites, but cells from AT patients override this control and continue to initiate In addition, the aforementioned γ-irradiation induced increases in p53 do not occur in AT

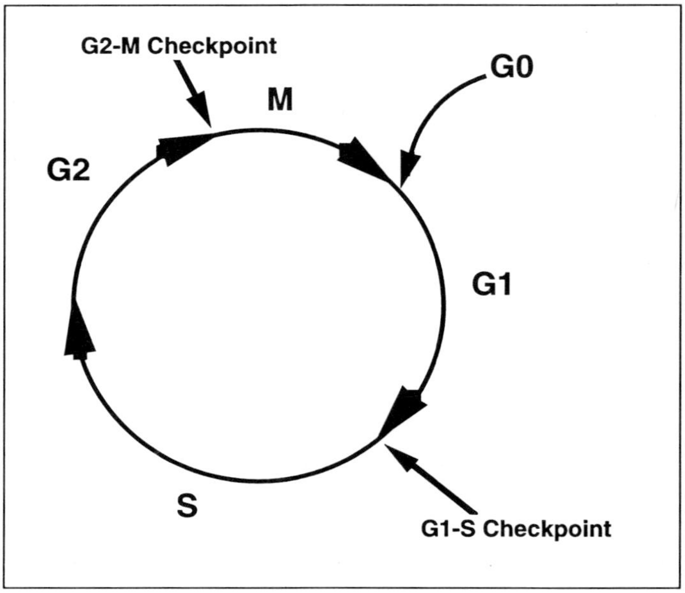

Fig. 3.6. The mammalian cell cycle checkpoints

cells.[61] This AT gene(s) is likely to be upstream of p53 in a pathway that controls the progression past the G1-S checkpoint.

v. Control at the G2/M Checkpoint

Very little is known of the G2/M checkpoint in mammalian cells but there are a number of genetic mutations which have been isolated in study of yeast cell biology. Aberrations at this point provide an obvious route for chromosome loss, duplication and recombination events. An example of a human lymphoma cell line with a defective G2/M checkpoint has been discovered[62] and a number cancer prone inherited syndromes show increased chromosome breakage at metaphase after γ-irradiation.[63] Cell lines derived from ataxia telangiectasia, Bloom's syndrome, Fanconi's anemia and xeroderma pigmentosum all exhibit an increase in chromosomal radiosensitivity in the G2 phase. Further studies indicate that the latter may also apply to apparently normal fibroblastic cells isolated from patients whose families have a history of cancer, suggesting a phenotypic convergence of inherited cancer prone diseases and the chromosome breakage syndromes. Considering our previous discussion, G2 phase chromosomal radiosensitivity could be either be due to a reduced fidelity of genomic surveillance at this checkpoint (G2/M) or a reduced ability to repair lesions at this point. In addition, in mammalian cells the G2/M checkpoint is abolished by treatment with caffeine.[64] Consequently, cells enter mitosis without repairing DNA strand breakage and hence loss or rearrangement of genomic material may occur. Caffeine is metabolized to theophylline, a stimulator of a phosphodiesterase responsible for elevation of cAMP levels.

References

1. Dexter TM, Garland JM, Testa NG. Colony stimulating factors: Molecular and cellular biology. New York: Marcel Diktel Inc, 1990.
2. Cowling CJ, Dexter TM. Erythropoietin and myeloid colony stimulating factors. TIB TECH 1992; 10:349-357.
3. Downward J, Yarden Y, Mayes E et al. Close similarity of EGF receptor and v-erb B oncogene protein sequences. Nature 1994; 307:521-527.
4. Gullick WJ. New developments in the molecular biology of breast cancer. E J Cancer 1990; 26:509-510.
5. Heldin CH. Structural and functional studies on platelet derived growth factor. EMBO J 1992; 11:4251-4259.
6. Ross R, Bowden-Pope DF, Rann EW. Platelet derived growth factor and its role in health and disease. Phil Trans Roy Soc (London) 1990; 327:155-169.
7. Heldin CH, Westermark B. Signal transduction by the receptors for PDGF. J Cell Sci 1990; 96:193-196.
8. Balkwill FR. In: Peptide regulatory factors. Edward Arnold (London) 1989:50.
9. Pelligrini S, Schindler C. Early events in signalling by interferons. TIBS 1993; 18:

338-342.

10. Klein B, Bataille R. The critical role of IL-6 in the pathology of multiple myeloma. J Exp Clin Cancer Res 1991; 10:275-279.
11. Kishimoto T, Shizuo A, Testuya T. Interleukin-6 and its receptor a paradigm for cytokines. Science 1992; 258:593-597.
12. Suematsu S, Matsusaka T, Matsuda T et al. Generation of plamacytomas with the chromosomal translocation t(12:15) in interleukin 6 transgenic mice. Proc Natl Acad Sci USA 1992; 89:232-5.
13. Randall TD, Lund FE, Brewer JW et al. Interleukin-5 (IL-5) and IL-6 define two molecularly distinct pathways of β-cell differentiation. Mol Cell Biol 1993; 13:3929.
14. Sporn MB, Roberts AB. Transforming growth factor β: Recent progress and new challanges. J Cell Biol 1992; 119: 1017-1021.
15. Cross M, Dexter TM. Growth factors in development, transformation and tumorigenesis. Cell 1991; 64:271-280.
16. Tracey KJ, Cerami A. Tumour necrosis factor, other cytokines and disease. Annu Rev Cell Biol 1993; 9:317-343.
17. Brach MA. The mitogenic response to tumour necrosis factor alpha requires c-Jun/AP-1. Mol Cell Biol 1993; 13:4284-4290.
18. Taga T, Hibi M, Hirata Y. Interleukin 6 triggers the association of its receptor with a possible signal transducer gp130. Cell 1989; 58:573-581.
19. Hibi M, Murakami M, Saito m et al. Molecular cloning and expression of an IL-6 signal transducer gp130. Cell 1990; 63: 1149-1157.
20. Gearing DR, Comeau MR, Friend DJ, et al. The IL-6 signal transducer gp130: An oncostatin M receptor and affinity converter for the LIF receptor. Science 1992; 255: 1434-1437.
21. Nishisuka Y. Intracellular signaling by hydrolysis of phospholipids and activation of protein kinase C. Science 1992; 258: 607-614.
22. Mire-Sluis A. Cytokines and disease. TibTech 1993; 11:74-76.
23. Cacace AM, Guadagno SN, Krauss RS et al. The epsilon isoform of protein kinase C is an oncogene when overexpressed in rat fibroblasts. Oncogene 1992; 8:2C95-2104.
24. Housey GM, Johnson MD, Hsiao D et al. Overproduction of PKC causes disordered growth control in rat fibroblasts. Cell 1989; 52:343-352.
25. Persons DA, Wilkinson WO, Bell RM, et al. Altered growth regulation and enhanced tumourigenicity of NIH 3T3 fibroblasts transfected with PKC DNA. Cell 1988; 52: 447-458.
26. Megidish T, Mazurek N. A mutant PKC that can transform fibroblasts. Nature 1989; 342:807-811.
27. Kolch W, Heidecker G, Kochs G, et al. Protein kinase Cα activates raf-1 by direct phosphorylation. Nature 1993; 364: 249-252.
28. Pardee AB. G1 events and regulation of cell proliferation. Science 1989; 246:603-608.
29. Lin BTY, Greunwald S, Morla AO et al. RB cancer suppressor gene product is a substrate of the cell cycle regulator CDC2 kinase. EMBO J 1991; 10:857-864.
30. Bukovich K, Duffey LA, Harlow E. The RB protein is phosphorylated during specific phases of the cell cycle. Cell 1989; 58: 1097-1195.
31. Koff A, Cross F, Fisher A et al. Human cyclin E, a new cyclin tht interacts with two members of the CDC2 gene family. Cell 1991; 66:1217-1228.
32. Dulic V, Kaufmann WK, Wilson SJ et al. p53-dependent inhibition of cyclin-dependent kinase activities in human fibroblasts during radiation induced G1 arrest. Cell 1984; 76:1031-1023.
33. Ohtsubo M, Roberts JM. Cyclin-dependent regulation of G1 in mammalian fibroblasts. Science 1993; 259:1908-1911.
34. Koff A, Ohtsuki M et al. Negative regulation of G1 in mammalian cells. Inhibition of cyclin E-dependent kinase by tgf-β. Science 1993; 260:536-538.
35. Laiho M, DeCaprio JA, Ludlow P et al. Growth inhibition by TGFβ linked to suppression of retinoblastoma protein phosphorylation. Cell 1990; 62:175-185.
36. Ewen M, Sluss Hk, Sherr CJ, et al. Functional interactions of the RB protein with mammalian D-type cyclins. Cell 1993; 73: 487-497.

37. Devoto SH, Mudrij M, Pines J et al. A cyclin-A protein kinase complex possesses sequence-specific DNA binding activity: P33 CDCK is a componenet of the E2F-cyclin A complex. Cell 1992; 68:161-167.
38. Pagano M, Draetta J, Piddle JD. Association of CDC2 kinase with the transcription factor E2F during S phase. Science 1992; 225:1144-1147.
39. Brechot C. Onogenic activation of cyclin A. Current Opinion in Genetics and Development 1993; 3:11-18.
40. Elledge SJ, Spottswood MR. A new human p34 protein kinase CDK2, indentified by complementation of a CDC28 mutation in S, Cerevisiae is a homolgue of Xenopus Eg1. EMBO J 1991; 10:2653-2659.
41. Hamaguchi JR, Tobey RA, Pines J et al. Requirement of p43 CDC2 kinase is restricted to mitosis in the mammalian CDC mutant FT210. J Cell Biol 1992; 117: 1041-1053.
42. Whitfield WG, Gonzalez C, Maldonaldo-Codina G, Glover DM. The A and B type cyclins of Drosophila are accumulated and destroyed in temporally distinct events that define separable phases of the G2-M transition. EMBO Journal 1990; 9:2563-72.
43. Moses HL, Yang EY, Pietenpol JA. TGFβ stimulation and inhibition of cell proliferation. New mechanistic insights. Cell 1990; 63:245.
44. Walker NA, Nicola D, Metcalf AN. Hierarchical down modulation of haemopoietic growth factor receptors. Cell 1985; 43: 269-276.
45. Wyllie AH, Rose KA, Morris RG et al. Rodent fibroblast tumors expressing human myc and ras genes: growth metastasis and oncogene expression. Br J Cancer 1987; 56: 251-259.
46. Dexter TM, Heyworth CM, Spooner E et al. The role of growth factors in self renewal and differentiation of haemopoietic stem cells. Phil Trans Roy Soc (London) 1990; 327:85-98.
47. Heyworth CM, Dexter TM, Kan O, et al. The role of haemopoietic growth factors in self renewal and differentiation of IL-3 dependent multipotential stem cells. Growth factors 1990; 2:197-211.
48. Gronwald RGK, Seifert RA, Bowen-Pope DF. Differential regulation of expression of two platelet derived growth factor recptor subunits by transforming growth factor β. J Biol Chem 1989; 264:8120-8125.
49. Wrann M, Fox CF. Modulation of epidermal growth factor receptors on 3T3 cell by platelet derived growth factor. Science 1980; 210:1363-1365.
50. Barnard JA, Lyons RM, Moses HL. The cell biology of transforming growth factor β. Biochim Biophys Acta 1990; 1031:79-84.
51. Sakela O, Rifkin DB. Release of basic growth factor-heparan sulfate complexes from endothelial cells by plasminogen activator mediated proteolytic activity. J Cell Biol 1990; 8:55-58.
52. Perry ME, Levine AJ. Tumour supressor p53 and the cell cycle. Current Opinion in Genet and Devl 1993; 3:50-54.
53. Kastan MB, Onyewere O, Sidransky D, et al. Participation of p53 protein in the cellular response to DNA damage. Cancer Research 1991; 51:6304-6311.
54. Kuerbitz SJ, Plunkett BS, Walsh WV et al. Wild-type p53 is a cell cycle checkpoint determinant following irradiation. Proc Natl Acad Sci 1992; 89:7419-7495.
55. Fritsche M, Haessler C, Brander G. Induction of nuclear accumulation of the tumour suppressor protein p53 by DNA damaging agents. Oncogene 1993; 8:317-318.
56. Khanna KK, Lavin MF. Ionizing radiation and UV induction of p53 by different pathways in ataxia-telangiectasia cells. Oncogene 1993; 8:3307-3312.
57. Livingstone LR, White A, Sprouse J. Altered cell cycle arrest and gene amplification potential accompany loss of wild-type p53. Cell 1992; 70:923-935.
58. Yin Y, Tainsky MA, Bischoff FZ. et al. Wild-type p53 restores cell cycle control and inhibits gene amplification with mutant p53 alleles. Cell 1992; 70:937-948.
59. Volgelstein B, Kinzler KW. p53 function and dysfunction. Cell 1992; 70:523-526.
60. Painter RB, Cramer P, Howard R. et al. In: Harris CC, Cerutti PC, eds. Mechanisms of chemical carcinogenesis. New York: Alan Liss, pp 383-387.
61. Kastan MB, Zhan Q, El-Deiry WS. et al. A

mammalian cell cycle checkpoint pathway utilising p53 and GADD45 is defective in AT. Cell 1992; 71:587-597.

62. O'Connor PM, Jackman J, Jondle D et al. Role of the p53 tumour suppressor gene in cell cycle arrest and radiosensitivity of Burkitt's lymphoma cell lines. Cancer research 1993; 53:4776-4780.
63. Parshad R, Sanford SK, Jones GM. Chromosomal radiosensitivity during the G2 cell-cycle period of skin fibroblasts from individuals with familial cancer. Proc Natl Acad Sci USA 1985; 82:5400-5403.
64. Busse PM, Bose SK, Jones RW. The action of caffeine on X irradiated Hela cells. Radiation Research 1978; 76:292-397.

CHAPTER 4

System Breakdown

1. INTRODUCTION

A transformed phenotype can result from cellular alterations which are a consequence of either a fixed change in the cell's DNA, i.e., a genetic event (mutation) or a potentially reversible alteration in gene expression, i.e., an epigenetic event. In the two stage initiator/promoter hypothesis model of carcinogenesis it has been proposed that these two events occur sequentially; however, this hypothesis is limited and although it can be applied to experimental situations its relevance to human carcinogenesis is at present unclear.

2. TUMOR INITIATORS

Certain chemicals and some types of radiation (UV, γ) are said to be tumor initiating agents as subcarcinogenic doses will give rise to irreversible yet latent genetic changes without inducing tumor formation. Carcinogens have been classified on this basis of being either complete or incomplete carcinogens, whereby a complete carcinogen is one which can act as both a tumor initiator and promoter.[1]

As carcinogenesis is a multistep process which involves both genetic and epigenetic changes, then the concept of a tumor initiator which causes mutations in the cellular DNA such that the whole organism becomes predisposed to cancer is entirely in keeping with what is observed both in vivo and in vitro. Alterations in diverse families of genes could be cancer predisposing, including mutations in tumor suppressor genes, activation of oncogenes, changes in cell adhesion molecules, the enhanced expression of cell surface receptors, aberrant expression of cell cycle control proteins and over expression of proteins that affect signal transduction pathways. When studying the genetic changes that are present in the fully developed tumor it is of course impossible to pinpoint which mutagenic event results from the cells exposure to the tumor initiator. For example, the first somatic cell mutation that was demonstrated to be relevant to carcinogenesis was a mutationally activated *H-ras* gene found in a human bladder cancer, i.e., at the end of the neoplastic process[2] although activated K-*ras* genes have been detected in premalignant neoplasms of the human colon[3] and in human preleukemia.[4]

3. TUMOR PROMOTERS

The second event in the classical two stage model of carcinogenesis is tumor promotion. It has been proposed that this is (at least in the early stages) a reversible process. Therefore, tumor promoting chemicals (e.g. phorbol esters and okadaic acid[5,6]), wounding by incision[7] and viral toxicity[8] cause epigenetic changes. Thus treatment with one of these agents in the absence of a mutagen will not give rise to cancer, nor will it predispose to cancer at a later stage. In general, whilst these agents do not promote tumors per se, they act in concert with initiators to increase the growth of a selected cell population by stimulating cell division. However, by sustaining proliferation, the cells which already contain a mutation, will have increased risk of accumulating additional mutations.[9] In certain experimental systems it has been shown that isolated oncogene expressing cells appear to be suppressed by their normal neighbors.[10,11] Promoters are required to expand the population of oncogene expressing cells in order to: (i) overcome the inhibitory effects of other cells and (ii) allow additional deregulation events to occur. In cellular terms many tumor promoting agents have a net effect of increasing phosphorylation and so stimulate pathways for cellular proliferation. This can be achieved in several ways; for example, phorbol esters such as phorbol 12-myristate 13-acetate directly activate protein kinase C whilst chemicals in the okadaic acid class are inhibitors of protein phosphatases types 1 and 2 A. These are the serine/threonine phosphatases that normally reverse the action of many cellular protein kinases including PKC.[5,6]

However, it is often difficult to reconcile the in vitro data from model systems of initiation and promotion with that which occurs in the clinical progression of the disease in vivo. If true tumor promotion is considered to result from epigenetic changes in the growth and differentiation pathways that lead to a selected clonal expansion of initiated cells, then this poses many different questions. For example, which compounds can be considered to be tumor promoting agents in vivo? It could be argued that cytokines, hormones and growth factors may act in this respect and many tumors do seem to progress through a period where their growth is dependent upon the presence of these compounds. Hence, in the early stages of multiple myeloma the malignant plasma cells require the presence of IL-6 for proliferation whilst in the latter stages of this disorder the cells become IL-6 independent[12,13] and indeed, the growth of breast cancers have been shown to be influenced by hormone levels. However, there are also many situations where tumor growth is not dependent upon growth factors and cytokines, for example, there is no evidence for their effect in the promotion of lung or colon cancers and in these cases it is more likely that tumor promotion occurs from additional mutational genetic events.

4. MALIGNANT CONVERSION AND PROGRESSION

The progression to a malignant phenotype results from sequential discrete changes to the genome of the premalignant cells, with each step creating an additional phenotypic aberration. There is evidence which suggests that there is an increase in the genetic instability in cells that are progressing towards a more malignant phenotype and it has been proposed that early events in tumorigenesis confer a mutator phenotype on the cells.[14] Four types of predisposition to genetic change are associated with progression. These include loss or gain of whole chromosomes, widespread loss of domains from within chromosomes, an increase in gene amplification events and an increase in the spontaneous mutation rate. The mutations which cause the malignant conversion and progression of a tumor are likely to include alterations in the genes that encode proteins which are important for: (a) growth and differentiation pathways since these could lead to the selective expansion of a particular cell population.

(b) prolongation of cellular life span, as this would create a greater risk of cumulative mutations. Where immortalization occurs this may represent a true increase in replication potential or a decreased differentiation potential[15] and (c) the ability of the cell to invade the adjacent tissue and metastasis.[16]

There is now much information that is available on the multiple genetic alterations that underlie various human cancers and it appears that multiple oncogenes from different functional classes can cooperate in this process, e.g., *c-myc* and *ras*. However, when reconstructing a temporal sequence in which genetic lesions produce the malignant phenotype it has become apparent that individual genes differ in their contributions to tumorigenesis. This is in part dependent upon the tissue of origin and thus mutations in *ras* and amplification events in *myc* appear to occur early in the development of some tumors and late in others.[17] Alterations in the genes that aid the process of metastasis are most likely to be late events and the expression of specific genes has been associated with the metastatic phenotype.[18] However, metastasis may also reflect a loss of function, e.g., the decreased expression of *nm23* has been linked with metastasis of breast cancer.[19] Efforts have been made towards reconstructing the molecular events that lead to clinical progression of several tumor types and several families of activated proto-oncogenes (e.g., *ras, raf, jun, neu* and *myc)* and tumor suppressor genes, e.g. Rb and p53 have been associated with human lung cancer. Moreover, k-*ras*, APC, DCC, MCC and p53 alterations are all associated with the progression to a more malignant phenotype in human colon and lung cancer (see chapters 7 and 9).

In conclusion, the progression of a tumor to a malignant phenotype results from distinctive combinations of genetic lesions although in many cases these have yet to be defined.

5. COOPERATIVE EFFECTS BETWEEN ONCOGENES, ANTI-ONCOGENES AND TUMOR SUPPRESSOR GENES

Cooperative effects between oncogenes have been observed in both in vivo and in vitro model systems, however, whether these data truly reflect the situation that is occurring in the genesis of a tumor has yet to proven.

It has been demonstrated that the incorporation of specific combinations of oncogenes into primary rat embryo fibroblasts results in transformation, whilst individually, the same oncogenes are impotent. These studies lead to the proposal that specific combinations of oncogenes were able to act in concert to promote the transformation process and in this respect c-*myc* appears to be able to cooperate with *ras* thus demonstrating that cooperation is most readily observed between oncogenes of different classes, i.e., those that exert their effects in the cytoplasm and those that act in the nucleus.[20,21] Transgenic mice have been produced which contain oncogenes under tissue specific or ubiquitous promoters and whilst most animals show an enhanced level of tumorigenesis, this is generally delayed to adulthood. However, if strains of mice expressing different classes of oncogenes are crossed, then tumors occur much more rapidly. Thus the rate of tumor formation in mice expressing c-*myc* is much slower than in those mice which coexpress c-*myc* and *ras*.[22] Although these types of experiment are important, one has to question whether the information that can be obtained from such studies reflects the situation in a naturally occurring tumor. However, these types of experiments do confirm that which has already been observed experimentally in vitro, i.e., (a) oncogenes can cooperate to cause tumor formation and (b) in the mouse strains that are carrying one oncogene, additional mutations are required for neoplasia.

How then do these oncogenes cooperate in the transformation processes and what information can be learnt about the progression to a malignant phenotype? Possible insights into these two questions can be gained if one examines the general effects that are observed in cells which contain a mutated/overe xpressed form of either a cytoplasmic or a nuclear oncogene. The nuclear category includes the *myc* family (*c-myc, N-myc* and *L-myc*), *fos, jun,* E1A, and SV40 large T antigen, whilst the cytoplasmic class includes the *ras* family (*H-ras, K-ras* and *N-ras*), *src erb*B, *ros* and *yes*. In general, cytoplasmic oncogene products are able to alter cell morphology, change growth factor and anchorage requirements, whilst in contrast many nuclear oncogene products act in the pathways that lead to cell immortalization. Although the initial oncogenic conversion events may be defined as nuclear and cytoplasmic, the cytoplasmic oncoproteins will, via signaling pathways, exert their effects in the nucleus and the ultimate target of cooperation events is likely to be the transcription of a specific population of genes, e.g., those that trigger G0-G1 progression of the cell or cell cycle regulatory genes such as cyclins. It is known that the protein products of many cytoplasmic oncogenes are capable of inducing the expression of nuclear proto-oncogene products; for example, v-*ras* induces both *c-fos* and *c-jun,* leading to an increase in AP1 activity[23] and *v-src* induces *c-fos.*[24] Hence, if the cytoplasmic cascade of events that is brought about by activation of a cytoplasmic oncoprotein results in the increased expression of more than one nuclear oncoprotein, this perhaps may in part explain why transformation with one cytoplasmic and one nuclear oncogene is more effective than two nuclear oncogenes. In general cytoplasmic oncogenes do not cooperate with each other in the transformation process and it has been proposed that this could either be due to either: (a) specific cytoplasmic inhibitors only allowing one signaling pathway to be stimulated at one time or (b) if the cytoplasmic oncoproteins induce in the same signaling pathways, then they will have an identical set of targets.[25]

How then do mutated forms of tumor suppressor genes affect the transformation process? These proteins function in a number of different ways and for example, the actions resulting from an increase in the level of a mutated form of an oncoprotein may be partially held in check by a wild type suppressor protein. Hence, there is evidence which suggests that the Rb protein may be able to interact directly with specific nuclear proteins and thus may be capable of sequestering some of the transcription factors that are required for G1-S progression. Loss of such a function in concert with an increase in the activity of an oncoprotein would certainly aid the ability of a cell to escape from normal cell cycle control. In addition, some tumor suppressor genes show significant homology to cell adhesion molecules, (e.g. DCC), and loss of such a function of this type in addition to an increase in the level/activity of an oncoprotein may also have the overall effect of increasing the transformation potential of the cell. Finally, the p53 protein appears to function to maintain the integrity of the genome and acts as a G1 checkpoint; if cellular DNA is damaged, the accumulation of this protein will cause a temporal halt to the cell cycle.[26] Cells which carry an inactive form of p53 will not be able to carry out this function; thus exposure of these cells to DNA damaging agents will probably result in an increased rate of mutation and chromosomal translocation.

6. APOPTOSIS: PROGRAMMED CELL SURVIVAL IN TUMORIGENESIS?

It is often said that the only inevitability of life is death. This applies as much to the individual cell as it does to the macrocellular organism and the avoidance of death is a key mechanism by which a tumor promotes its own survival at the expense of its neighbors. Cell death is an integral part of the formation and function of many tissues. Amongst many examples, it is responsible for the acquisition of the correct balance of cell types during embryo-genesis, for formation of the vast number of precise connections between nerve cells and for the protection of the organism against cells involved in autoimmunity.

Cells have an inbuilt mechanism which triggers the death pathway, which varies between cell types. The signal to die may be of extracellular origin, e.g., in the absence of androgenic hormones, prostate cells undergo programmed cell death, as do particular cells of the immune system when deprived of IL-2.[27,28] This implicates a higher level control, that is, the fate of a cell is dependent upon other local and global changes in the organism, even though the death program is inbuilt. Some cells, however, appear to have an autonomous internal clock which controls the onset of cell death, for example, turnover of neutrophils in the hematopoietic system. Whilst the pathways which lead to cell death may vary according to cell type, these mechanisms may converge onto a single common pathway. It is, however, important to differentiate between pathways which are specific to the metabolism of a cell from those which are directly related to cell death. The intriguing prospect is that in a cancer cell, a degree of suppression of the cell death pathways occurs, thus prolonging the life of the cell.

Programmed cell death has been given the name *apoptosis,* which is derived from a Greek work describing defoliation. Apoptosis is distinguished from cell necrosis by the preprogramming element, although both processes may still be stochastic. Necrotic injury is a specific response to physical or chemical trauma, which has been referred to as 'accidental cell death'. This is first characterized by changes in the morphology of the mitochondria and a loss of osmotic homeostasis. Cell rupture releases the cell contents into the environment and usually involves an inflammatory response, necessary for the efficient removal of debris. The morphological changes which occur during apoptosis differ from those of necrosis.[29] Upon initiation of the cell death program, the cell membrane undergoes ruffling and blebbing, but without release of intracellular components and without an inflammatory response. The cell then shrinks in size, the chromatin condenses and synthesis of RNA and protein decreases. The nucleus eventually collapses and fragments (Fig. 4.1). This may be accompanied by double strand DNA chain interruptions in the linking regions between nucleosome cores.

Three different mechanisms can be identified and associated with apoptosis and are dependent upon the effect upon macromolecular synthesis: (a) the transduction mechanism (no effect), (b) the induction mechanism (new synthesis of RNA and protein required) and (c) the release mechanism (depends on an inhibition of the synthesis of RNA and protein). Each one of these are likely to have a different pathway of activation and require different gene products to be involved, although the precise effect upon survival of given tumor types in particular tissues remains to be elucidated (Table 4.1). The first important gene to be identified and associated with apoptosis was the *bcl*-2 gene, a gene product which is often over expressed human in B-cell follicular lymphoma.[30] B cells should normally die in the absence of exogenous cytokines but if transfected with the *bcl*-2 gene, the cells survive. These experiments have been repeated in transgenic animal models thus demonstrating the profound effect of over expression of this gene upon B-cell survival in vivo.[31] The expression of *bcl*-2 occurs in a wide variety of cell types, but it does not work in every cell lineage and cannot protect from cytotoxic T cells. The *bcl*-2 gene product cooperates with the c-*myc* gene product in tumor formation and indeed, the rate is considerably increased compared to that of B cells which over express c-*myc* alone and in addition, *c-myc* mediated apoptosis is blocked by the over expression of *bcl*-2.[31,32] The role of c-*myc* in apoptosis is intriguing given its undoubted role in cell proliferation. It may be that

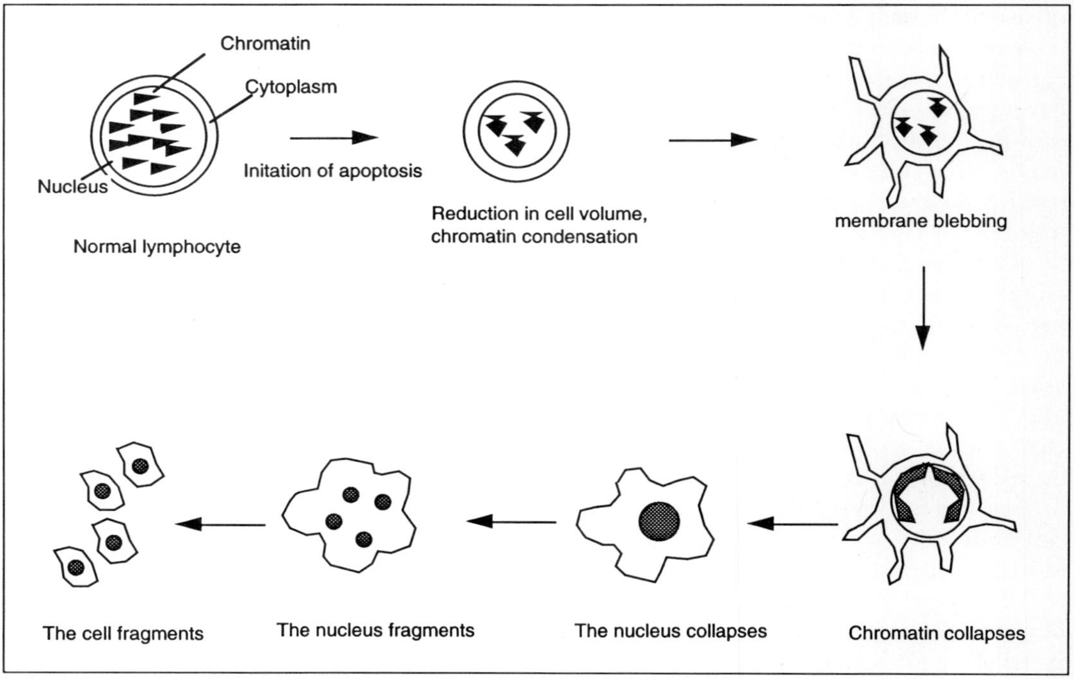

Fig. 4.1. Morphological changes due to apoptosis in lymphocytes.

Table 4.1. Genes involved in apoptosis

Gene	Effects upon Apoptosis	Location within the cell
APO - 1/fas	Stimulation	Cell membrane
bcl -2	Inhibition	Endoplasmic reticulum Mitochondrial membrane Nuclear envelope
c-myc	Stimulation	Nucleus
p53	Stimulation (wild type) Inhibition (mutant)	Nucleus

c-*myc* is involved in the determination of the choice between proliferation and cell death, such that if cooperating factors which are required for proliferation are absent, then apoptosis may ensue.[33] In lymphocyte apoptosis other gene products may be involved, one of which is a cell surface molecule known as APO-1 or *fas*, a protein homologous to the TNF and NGF receptors. Monoclonal antibodies directed against APO-1 trigger apoptosis and can stimulate tumor regression.[34] The apparent proliferation of lymphocytes in leukemia may thus have an element of lympho-accumulation associated with it. The tumor suppressor gene p53 may also be implicated in that the mutant p53 protein inhibits apoptosis in a manner akin to that of *bcl*-2.[35] The over expression of *bcl*-2 has been shown to block p53 dependent apoptosis and *c-myc* and *bcl*-2 appear to be able to modulate the function of p53 by altering its subcellular trafficking during the cell cycle.[36,37] As we have discussed previously, the role of wild type p53 protein may be to arrest damaged cells at the G1/S checkpoint and if this system is in danger of being circumvented, then the cell may resort to programmed cell death as a means of altruistic suicide.[38]

The organism has thus perfected methods for the elimination of cells that are either surplus to requirements or have entered a pathway that may be deleterious, e.g., steps leading towards transformation. Clearly, overriding these pathways could have very important consequences for the cancer process.

References

1. Boutwell RK. In: Slaga TJ, Sivak A, Boutwell RK, eds. Carcinogenesis: Mechanisms of tumor promotion and cocarcinogenesis. New York: Raven Press, 1978; 2:49-599.
2. Tabin C, Bradley S, Bargmann C et al. Mechanism of activation of a human oncogene. Nature 1982; 300:143-148.
3. Bos JL. The ras family and human carcinogenesis. Mut Res 1987; 195:255-271.
4. Lui E, Hjelle B, Morgan R. et al. Mutations of the K-ras proto-oncogene in human preleukemia. Nature 1987; 330: 186-188.
5. Suganuma M, Fujiki H, Suguri H et al. Okadaic acid: an additional non phorbol 12 teradacanoate-13 actetate type promoter. Proc Natl Acad Sci 1988; 85:1768-1771.
6. Nishizura Y. Studies and perspectives of protein kinase C. Science 1986; 233: 305-312.
7. Dolberg DS, Hollingsworth R, Hertle M. et al. The role of wounding in RSV mediated tumor formation. Science 1985; 230: 676-678.
8. zur Hausen H. Viruses in human cancers. Science 1991; 254:1167-1172.
9. Ames BN, Gold LS. Too many rodent carcinogens:mitogenesis increases mutagenesis. Science 1990; 249:970-971.
10. Stoker AW, Hatier C, Bissell MJ. The embryonic environment strongly attenuates v-src oncogenesis in mesenchymal and epithelial tissues but not in endothelia. J Cell Biol 1990; 111:217-228.
11. Dotto GP, Weinberg RA, Ariza A. Malignant transformation of mouse primary keratinocytes by HaSV and its modulation by surrounding normal cells. Proc Natl Acad Sci 1988; 85:6389-6393.
12. Hata H, Xiao H, Petrucci MT et al. Interleukin-6 gene expression in multiple myeloma: A characteristic of immature tumour cells. Blood 1993; 81:3357-3364.
13. Caligaris-Cappio F, Bergui L, Gregoretti MG, et al. The role of bone marrow stromal cells in the growth of human multiple myeloma. Blood 1991; 77:2688-2693.
14. Meuth M. The strucutre of mutation in mammalian cells. Biochim Biophys Acta 1990; 1031:1-17.
15. Harris H. The role of differentiation in the supression of malignancy. J Cell Sci 1990; 97:5-10.
16. Newbold RF. Multistep malignant transformation of mammalian cells by carcinogens: induction or immortatlity as a key event. Carcinogenesis 1985; 9:17-28.
17. Sukumar S. Ras oncogenes in chemical carcinogenesis. Corr Topics Microbiol Immunol 1989; 148:93-114.
18. Hart IR, Goode NT, Wilson RE. Molecular aspects of the metastatic cascade. Biochim Biophys Acta 1989; 989:65-84.
19. Liotta LA, Steeg Ps, Setler-Stevenson WG. Cancer metastasis and angiogenesis: an imbalance of positive and negative regulation. Cell 1991; 64
20. Land H, Parada LF, Weinberg RA. Tumorigenic conversion of primary embryo fibroblasts requires at least two cooperating oncogenes. Nature 1983; 304: 596-602.
21. Weinberg RA. The action of oncogenes in the cytoplasm and nucleus. Science 1985; 230:770-776.
22. Cory SJ, Adams JM. Transgenic mice and oncogenesis. Ann Rev Immunol 1988; 6: 25-48.
23. Imler JL, Schatz C Wasylyk C et al. A harvey-ras responsive transcription element is also responsive to a tumour promoter and to serum. Nature 1988; 332:275-278.
24. Fujii M, Shalloway D, Verma IM. Gene regulation by tyrosine kinases:src protein activates various promotors, including c-fos. Mol Cell Biol 1989; 9:2493-2499.
25. Hunter T. Cooperation between oncogenes. Cell 1991; 64:249-270.
26. Kastan MB, Onyinye O, Sidransky D et al.

Participation of the p53 protein in the cellular response to DNA damage. Cancer Res 1991; 51:6304-6311.
27. Ashwell JD, Berger N, Cidlowski JA et al. Coming to terms with death:apoptosis in cancer and immune development. Immunol Today 1994; 15:147-150.
28. Collins MK, Rivas L. The control of apoptosis in mammalian cells. TIBs 1993; 18:307-309.
29. Williams GT, Smith A, McCarthy J et al. Apoptosis: final control point in cell biology. Trends in Cell Biol 1992; 2:263-267.
30. Hockenbery D, Nunez G, Milliman C. et al. Bcl-2 is an inner membrane mitochonbdrial protein that blocks programmed cell death. Nature 1990; 348:334-336.
31. McDonnell TJ, Korsmeyer. Progression from lymphoid hyperplasia to high-grade malignant lymphoma in lice transgenic for the t(14;118). Nature 1991; 349:254-256.
32. Vaux DL, Cory S, Adams JM. Bcl-2 gene promotes haemopoietic cell survival and cooperates with c-myc to immortalise pre-B-cells. Nature 1988; 335:440-442.
33. Wagner AJ, Small MB, Hay N. Myc-mediated apoptosis is blocked by ectopic expression of Bcl-2. Mol Cell Biol 1993; 13: 2432-2440.
34. Evan GI, Wyllie AH, Gilbert CS et al. Induction of apoptosis in fibroblasts by c-myc protein. Cell 1992; 69:119-128.
35. Yonish-Rouach ED, Resnitzky J, Lotem L et al. Wild-type p53 induces apoptosis of myeloid leukaemic cells that is inhibited by IL-6. Nature 1991; 352:345-347.
36. Chiou SK, Rao L, White E. Bcl-2 blocks p53 dependent apoptosis. Mol Cell Biol 1994; 14:2556-2563.
37. Ryan JJ, Prochownik E, Gottlieb CA et al. c-myc and bcl-2 modulate p53 function by altering p53 subcellular trafficking during the cell cycle. Proc Natl Acad Sci 1994; 91: 5878-5882.
38. Kuerbitz SJ, Plunkett BS, Walsh VW et al. Wild-type p53 is a cell cycle checkpoint determinant following irradiation. Proc Natl Acad Sci 1992; 89:7941-7945.

CHAPTER 5

Mechanisms for Protection Against Cancer and Their Influences on Treatment of the Disease

1. INTRODUCTION

In this chapter we discuss those mechanisms which have evolved to prevent the accumulation of mutations. Contrary to popular belief, DNA has a relatively unstable structure, and like all other biological molecules, decomposes at an appreciable rate. It is susceptible to damage resulting from insult by exogenous agents such as radiation and chemicals and there are a number of mechanisms to prevent DNA damage. The first of these is to prevent endogenous reactive species from reaching the DNA. The second is to repair the lesions which are introduced as a result of both spontaneous decomposition and environmental insult. Thirdly, an immune surveillance system is available to recognize and remove malignant cells. All of these processes are extremely complex and it is likely that there will be interindividual variation. Thus deficiencies in the enzymes that prevent or repair DNA damage could predispose to cancer. This has particular relevance to a number of inherited cancer prone conditions, in which the operative defects are thought to involve the DNA repair machinery. Since the DNA repair process is not completely efficient, mutations in the DNA will accumulate, contributing towards carcinogenesis and aging.[1] We will examine some of the mechanisms by which DNA can be damaged and the methods available for its repair. Since many of the chemicals/agents which damage DNA are also used for treatment of cancer, we will also discuss the effects that genetic variation in the repair processes may have on the efficacy of treatment.

2. OXIDATIVE DAMAGE TO DNA AND MECHANISMS FOR PREVENTION

Reactive species such as hydrogen peroxide, hydroxyl radicals ($\cdot OH$) and superoxide ($O_2^{-}\cdot$) are produced during metabolism, and singlet oxygen is produced by lipid peroxidation or neutrophil activity. Lipid peroxidation may also give rise to lipid epoxides, α,β, unsaturated aldehydes, lipid hydroperoxides and alkylated peroxyl radicals, all of which are potentially mutagenic. Several defense mechanisms have evolved to combat such lesions but these are not 100% efficient, such that oxidative lesions accumulate with age. Indeed, a 2 year old rat may have up to 2 x 10^6 lesions/cell, approximately double that of a neonate. Similarly, in humans the mutation frequency is approximately nine times higher in lymphocytes derived from elderly people compared to those of children. The production of reactive oxygen species is thus probably proportional to the metabolic rate which will of course be related to species and age. The progressive addition of electrons to oxygen (e.g. via mitochondrial cytochrome oxidase or as a by product of metabolism) provides one route towards the generation of DNA damaging oxidation products which then become targets for antioxidants. Endogenous and exogenous sources of oxidants are indicated (Table 5.1). There is thus a compromise between the production of reactive species during metabolism and their removal. Antioxidants in the diet play a crucial role in this process. Several studies and lines of evidence indicate a correlation between an increased cancer risk and a low intake of fresh fruit and vegetables.[2] However, the precise effects of the specific antioxidants such as ascorbate (vitamin C), carotenoids (β carotene, vitamin A) and tocopherol (vitamin E) are difficult to determine. For some, there is in vitro evidence for anti-oxidant effects, such as the action of carotenoids upon singlet oxygen. We cannot however, exclude the potential contribution of several hitherto neglected compounds such as ubiquinol, which may act as an antioxidant in membranes.

There are also endogenous defenses against the effects of reactive oxidative compounds which in general fall into two categories, structural and enzymatic. These are inducible in response to the degree of oxidative damage and indeed, may confer protective effects. For example, many fruits and vegetables contain other nutrients which may help protect against mutation; niacin is important in synthesis of poly ADP-ribose, and folate is required for nucleotide synthesis. Reduced levels of folate are associated with an increase in cancer risk and indeed, may be a factor which contributes to chromosome breakage.

A number of mechanisms have evolved to combat reactive oxygen species, predominantly of a structural and enzymatic nature. Structural defenses include: (a) the peroxisome mediated sequestration of enzymes involved in the generation of hydrogen peroxide and (b) chelation of iron and copper by transferrin, ferritin or ceruloplasmin. Iron and copper aid in free radical generation via the Fenton reaction, and indeed, excess absorption of these ions is a significant cancer predisposing factor in

Table 5.1. Endogenous and exogenous sources of oxidants

Endogenous	Oxidant
Mitochondrial respiration	hydrogen peroxide, superoxide, hydroxyl radical
Phagocytosis*	hydrogen peroxide, superoxide, chlorate, nitrous oxide
Peroxisomes^	hydrogen peroxide
Cytochrome p450	oxidant by products
Exogenous	
Cigarette smoke	nitrous oxides
Dietary iron	oxidants from peroxides
Natural phenols	redox cycling from caffeic acid

* From chronic viral infections; may result in inflammation
^ From fatty acid degradation

hemochromatosis disease. Enzymatic defenses involve: (a) enzymes involved in free radical scavenging such as superoxide dismutase, catalase, glutathione peroxidase and glutathione-S-transferase. The latter aid in the inactivation of mutagenic electrophiles, found as a result of lipid peroxidation, (b) a series of DNA glycosylases and other enzymes for the direct repair of DNA and (c) proteases which detect and destroy oxidized proteins. The level of these defenses will increase in relation to the amount of damage, so, for example, low doses of radiation can induce the defenses such that there is increased protection against higher levels of radiation.

3. SPONTANEOUS DNA DAMAGE

Hydrolysis of the base-sugar bonds in DNA results in the generation of apurinic/pyrimidinic (AP) sites in the DNA with the loss of the purines (adenine and guanine) occurring at a 20-fold increased rate when compared to the pyrimidines (cytosine and thymine). At such a site, the action of AP endonucleases activate a repair process by cleaving the DNA chain at the 5' side of the AP site, making it accessible for the action of a phoshophodiesterase, a DNA polymerase and a DNA ligase, in that order. Each human cell has a purine turnover of between 2×10^3 and 1×10^4 bases per day due to base hydrolysis and repair.[3] However, the capacity of the system far exceeds that required for the repair of spontaneous lesions and it is also used to correct the action of exogenous agents.

5-methyl cytosine residues are preferred sites for mutagenesis due to spontaneous hydrolytic deamination reactions, which occur at a 3- to 4-fold increased rate when compared to the equivalent cytosine residue. The effects of this difference in rate are multiplied by differences in the DNA repair systems available. Uracil DNA-glycosylase rapidly removes deaminated cytosine (i.e. uracil) to generate a base free site which is restored by a mechanism which begins with AP endonuclease action. However, deaminated 5-methyl cytosine (i.e. thymine) leaves a G:T mismatch for repair by specific mismatch correction systems which are considerably slower than repair of the corresponding G:U mismatches. It has been suggested that up to 40% of all germline point mutations in mammalian cells could be the result of methylation at CpG dinucleotides[4] which thus serve as hot spots for mutation. A number of other such reactions may produce premutagenic lesions, e.g., the action of DNA methyltransferase upon 5-methylcytosine or the action of hypoxanthine DNA glycosylase upon the deamination product of adenine (hypoxanthine).[1] The precise role played in in vivo mutagenesis must await further experimentation.

Exposure to active oxygen is again an important source of genome damage. Hydroxyl free radicals cause the production of 8-hydroxy guanine which mismatches with adenine whilst superoxide radicals are responsible for the generation of formamidopyrimidines.[5] Both residues are removed by a specific DNA glycosylase. Generation of 8-hydroxy-dGMP from oxidation of dGTP creates a residue that can be misincorporated adjunct to adenine during replication, although a specific DNA glycosylase does exist. Other lesions which are of uncertain importance include the formation of pyrimidine hydrates and of thymine and cytosine glycols. The lesions are noncoding due to ring saturation. Oxidative damage may also generate 8,5' cyclopurinedeoxyribonucleosides, again of uncertain of mutagenic potential.

A potentially significant endogenous source of DNA damage is the action of S-adenosylmethionine, which besides its role in protein methylation, is present in the mammalian cell nucleus and is required as a cofactor for enzymatic DNA methylation. The latter generates 5-methyl cytosine which forms part of an important mechanism for regulation of transcription. This site is a poor receptor for alkylating agents and the cell may thus avoid DNA repair mechanisms designed to remove these lesions. S-adenosylmethionine, however, has a significant nonenzymatic methylation rate upon DNA and as such, mimics the action of simple alkylating agents, thus generating 7-methyl guanine and 3-methyl adenine. The former does not disrupt coding specificity whilst the latter blocks DNA replication and is thus cytotoxic.

DNA repair systems have evolved to correct spontaneous DNA damage due to oxidative effects of methylation. These systems are probably equipped to cope with most of the DNA lesions likely to occur as a result of such damage,[6] but they are not 100% efficient. Thus damage to the primary structure of DNA may be expected to make a major contribution to the accumulation of mutations in the genome.[7] This may be either due to damaged nucleotides in the DNA templates including mismatches or to misreading of the template due to infidelity of the DNA polymerase. Either way, the mutations so generated may contribute to carcinogenesis.[8] However, it is likely that the two main mutagenic lesions to DNA which result from spontaneous degradation are 5-methyl cytosine and 8-hydroxyguanine.

Depending upon the mechanism involved, there is a wide variation in the rate of mutation across the human genome. If gene sequences are unique, then they appear to change infrequently, e.g. at a rate of 1 out of 400 amino acids in 200,000 years. These mutations are referred to as *static* since the mutant has the same mutation rate as the preceding generation. However, the repeated sequence represents a class of genetic element which demonstrates constant instability. These sequences are often inconsequential to the phenotype since being associated with heterochromatin, they are generally remote from the euchromatin associated gene coding sequences. A second class of element is the microsatellite or interspersed repeated DNA sequence which can often occur in or near gene coding sequences. These may be related to increased mutation rates, via a mechanism which depends upon a change in copy number. This is referred to as *dynamic* mutation. Several human genetic diseases have been linked to mutations which arise through a dynamic mechanism which involves variation in the copy number of a trinucleotide repeat (see Huntingtons disease, Kennedys disease, myotonic dystrophy and fragile X syndrome). Whilst there are not yet any cancer prone inherited diseases which exhibit such mutations, trinucleotide repeats have been found in several proto-oncogenes, e.g., $p(CGG)_n$ is present in the 5' untranslated region of *c-cbl* and $p(CAG)_n$ in the *pim*-1 proto-oncogene. There is currently much speculation regarding the involvement of such repeats in the development of breast cancer.

4. DAMAGE AND REPAIR OF DNA BY ENVIRONMENTAL AGENTS

It has been estimated that there may be between 100 and 200 genes involved in mammalian DNA repair[9] although these figures should be regarded as minimal. There are several pathways for the repair of damaged DNA: (a) nucleotide excision repair, (b) base excision repair via the action of DNA glycosylases, (c) recombination repair, (d) mismatch repair and (e) direct reversal of lesions such as O^6-methylguanine. We will discuss the types of ways in which DNA can be damaged and how these processes are used in repair pathways.

i. Radiation Damage to DNA

It can be argued that carcinogenesis due to radiation is a 20th century phenomenon. We are increasingly exposed to diagnostic radiology, medical treatment, nuclear fallout and the uncertain effects of possible increases in cosmic radiation due to depletion of the ozone layer. There has of course always been exposure to natural sources of radiation, for example, ultraviolet radiation from the atmosphere or radon gas from geological sources; the task now facing us is to identify the magnitude of the excess cancer incidence due to new sources or increases in those already existing. This is an extremely complex task due to two factors: (a) that radiation induced cancers are indistinguishable from any other and (b) frequencies may be increased due to a plethora of other environmental causes. However, there are three groups of patients that are now giving significant information: (a) the life span study of the victims of Hiroshima and Nagasaki, (b) those close to the reactor meltdown in Chernobyl and (c) studies on patients with ankylosing spondylitis who have been treated with significant radiation doses in an effort to cure this condition. As with other models, radiation carcinogenesis can be divided into initiation and promotion stages. However, as is a central theme of this book, the effects of radiation cannot be considered in isolation and plays a part in the accumulation of mutations in conjunction with other environmental, chemical, hormonal and inherited factors. What we must judge is the extent to which radiation accelerates the accumulation of mutation. Before we dissect the molecular events associated with radiation damage and the consequences of an inability to repair these lesions, we will firstly summarize some of the basic characteristics of radiation and the damage which it causes.

a. Ionizing radiation

Radiation occurs in many forms, but is always deposited in discrete packets, the nature of which depends on the type of radiation, the absorbing medium and its energy. Radiations are characterized according to their linear energy transfer (LET) which reflects the rate of transfer of energy to the absorbing medium over a given distance. High LET radiations (alpha particles, neutrons and protons) are very damaging in terms of mutagenic and carcinogenetic potential when compared to either X or γ rays (Fig. 5.1). When radiation hits a given atom, an electron is released which polarizes water in the environment to form a hydrated electron, similar in activity to a free radical in that it is free to diffuse. Since in biological tissues the deposited radiation is equipartitioned according to the proportions of the atomic populations, 80% of the radiation has its effect within the aqueous environment of the cell or tissue. The ionized water molecule forms hydroxyl free radicals (OH·) and reactive hydrogen (H·), both of which can interact to form H_2O_2 and H_2, but others are free to diffuse away.

High radiation doses may have severe effects upon the integrity of plasma membrane including a disruption to protein permeability.[10] Lower doses reveal more effects including a cessation of DNA replication, DNA repair inefficiencies, chromosomal translocation, mutation and a block to cell division. Base substitutions are the most common types of radiation induced mutational events, with both transitions and transversions being found at AT as well as GC base pairs.[11] In tissues, the most sensitive to radiation are those undergoing replacement (i.e. DNA replication and cell division) such as the cells in the gut epithelium and bone marrow.

Radiation causes single and double strand breaks in DNA, the relative proportions of which depend upon the LET of the radiation. These lead to a wide variety of chromosomal abnormalities and mutations whilst the cell attempts to repair the damage. In replicating cells DNA damage must be repaired before proceeding.

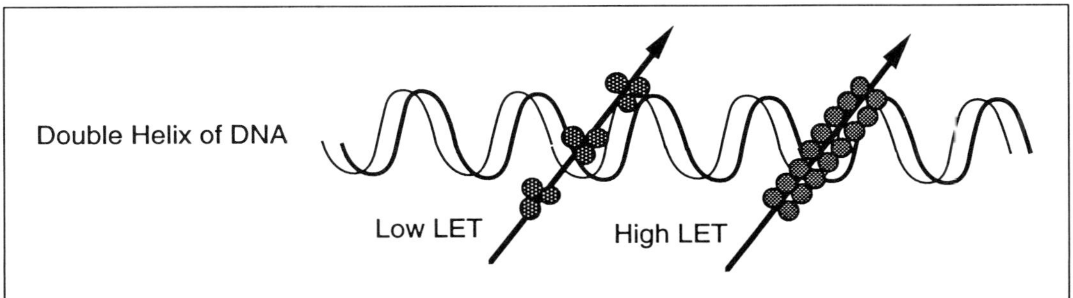

Fig. 5.1. Radiation damage to the double helix.

One clue as to the relevance of radiation carcinogenesis is given by the human cancer prone inherited disease, ataxia telangiectasia (section 3). These patients are both prone to a wide variety of cancers and are hypersensitive to the effects of X-irradiation.

b. Repair of DNA damage induced by ionizing radiation

Free radicals

Cells have evolved protective mechanisms against free radicals, the first being the ability to transfer an electron to a sulphydryl moiety. The second is in use of the enzyme superoxide dismutase for removal of anionic superoxide radicals, a molecule of frequent occurrence in cellular electron transfer. As indicated in a previous section, the phorbol ester tumor promoting agents act via protein kinase C to activate cellular signaling. Superoxide dismutase prevents this tumor promoting effect by an as yet unknown mechanism.

Strand break repair

The cell must be able to directly repair the double and single DNA strand breaks that result from their exposure to ionizing radiation. Certain genes that are directly involved in mammalian and strand break repair, XRCC 1-2 (X-ray repair cross complementing) have been identified. Both XRCC 1 and 2 provide increased resistance to ionizing radiation and in the case of XRCC 1, also to ethyl methane sulphonate.[13] Over expression of XRCC 2 is also associated with increased resistance, but this time to a broad range of damaging agents such as mitomycin C and ultraviolet radiation. This suggests that these proteins also participate in the more general excision repair pathway. Enzymes that are central to normal DNA metabolism (e.g. polymerases and ligases in DNA replication) are also likely to be involved at the end stages of these processes and they will be required to fill in the gaps in the DNA duplex. However, the excision repair pathways that correct damage to DNA which is caused by ionizing radiation are not well understood and most of the proteins that are associated with this process have yet to be defined.

Repair of ionizing radiation-type base damage

There are various forms of direct base damage caused by ionizing radiation and which can be repaired utilizing a number of different glycosylases. These enzymes act by catalyzing the hydrolysis of the N-glycosidic bond that links the altered base to the deoxyribose-phosphate backbone of the DNA and thus causes the release of free bases (Fig. 5.2). Enzymes with these activities were initially discovered in *E. coli* but similar activities have also been found to exist in mammalian cells.

Urea DNA glycosylase

Thymine can be converted into thymine glycols by ionizing radiation. These further degrade to give formylpyruvyl urea and urea. An enzyme with this activity has been described in mammalian cells.[14]

DNA glycosylase that releases purines with opened imidazole rings.

Substituted diaminopyrimidines can occur in DNA as a consequence of exposure of cells to ionizing radiation. A DNA glycosylase which excises formaminopyrimidine has been identified in calf thymus and human fibroblasts.[15]

c. Ultraviolet radiation

Exposure of cells to light of wavelength 260 nm (UV) results in several types of damage to DNA which, dependent upon the dose received, can result in mutation, carcinogenic transformation or cell death. There are numerous lesions that are produced in the DNA after exposure to UV, however, only those which have been shown to have significant biological effects will be discussed herein.

Cyclobutane pyrimidine dimers

These occur when adjacent pyrimidines become covalently linked by the formation of a four membered ring structure. These are very stable and can even survive the

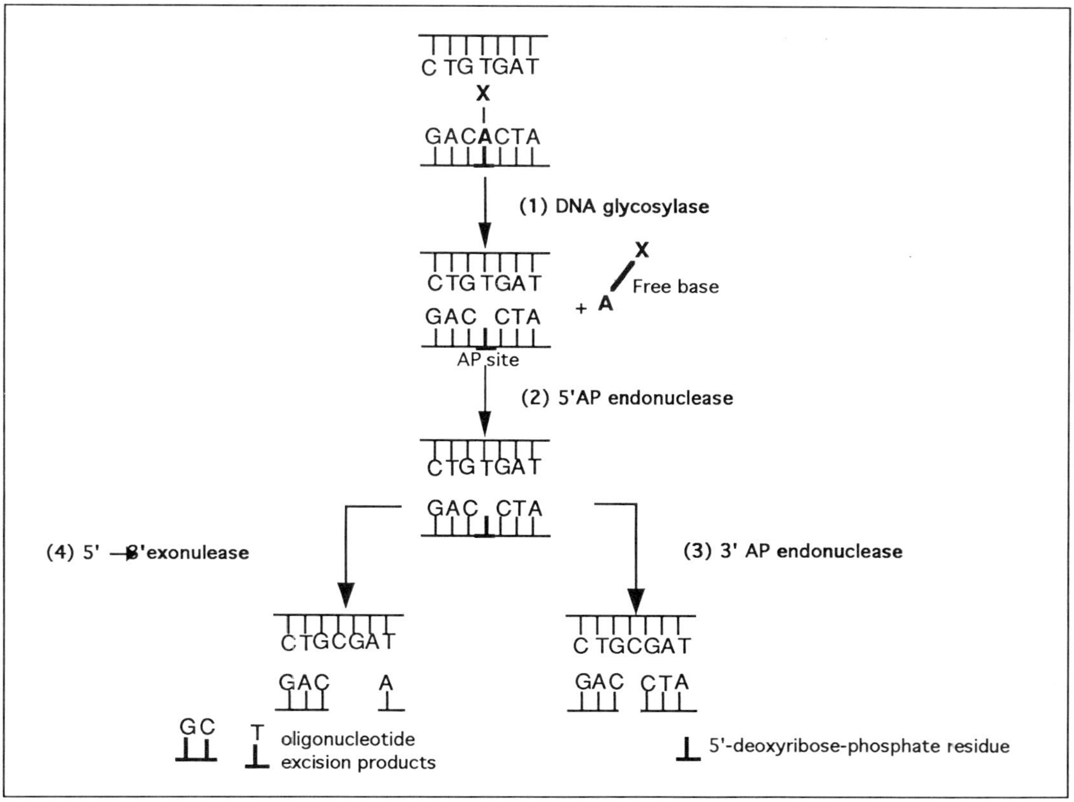

Fig. 5.2. General method of action of DNA glycosylases. Removal of modified base by a DNA glycosylase. (1) DNA glycosylase removes the modified guanine base, leaving an apurinic site (AP). (2) A 5'AP endonuclease makes an incision in the DNA strand. Two different routes are then possible: (3) A 3'AP endonclease cleaves the DNA on the opposite side of the AP site, removing the apurinic sugar moiety, or (4) A 5'to 3'exonuclease removes nucleotides, which include the AP site. The resulting gap in the duplex is sealed by the actions of DNA polymerase and DNA ligase.

total acid hydrolysis of DNA. Their formation is influenced by the composition of the adjacent nucleotide with TT dimers occurring more frequently than CC and the surrounding DNA sequence; for example, ATTA dimerizes more easily than ATTG. These dimers do not cause mutation per se but they do block the progression of DNA polymerases during replication and if left unrepaired, cell death will ensue.

Pyrimidine-pyrimidone (6-4) lesions

These are probably the most biologically relevant lesions which result from UV DNA damage. The number produced is directly proportional to the dose of UV received and moreover, there is a good correlation between the frequency of nonsense mutations and 6-4 photoproduct induction.[16,17] These are therefore the types of alteration which would result in the accumulation of mutations.

d. Repair of UV induced DNA damage

In mammalian cells UV damaged DNA can be repaired by: (a) direct reversal of the damage and (b) excision of the damage. The effect of a deficiency in the excision repair pathways is observed in the human cancer prone inheritable syndrome xeroderma pigmentosum where patients with this disease are unable to repair UV induced DNA damage and as a result, have a very high incidence of skin cancer.

Direct Reversal of UV damage

A photoreactivating enzyme (DNA photolyase) has been discovered in cell extracts from several mammalian cell types. This enzyme is able to reverse pyrimdine dimers, although the mechanism of the reaction in eukaryotic cells has yet to be defined.[18,19] However in prokaryotes it is thought to involve an electron transfer from the excited ring of tryptophan within the enzyme to the dimer, resulting in the photosensitized splitting of this dimer (Fig. 5.3).

Excision repair pathways

In mammalian cells there are complex excision repair pathways that can be utilized to repair DNA which contains bulky adducts; this includes damage caused to DNA by both UV and DNA cross-linking agents. The repair takes place in large transcription units and thus it can be rather difficult to assign specific functions to the individual proteins that have been isolated. Three methods have been utilized to identify those proteins which act in the mammalian systems; these include (a) the microinjection of partially purified material into repair deficient cells lines derived from the human chromosome breakage disorders, e.g., xeroderma pigmentosum, (b) the purification of proteins that are capable of binding to stretches of DNA which contain a damaged base and (c) the correction of the UV sensitivity phenotype of either XP cell lines or artificially generated rodent mutant cell lines by DNA transfection.[20] These approaches have led to the discovery of a number of relevant protein products, although in some cases their functions have yet to be elucidated. The DNA in mammalian cells is a tightly coiled condensed structure held together by a number of different proteins which includes histones. Therefore, the initial stages of the repair pathways must require the actions of helicases to unwind the DNA such that the damage becomes accessible. In this respect, three putative DNA helicases have been discovered which are the products of the excision repair cross complementing genes (ERCC) 2, 3 and 6.[21-23] ERCC 2 has a nucleotide binding domain and shows a strong homology to the RAD 3 repair helicase.[21] This protein appears to have an essential cellular function since frame shifts in the ERCC 2 genes are lethal. This gene corrects the defect that is observed in cell lines derived from patients with XP type D.[22] ERCC 3 contains a helix-turn helix DNA binding motif and nuclear location signal and it has been proposed that it functions as a DNA and chromatin binding helicase. This gene complements the defect in XP-B cells. The third protein which has putative helicase activity in conjunction with chromatin and nucleotide binding domains is the protein product of the ERCC 6 gene. There are data which suggest that the ERCC 2 and ERCC 3 genes fulfill complementary functions, with these enzymes unwinding the DNA in opposite directions and perhaps cooperating in scanning for structural distortions in the DNA. It has been proposed that ERCC 6 is required for specifically opening segments of DNA that are being actively transcribed.[23] Additional proteins must be necessary to bind to the damaged region of DNA and finally to excise the defective bases. The products of the XP-A and XP-C genes both bind DNA and moreover, the XP-A gene product which contains a zinc finger motif is able to specifically bind to UV damaged DNA.[25,26]

A candidate protein for the excision of the damaged bases has been identified in human cells and removes thymine dimers from DNA by incising the 22nd phosphodiester bond 5' to the photodimer and the 6th phosphodiester bond 3' to the photodimer.[27] It has been proposed that the products of ERCC 1, ERCC 4 and XP-11 also participate in the incision process.[28] However, it appears that these proteins may be specifically involved in the repair of damage caused by DNA cross linking agents since ERCC 1 and ERCC 4 mutant cell lines are hypersensitive to these agents.[29] Interstrand cross links may require additional recombination steps for their complete removal. The human single stranded binding protein is also required for excision repair and may function to displace the nucleotides or protect the gapped region of the duplex from damage by nucleases[30] (Fig. 5.4). Finally, the resultant gap must then be filled in by a DNA polymerase. Since proliferating cell nuclear antigen (PCNA) is required, this implies that synthesis is probably carried out by either DNA polymerase δ or ε.[31] The final step in this process is the sealing of the gap in the duplex structure by the action of DNA ligases (Fig. 5.5).

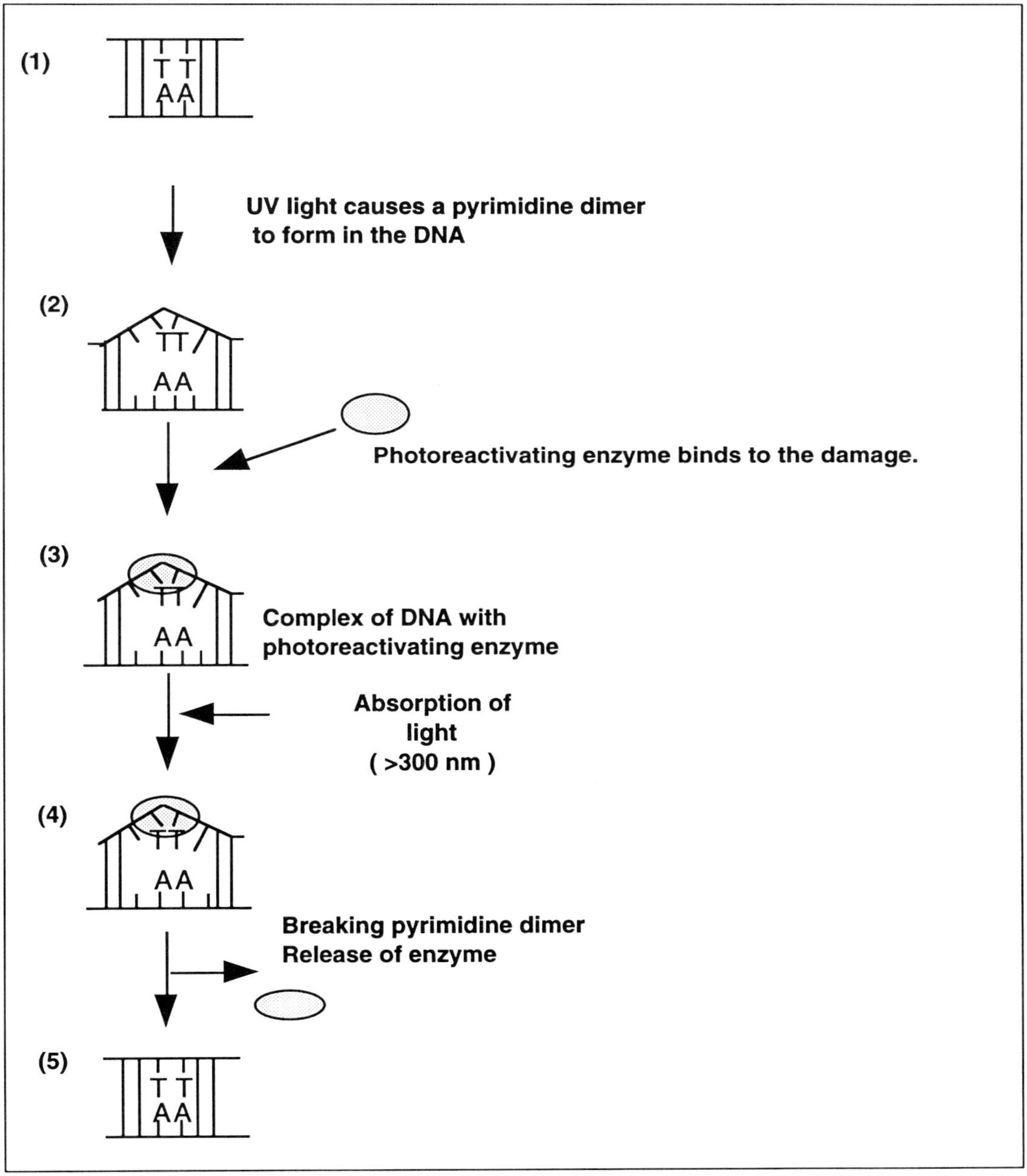

Fig. 5.3. Model for photoreaction by DNA photolyase. (1) and (2) Ultraviolet radiation causes the formation of a cyclobutane pyrimidine dimer. (3) The photoreactivating enzyme binds to the DNA. (4) The enzyme absorbs visible light, splits the dimer and (5) finally dissociates.

ii. Chemical Damage to DNA

a. Introduction

The genotoxic effects of chemical agents are determined largely by their reactivity with DNA. Much of the information on the effects that certain classes of chemicals (including alkylating agents and DNA crosslinking agents) have on DNA, has come from the field of cancer biology where these chemicals are frequently used to kill rapidly dividing tumor cells. However, treatment of cells with noncytotoxic doses of chemotherapeutic agents can result in a spectrum of mutation.

b. Alkylating agents

These are electrophilic compounds with affinity for nucleophilic centers in organic macromolecules. The sites of reaction in DNA include adenine at positions N1, N3, N6, N7; guanine at positions N1, N2, N3, N7 and O6; cytosine in positions N3, N4, O2 and thymine in positions N3, O2 and O4.[32,33] Alkylation of oxygen in linkages results in the formation of phosphotriesters. The extent to which each residue is alkylated is dependent upon a number of factors including the reactivity of the chemical used. For example, methylmethanesulphonate has a much lower affinity for the O^6 position of guanine than ethylmethanesulphonate.

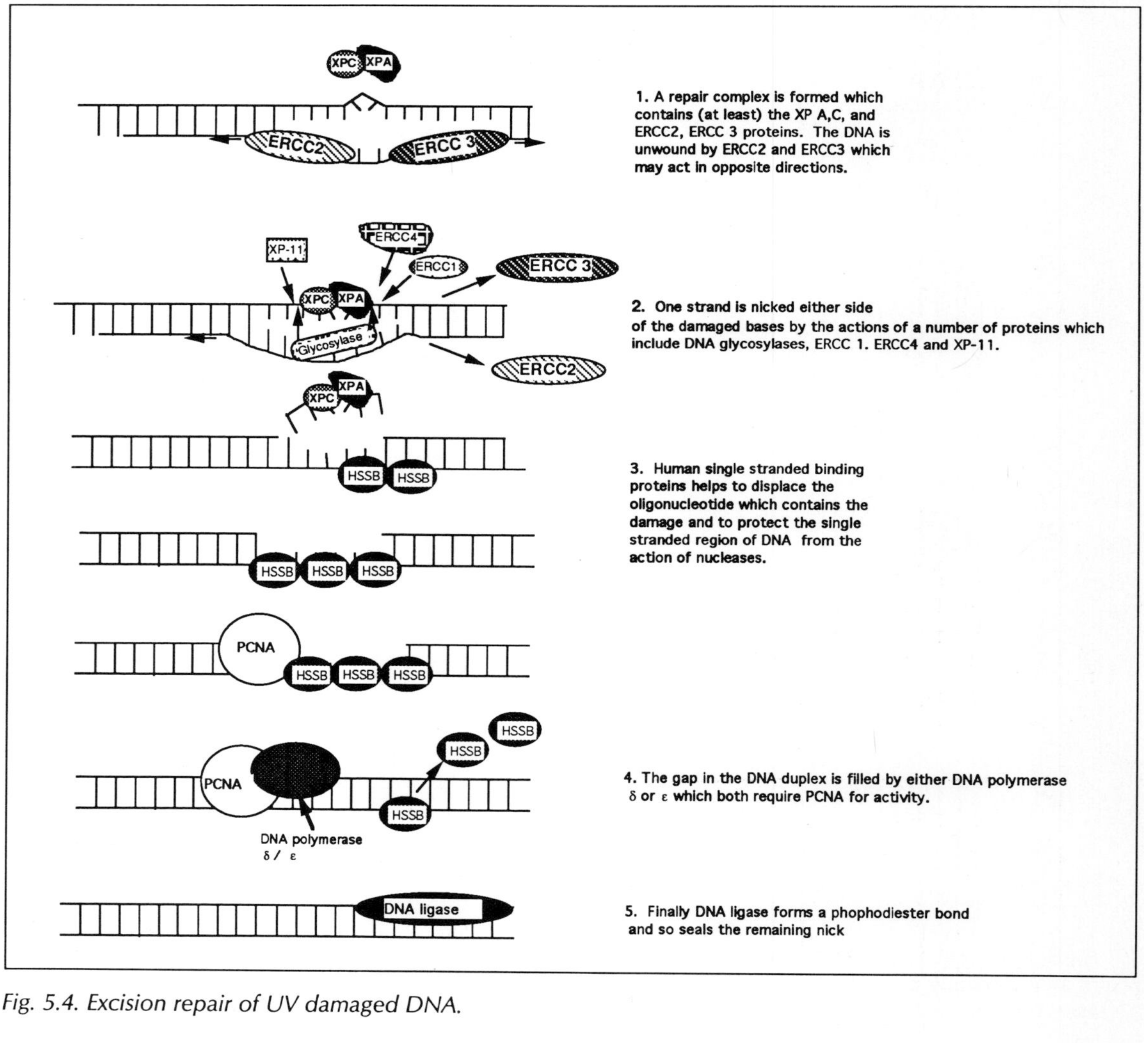

Fig. 5.4. Excision repair of UV damaged DNA.

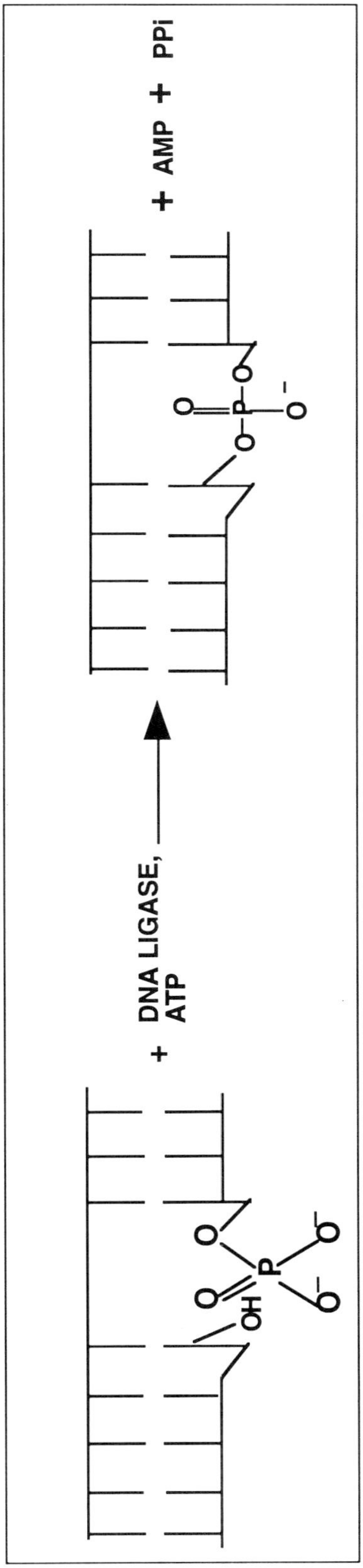

Fig. 5.5. Direct joining of DNA strands can be catalyzed by DNA ligase.

c. Repair of DNA damage caused by alkylation

O⁶ methylguanine DNA methyl transferase

This enzyme removes alkyl groups from the O^6 position of guanine with a slower rate of reaction for ethyl groups than methyl groups.[34,35] The mechanism of action of this enzyme is virtually identical in both prokaryotes and eukaryotes whereby the O^6 from the guanine is transferred to a cysteine residue in the enzyme; each methyltransferase can only repair a single O^6 methylguanine residue (Fig. 5.6).[36] Uncorrected O^6 methylguanine residues are mutagenic and in rat tissues there is an inverse relationship between methyltransferase activity and the organs in which the tumors are induced by methylating carcinogens.[34,37]

3-methyl adenine-DNA glycosylase

This enzyme has been purified from a variety of mammalian sources and two different species have been discovered in calf thymus. Both enzymes are capable of releasing 3-methyl adenine, and 3-methylguanine from DNA . The degree to which the levels of both of these enzymes varies between different individuals may be worth considering in any model of cancer predisposition. However, it is extremely difficult to separate those effects due to environmental factors, i.e., diet and unknown exposure to alkylating agents, from those that are inherited.

d. The cellular consequences of mutations caused by alkylating agents

Activation of Ha-ras by N-methyl-N-nitrosourea

As previously discussed, N-methyl-N-nitrosourea (MNU) causes the formation of both noncoding and miscoding lesions, predominantly by methylation of the O^6 position of guanine and less so at the O^4 position of thymine. This results in GC to AT and AT to GC transitions respectively.

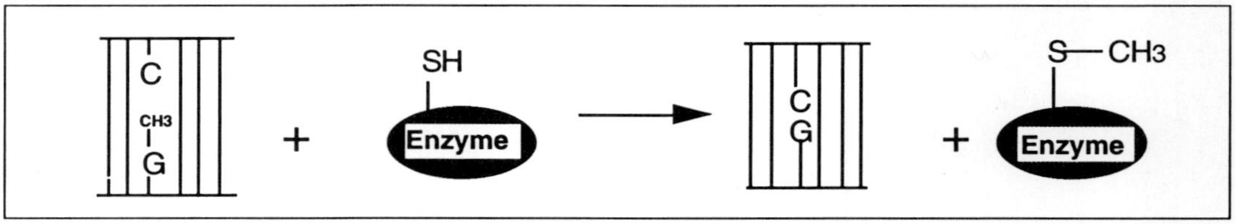

Fig. 5.6. Mechanism of action of O^6-methylguanine DNA methyltransferase. The enzyme removes a methyl group from the O^6 position of guanine and transfers it to one of its own cysteine residues. The reaction mechanism is stochiometric and each methyltransferase molecule can repair only a singe O^6 methyl guanine residue.

It is of great interest that MNU shows a strong bias for mutation of a particular region of the Ha-*ras* genome, in particular the second G of codon 12 (GGA) (Table 5.2). Other chemicals show a similar bias in mutational spectrum in the Ha-*ras* gene (Table 5.2), when compared to the frequencies of transformation expected from studies of transfection into established rat fibroblasts. Thus (a) some sequences may present particular bases as more accessible targets for mutation, perhaps as a result of chromatin conformation, (b) some damaged DNA sequences may be protected from repair activities by both the nature of the surrounding sequences and chromatin folding or (c) there is an inadequacy in comparing rat tissues and in vitro cell based systems. The site specific preference of certain chemicals for mutation of particular genes has profound implications for Ha-*ras* carcinogenesis and evidence is accumulating for similar effects in other genes, e.g., mouse N-*ras* and rat *neu*. It would not be wise to discount more subtle effects on other growth enhancing genes, such as the inactivation of tumor suppressor genes.

e. DNA crosslinking agents

Intrastrand DNA crosslinks are an important type of chemical damage to DNA, as by preventing DNA strand separation, they cause complete blocks to DNA replication and transcription. Chemicals that form part of this class of compounds include, nitrous acid, sulphur mustard, mitomycin C, cis-diamminedichloroplatinum and photoactivated psoralens.[32] The structures that are formed are not well defined, with the exception of nitrogen mustard. In this case the DNA bound mustard molecules form interstrand cross links between the N7 positions of guanine on opposite DNA strands. If left unrepaired, then the lesions caused by such DNA crosslinking agents are cytotoxic by prevention of replication.

f. Repair of DNA crosslinks

The repair of DNA crosslinks is a complex process and this type of damage is probably removed by the concerted actions of the proteins that form part of the short patch excision repair pathways. This is thought to be achieved in a manner which is similar to the repair damage caused to DNA by UV and indeed, many of the same proteins appear to be used in this process (see above).

iii. Enzymes That Are Induced by DNA Damage But Are Not Directly Involved in the Repair Process

In addition to the enzymes that repair DNA damage, a host of other proteins are induced by DNA damaging agents. As discussed previously, damage to cellular DNA causes growth arrest in both the G1 and G2 phases of the cell cycle and cessation of DNA synthesis. This is presumably to allow time for the repair of such damage and thus helps prevent mutations from being transferred into subsequent generations. Therefore, one would expect that the proteins which are involved in the regulation of the cell cycle and in signal transduction pathways would be associated with this process. In this regard DNA damage to Chinese hamster ovary cells has lead to the

Table 5.2. Mutational preference for carcinogen action in the Ha-ras gene

Tumor	Codon	Position	Change	Carcinogen
Rat mammary	12 (CGA)	2	G to A	MNU
Mouse hepatic	61 (CGA)	2	A to T or G	VC, HO-DHE
		1	C to A	HO-AFF
Mouse skin	61 (CAA)	2	A to T	DMBA

MNU, N-methyl-N-nitrosourea; VC, vinyl carbamate; HO-DHE, 1'-hydroxy-21, 31 dehydroestradial; HO-AFF, N-hydroxy-2 acetylaminofluorene; DMBA, 7, 12-dimethylbenz[a]anthracene

identification of 49 independent damage associated cDNA clones, although the total number of proteins that are involved in these processes are likely to be much greater than this.[38] Five of these cDNA clones encode transcripts that are increased by other growth cessation signals, e.g., serum reduction, medium depletion and contact inhibition and experimental evidence indicates that they probably represent part of a novel regulatory pathway involved in the negative control of mammalian cell growth.[38] These genes are termed growth arrest and DNA damage inducible or GADD genes. One such gene product, that of GADD 45, is particularly interesting as it specifically induced by ionizing radiation and it appears that it is not activated by signal transduction pathways that involve protein kinase C.[39]

After exposure to γ or UV irradiation or DNA cross linking agents (cisplatin, mitomycin C), the levels of p53 are increased.[40-43] The type of induction depends upon the nature of the DNA damaging agents used, suggesting that p53 may be involved in two separate repair pathways. This is not perhaps surprising, since as discussed earlier, the excision repair pathways for damage caused by DNA cross linking agents and UV differ to those that are utilized to repair damage cause by γ irradiation.[44] In the case of γ irradiation the level of the p53 protein is increased transiently for up to 2 hours and this appears to have a critical role in G1 arrest.[42,45] This arrest seems to utilize the signaling pathways which involve protein kinase C.[46] Following exposure to UV there is a greater increase in the amount of p53 compared to that observed with γ irradiation and it appears that the G1 arrest may in part be due to p53 mediated induction of a CDC kinase inhibitor which blocks the action of both cyclin A and cyclin E dependent kinase 2.[43,47] An additional role for p53 in the repair response has also been proposed. This protein is able to bind to single stranded DNA and catalyze DNA renaturation and strand transfer. Thus p53 may take a direct part in the repair of DNA strand breaks, including the joining of complementary single stranded DNA ends.[48]

Some of the early response genes are also transiently induced by DNA damage. These include *c-fos, c-myc, c-jun, junB, junD* and *erg I*.[49-51] This suggests that perhaps a number of distinct signaling cascades can be induced by DNA damage. It is perhaps rather surprising to find that the levels of the *c-myc* protein are induced by DNA damage since it is normally associated with cellular proliferation. However, these observations are in keeping with the demonstration of a role for *c-myc* in programmed cell death in certain cellular contexts. It appears that in addition to the induction of *c-myc* by a signaling cascade in which an increase in the protein levels are observed only after 2 hours, there is an additional mechanism whereby the level of the *c-myc* protein is tightly linked to the number of DNA strand breaks per genome with maximal induction of *c-myc* caused by approximately 3000 genomic breaks.[51] One could postulate that the *c-myc* protein may, in a similar fashion to p53, have a dual function whether this be direct or indirect in DNA repair/apoptosis processes. For example, *c-myc* may be simply acting as a transcription factor, thus a rapid increase in its level would allow the cell to respond to the damage by transcribing those genes that are required for the repair. Alternatively the *c-myc* protein may be directly interacting with the DNA strand breaks to aid their repair.

Poly ADP-ribose polymerase (PADPR) plays an adjunct role in the repair of DNA damage, most likely as a protection against protein degradation if, due to the size of the insult, transcription is arrested. It may also play a role in the modulation of enzyme activity in the normal cell, for the purposes of proliferation, differentiation or recombination.[52] PADPR is activated by DNA strand breakage whereby it attaches ADP-ribose from nicotinamide adenine dinucleotide into acceptor proteins in the cell nucleus. These are then polymerized by further similar additions to leave either a straight or branched chain of poly ADP-ribose. The length of the chains is maintained by the balance between poly ADP-ribose polymerase and a specific poly ADP-ribose glycohydrolase. Whilst the polymerase has a general DNA binding capability, its catalytic activity is dependent upon DNA chain interruptions, either single or double stranded. Several domains have been identified within the protein, and in particular a run of glutamic acid residues which are involved in auto-poly ADP-ribosylation, together with two zinc fingers domains which are involved in the recognition of DNA strand breaks.[53,54] Of the two sites, in vitro DNA binding is considerably reduced if the metal binding activity of the second, but not the first, is disrupted. Wild type and mutant forms of the poly ADP-ribose polymerase DNA binding domain have been introduced into living cells and shown to block repair of MNNG alkylation damage, but not that of damage due to UV irradiation.[55] The latter is perhaps not surprising since UV damage is a poor activator of the enzyme due to a low steady state level of DNA chain breaks post-UV irradiation.

These data illustrate the importance of poly ADP-ribose polymerase to the repair of alkylation damage although the mechanism of action has not yet been resolved. Poly ADP-ribosylation may either facilitate access to repair enzymes or may protect free DNA ends from this machinery until it is itself activated and is auto-ribosylated to prevent rebinding to the substrate. Consistent with this, inactive polymerase actually inhibits DNA repair in a novel in vitro assay and removal of the polymerase from crude extracts was found to be equivalent to provision of nicotinamide adenine dinucleotide.[56] A genetic polymorphism in the poly ADP-ribose gene has been associated with a 2- to 3-fold increased cancer incidence in endemic Burkitts' lymphoma, B-cell follicular lymphoma, colorectal carcinoma, breast and small cell lung carcinomas, when compared to appropriately matched noncancer controls.[57] The same study indicated that this deletion, which maps to 13q33-qter, is 3-fold more common in Blacks as compared to Caucasians.

Preferential Repair of Transcribed Regions and the Coupling of Transcription and DNA Repair

Lesions to DNA immediately affect the rate of transcription. To cope with this, mammalian cells have evolved a special system of nucleotide excision repair which preferentially removes certain lesions from the transcribed strand of active genes. Human cells are particularly proficient in this activity when compared to rodent cells; the latter remove only a small proportion of cyclobutane pyrimidine dimers after UV irradiation, but are equally UV resistant. The difference lies in the ability of rodent cells to undertake strand selective repair which probably helps prevent the accumulation of mutations on the transcribed strand. The cancer prone inherited disease xeroderma pigmentosum (complementation group C) shows a deficiency in the repair of the nontranscribed strand at the 5' end of two marker genes, which suggests that the XP-C gene product is involved in the processing of damage to transcriptionally inactive genomic regions.[58] For eukaryotes in general, enhanced repair does occur on both strands, but transcription blocking lesions are repaired faster in the template strand. In *Escherichia coli* a gene (*mfd*: mutation frequency decline) has been identified as necessary for strand specific repair[59] and it will be interesting to see if mammalian equivalents can be identified. In a UV irradiated mouse fibroblast cell line, pyrimidine dimers are removed more efficiently from a transcriptionally active gene (c-*abl*) than from a nonexpressed gene (c-*mos*) in a mechanism which is independent of both the cellular growth state and replicative DNA synthesis.[60] Whether this retarded repair contributes to the mutation frequency within the nontranscribed region is not yet clear. Transcriptional initiation requires RNA polymerase II and transcription factors which control both activated and basal levels of transcription. The latter category can function with a minimal promoter to initiate transcription in the presence of nucleoside triphosphates. The binding of one of these factors, TFIID, is probably the first step in formation of a multienzyme complex with at least six other members (TFIIA, B, E, F, J, H). TFIIH has recently been demonstrated to exhibit both a protein kinase and an ATP dependent DNA helicase activity; upon tryptic digestion and microprotein sequencing TFIIH has revealed homology to ERCC 3.[61] This nucleotide excision repair protein is mutated in xeroderma pigmentosum (Group B) and Cockayne's syndrome and thought to be a helicase involved at an early stage in the excision repair process. These data raise interesting questions concerning the relationship between nucleotide excision repair and transcriptional initiation. For example, for initiation to occur, local DNA melting is required in order for RNA polymerase II to gain access to the transcribed strand. For repair, local DNA unwinding has been implicated in scanning for lesions and in release of the injured strand, at least in *Escherichia coli*. It is unlikely that these processes are independent, given that there is preferential repair of the transcription template. In returning to the aforementioned bacterial mutant (*mfd*), the gene product involved may function as a factor which recognizes and displaces stalled RNA polymerases, i.e. those that have reached a lesion. This factor may then make the region accessible for repair and/or recruit the repair machinery to the site. In this respect, the *mfd* gene product and ERCC 3 have similarities, i.e., are both DNA dependent ATPases, contain helicase motifs and confer sensitivity to UV irradiation. Alternatively, TFIIH/ERCC 3 may precede the initiation complex scanning for lesions and upon meeting an abnormality, recruits repair enzymes. In both cases, ERCC 3 is involved in detection of lesions rather than nucleotide excision repair per se.

A CONTINUUM OF SUSCEPTIBILITY

The steady state number of DNA lesions in any given cell is remarkably high. It has been estimated that up to 90,000 8-hydroxydeoxyguanosine residues are present per rat cell due to endogenous oxidative damage at any one time.[62,63] This is only one of at least 20 oxidative DNA adducts that have been identified. This high rate of endogenous damage may mean that acute exposure to low doses of exogenous mutagens (i.e. nonmitogenic doses) may not have a significant effect upon total DNA damage.[64] However, in the development of the majority of human cancers, the accumulation of neoplastic mutations occurs over the lifetime of the organism and is equivalent to low level chronic exposure. Exposure to environmental carcinogens must therefore be considered to be a continuum whereby the boundaries are marked by the level of endogenous DNA damage, i.e., the hypothetical "no exposure to carcinogens whatsoever" and acute high dose exposure, e.g., the Chernobyl incident. In the former case growth enhancing mutations may be accumulated by the natural age dependent breakdown of the cellular processes such as the DNA repair and immune surveillance mechanisms. This continuum is probably in part reflected in the time that it takes to develop cancer. This process can be accelerated by genetic predisposition and those cancer prone syndromes which are thought to harbor defects in the DNA repair machinery. It should be noted that mutagens are effective at both killing cells by damaging DNA and also by causing inflammatory reactions and cell proliferation; it has been argued that although the effect of mutagens at low doses can be detected[65] carcinogenicity after acute exposure may be due primarily to mitogenesis.[64]

4. EFFECTS THAT DNA REPAIR ENZYMES AND OTHER DETOXIFICATION SYSTEMS MAY HAVE ON CANCER TREATMENT

i. Mechanisms of Resistance to Alkylating Agents

Alkylating agents form the front line of cytotoxic drugs used in treatment of leukemia and lymphoma. However, resistance to these agents occurs and in some cases (e.g. myelodysplastic syndromes) may even potentiate the condition. Alkylating agents may react with any cellular macromolecule, but the important target is undoubtedly DNA. Common drugs such as cyclophosphamide and chlorambucil are bifunctional alkylating agents and after the primary reaction with DNA, the second arm of the molecule may react with another moiety; if this is DNA, then either inter- or intra-DNA strand cross links may occur. This second reaction produces a significant increase in toxicity compared to the monofunctional agents, perhaps as a result of the difficulties in removing intrastrand cross links (via two alternate cycles of excision repair?) and loss of a second strand template for the repair reaction. Clinically speaking, there is a highly significant occurrence of resistance to alkylating agent therapies, which most likely arises by clonal selection of a pre-existing variant. Clearly, in the absence of selective pressure (i.e. the variant is vastly outnumbered by living nonresistant cells), there is no reason for a resistant variant to expand in numbers. However, due to their mutagenic action, alkylating agents could introduce mutations which increase the heterogeneity in that population of cells which survives the chemotherapy, for whatever reason. There are many mechanisms which could participate in drug resistance, the most well known of which is acquisition of the multiple drug resistance phenotype. There are at least seven other mechanisms to be considered.

ii. Pharmacokinetic Effects

Firstly, individuals vary in the extent to which drugs are either metabolized or activated via the phase I/II detoxification systems. A variety of nonpolar and hence unreactive compounds undergo metabolic activation to reactive forms which are capable of interacting with nucleophilic centers in DNA. This is affected by induction of tissue specific enzymes for detoxification of potentially cytotoxic nonpolar chemicals via conversion into water soluble forms suitable for excretion. Using this method, many compounds are removed in an innocuous way, but unfortunately some are converted into reactive electrophiles and are hence genotoxic. This, in part, explains carcinogenicity at remote sites of administration, e.g., bladder cancer due to administration of certain aromatic amines. The enzymes responsible for the first state of such detoxification (phase I) are the flavoprotein reductases, or cytochrome p450 complexes of the endoplasmic reticulum. These are dependent upon dissolved oxygen and NADPH for activity. A second set of reactions (phase II) are then responsible for the formation of conjugated esters, suitable for excretion (Table 5.3).

Other clinical variations could arise from differences in the levels of the cytochrome p450 enzymes. Other drugs, e.g., melphalan are administered in an active form and as such, are likely to undergo extensive metabolic activation.

In addition, alkylating agents may show differences in absorption through the gut; in particular, melphalan shows a wide variation. Similarly, there is evidence to suggest that tumor cell derived factors may affect drug clearance in rodent models.

iii. Reduced Drug Activation

In a similar vein, cellular metabolism may be required to activate other drugs and a reduction in the level of such enzymes may in part be responsible for drug resistance. For example, a reduction in deoxycytidine kinase may be involved in acquisition of resistance to cytosine arabinoside.

iv. Detoxification by the Cell

Tumor cells may have enhanced expression of enzymes which would normally protect against foreign compounds or are involved in intermediary metabolism. Melphalan resistance is associated with the level of glutathione, which inactivates it. This may be enhanced by the action of glutathione S-transferases, elevation of the latter thus contributing to drug resistance. There are three isoforms of glutathione S-transferase (α, π, μ) of which α appears to be most relevant to detoxification, whilst the π form is dominant in amount.

v. Biochemical Changes

Resistance to some drugs, e.g., methotrexate can be mediated by molecules to which it binds, which in this case is dihydrofolate reductase.

vi. Cytotoxic Drugs

Enzymes which bypass cytotoxic metabolic pathways may be induced to mediate resistance, or in the case of alkylating agents, there may be a general increase in the DNA repair machinery. This could in turn increase resistance to cytotoxic effects.

vii. Apoptosis

Since cells may vary in their ability to repair DNA, then they may also differ in the amount of DNA damage they can tolerate before activating an apoptotic pathway. Less apoptosis implies increased resistance.

viii. Drug Uptake

Poorly lipid soluble drugs can be taken into the cell using an ATP dependent

Table 5.3. Cancer predisposing genetic polymorphisms

Allele	Comment
Phase I	
cyp1A1	Involved in metabolism of a number of procarcinogens Some studies have linked polymorphisms with lung cancer
cyp1A2	Metabolism of nitrosamines, aromatic hydrocarbons and arylamines
cyp2A6	Activation of procarcinogens, including NNK* and aflatoxin B1
cyp2C	Benzo[a]pyrene activation
cyp2D6	1.8 fold increased susceptibility to lung and bladder cancer in 'extensive' metabolizers
cyp2E1	Metabolizes nitrosamines and benzene
cyp3A4	Activates benzo[a]pyrene and aflatoxin B1
ALDH1	Involved in cyclophosphamide metabolism
Epoxide hydrolases	Activates benzo[a]pyrene
Phase II	
GSTμ	Metabolism of benzo[a]pyrene
Acetyl transferase	Metabolism of thiopurine cancer chemotherapeutics
Methyl transferase	Metabolism of various carcinogens

NNK, 4 (methyl nitrosamine)-1-(3 pyridyl)-1-(butanone); ALDH1, aldehyde dehydrogenase; GST, glutathione-S-transferase transporter, on the basis of structural similarities to compounds which are normally taken up by this route. Should the carrier proteins be altered such that drug uptake is reduced, then resistance to the drug may be apparent.

ix. The Multiple Drug Resistance Phenotype

In several cases, treatment with one drug will lead to resistance to a second unrelated drug and this is one of the greatest problems facing successful cancer chemotherapy.[66] This is in part due to the upregulation of the multiple drug resistance (*mdr*1) gene or P glycoprotein. This gene encodes a transmembrane efflux pump which leads to a reduction in the intracellular levels of the drug and hence resistance to a variety of lipophillic drugs.

6. GENETIC INFLUENCE, CANCER PREDISPOSITION AND DRUG METABOLISM

There are clearly many environmental influences which impact upon an individual's predisposition to cancer. But to what extent is this also related to genetic makeup? Is there sufficient genetic polymorphism within the population to impact upon cancer frequencies? The answer is undoubtedly yes.

Examples of cancer predisposing polymorphisms appear in the xenobiotic metabolizing enzymes, both for phase I (the cytochrome p450 or *cyp* enzymes) and phase II detoxification (Table 5.3). Four cases are worthy of mention. In particular, two populations of *cyp*2D6 have been identified and designated: extensive drug metabolizers (EMs, 'normal' levels of metabolism) and poor drug metabolizers (PMs). There are at least 30 drugs which are metabolized by this route[67] and the literature reveals that there is an overall 1.8-fold decreased incidence of the PM genotype in lung cancer patients.[68] Whilst a number of mechanisms are possible, it is interesting to note that *cyp*2D6 can activate NNK, the tobacco specific nitrosamine.

Metabolic detoxification applies to cyclophosphamide and ifosfamide which both undergo a complex series of metabolic transformations catalyzed by microsomal mixed function oxidizations, usually in the liver. The intermediate species, aldophosphamide, enters the cell and can be further metabolized to the active alkylating agent, phosphoramide mustard and acrolein, the probable mediator of hemorrhagic cystitis which is a side effect of the treatment. In particular, the efficacy of these drugs could be determined by the level of aldehyde dehydrogenase (ALDH1[69]) in different individuals, perhaps helping to explain the variations within the clinical response. It is interesting to note that bone marrow progenitor cells (stem cells) have a high level of this enzyme and are relatively resistant to cyclophosphamide. These data are of profound importance to cancer chemotherapy since the extent of drug activation by this pathway, i.e., the extent of genetic polymorphism, will be proportional to the amount of phosphoramide mustard produced and hence will be related to the efficacy of the drug.

In a similar fashion, epoxide hydrolases acting in concert with cytochrome p450 enzymes may play a role in activation of benzo[a]pyrene to the mutagenic 7,8 diol, 9,10 epoxide form. Again, genetic polymorphism at these loci may be important in susceptibility to cancer.

Regarding phase II detoxification, there may be an association between a lack of glutathioneS-transferase and an increased risk of lung cancer amongst smokers, although the available evidence is far from convincing.

7. IMMUNE SURVEILLANCE MECHANISMS

It has been proposed that mammalian systems contain immune surveillance mechanisms whereby there exists a pool of lymphocytes which migrate through somatic tissues recognizing certain neoplastic antigens or malignantly transformed cells. There is not as yet a great deal of experimental evidence which supports the existence of such systems, although in patients undergoing long-term immunosuppressive therapy or those with HIV there is a greatly increased risk of tumors formation. This may in part be due to reduced immunosurveillance. In immunocompromised patients which receive high doses of sunlight, e.g., Australia and South East Asia, there is a significantly higher frequency of skin cancer.[70] If it is demonstrated unequivocally that immune surveillance mechanisms are important in cancer formation they will no doubt be shown to contribute towards the genetic influences upon cancer predisposition.

References

1. Lindahl T. Instability and decay of the primary structure of DNA. Nature 1993; 362: 709-714.
2. Ames B, Shigenaga M, Hagen T. Oxidants, antioxidants and the degenerative diseases of aging. Proc Natl Acad Sci USA 1993; 90:7915-7922.
3. Lindahl T, Nyberg B. Biochemistry 1972; 11:3610-3618.
4. Cooper DN, Youssoufian M. The CpG dinucleotide and human genetic disease. Human Genetics 1988; 78:151-155 .
5. Tchou J. 8-Oxoguanine (hydroxyguanine) DNA glycosylase and its substrate specificity. Proc Natl Acad Sci 1991; 88: 4690-4694.
6. Snowden A, Kow YW, van Houten B. Damage Repertoire of the E. *coli* Uvr ABC nuclease couplex includes A-basic sites, base damage analogues and lesions containing adjacent 5' or 3' nicks. Biochemistry 1990; 29:7251-7259.
7. Lutz WK. Endogenous genotoxic agents and processes as a basis of spontaneous carcinogenesis. Mutation Research 1990; 238: 287-297.
8. Smith KC. Spontaneous mutagenesis, environmental genetic and other factors. Mutation Research 1992; 2777:139-162.
9. Hickson ID, Harris A. Mammalian DNA repair using mutants hypersensitive to cytotoxic agents. TIG 1988; 4: 101-106.
10. Iliakis G. The role of DNA double strand breaks in ionising radiation-induced killing of eukaryotic cells. Bioessays 1991; 13: 641-6444.
11. Breimer LH, Lindahl T. Ehzymatic excision of DNA bases damaged by exposure to ionising radiation. Mut Res 1985; 150: 85-89.
12. Jacobs A, Bopp A, Hagen U. In vitro repair of single stand breaks in g irradiated DNA by polynucleotide ligase. In J Radiat Biol 1972; 22:431-433.
13. Boothman DA, Bouvard I, Hughes EN. Identification of x-ray induced protein in human cells. Cancer Res 1989; 49: 2871-2878.
14. Breimer LH. Urea-DNA glycosylase in mammalian cells. Biochemistry 1983; 22: 4129-4997.
15. Chetsanger CJ, Lozon M, Markoff C et al. Purification and characterisation of E. C*oli* formamidopyrimidine-DNA gylcosylase. Biochemistry 1981; 20:5201-5205.
16. Brash DE, Haseltine WA. UV induced mutation hot spots occur at DNA damage hot spots. Nature 1982; 298:189-192.
17. Tornaletti S, Rozek D, Pfeifer GP. The distribution of UV photoproducts along the human p53 gene and its relaticn to mutations in skin cancer. Oncogene 1993; 8:2051-2057.
18. Sutherland BM. Photoreactivating enzyme from human leukocytes. Nature 1974; 248:109.
19. Hamilton KK, Kim PH, Doetsch PW. A eukaryotic DNA glycosylase/lyase recognizing UV-light induced pyrimidine dimers. Nature 1992; 356:725-728.
20. Hoeijmakers JH, Eker APM, Wood RD et al. Use of in vivo and in vitro assays for the characterisation of mammalian excision repair and isolation of repair proteins. Mut Res 1990; 236:223-238.
21. Weeda G, Ma L, vanHam RCA. Structure and expression of the human ERCC3 gene involved in DNA repair disorders xp and Cockayne's syndrome. Nucleic Acid Res 1991; 19:6301-6308.
22. Flejter WL, McDaniel LD, Johns D et al. Correction of xp group D by chromosome and gene transfer. Involvement of the human ERCC2 DNA repair gene. Proc Natl Acad Sci 1992; 89:261-265.
23. Troelstra C, Odijik H, deWit J et al. ERCC6 a member of a subfamily of putative helicases is involved in Cockayne's syn-

drome. Cell 1992; 71:939-953.
24. Weber CA, Salazar EP, Stewart SA, et al. ERCC2: cDNA cloning and molecular characterization of a human nucleotide excision repair gene with high homology to RAD 3. EMBO J 1990; 9:1437-1447.
25. Robbins P, Jones CJ, Biggerstaff M et al. Complementation of DNA repair in XPA cell extracts by a protein with affinity for damaged DNA. EMBO J 1992; 10: 3913-3921.
26. Tanaka K, Miura N, Satokata I, et al. Analysis of a human DNA excision repair gene involved in group A XP and containing a zinc finger domain. Nature 1990; 348: 73-76.
27. Huang J, Svoboda DL, Reardon JT et al. Human nucleotide excision repair nuclease removes thymine dimers from DNA by incising the 22nd phophodiester bond 5' and the 6th phosphodiester bond 3' to the photodimer. Proc Natl Acad Sci 1992; 89:3662-3668.
28. Biggerstaff M, Szymokowski DE, Wood RD. Co-correction of the ERCC1 and ERCC4 and XP group F DNA repair defects in vitro. EMBO J 1993; 12:3685-3692.
29. Van Vuuren AJ, Appeldoorn E, Odijk H et al. Evidence for a repair enzyme complex involving ERCC1 and completmenting activities of ERCC4 and ERCC1 and XP group F. EMBO J 1993; 12:3693-3701.
30. Coverley D, Kenny MK, Munn M et al. Requirement for the replication protein SSB in human DNA excision repair. Nature 1991; 349:538-541.
31. Shivji MKK, Kenny MK, Wood RD. Proliferating cell nuclear antigen is required for DNA excision repair. Cell 1992; 69:367-374.
32. Friedberg EH. In: DNA repair. New York: WH Freeman and Company, 1985.
33. Shapiro R. Damage to DNA caused by hydrolysis. In: Seeberg E, Kleep, eds. Chromosome damage and repair. New York: Plenum, 1981.
34. Pegg AE. Reviews in Biochemical toxicology. New YorK: Elsevier Biomedical, 1983:83-133.
35. Brent TP Dolan ME, Fraenkel-Conrat H et al. Repair of o-alkylpyrimidine in mammalian cells: A present consensus. Proc Natl Acad Sci 1988; 85:1758-1762.
36. Lindahl T, Sedgewick B, Sekiguchi M et al. Regulation and expression of the adaptive response to alkylating agents. Annu Rev Biochem 1988; 57:133-157.
37. Pegg AE. Mammalian O6 alkylguanine DNA alkyltransferase: Regulation and importance in the response to alkylating carcinogenic and therapeutic agents. Perspectives in Cancer Research 1990; 50: 6119-6129.
38. Fornace AJ, Nepert DW, Hollander C. Mammalian gene coordinately regulated by growth arrest signals and DNA damaging agents. Mol Cell Biol. 1989; 9:4196-4203.
39. Papathanasiou MA, Kerr NC, Robbins JH et al. Induction of ionizing radiation of the GADD 45 gene in cultured human cells: Lack of mediation by protein kinase C. Mol Cell Biol 1991; 11:1009-1016.
40. Kastan MB, Onyinye O, Sidransky D et al. Participation of the p53 protein in the cellular response to DNA damage. Cancer Res 1991; 51:6304-6311.
41. Kuerbitz SJ, Plunkett BS, Walsh W et al. Wild-type p53 is a cell cycle checkpoint following irradiation. Proc Natl Acad Sci 1992; 89:7491-7495.
42. Zhan Q, Carrier F and Fornace AJ. Induction of cellular p53 activity by DNA-damaging agents and growth arrest. Mol Cell Biol 1993; 13:4242-4250.
43. Lu X, Lane DP. Differential induction of transcriptionally active p53 following UV or ionising radiation: Defects in chromosome instability syndromes. Cell 1993; 75: 756-778.
44. Khanna KK, Lavin MF. Ionising radiation and UV induction of p53 by different pathways in AT cells. Oncogene 1993; 8: 3307-3312.
45. O'Connor PM, Jackman J, Jondle D et al. Role of the p53 tumour suppressor gene in cell cycle arrest and radiosensitivity. Cancer Res 1993; 53:4776-4780.
46. Price BD, Calderwood SK. Increased sequence specific p53-DNA binding activity after DNA damage is attenuated by phorbol esters. Oncogene 1993; 8:3055-3062.
47. Dulic V, Kaufmann WK, Wilson SJ et al.

p53 dependent inhibition of cyclin dependent kinase activities in human fibroblasts during radiation induced G1 arrest. Cell 1994; 76:1013-1023.

48. Bakalkin G, Yakovleva T, Galina S et al. p53 binds single stranded DNA ends and catalyzes DNA renaturation and strand transfer. Proc, Natl. Acad. Sci. 1994; 91: 413-417.
49. Wilson RE, Taylor SL, Atherton GT et al. Early response gene signalling cascades activated by ionising radiation in primary human B cells. Oncogene 1993; 8: 3229-3237.
50. Fritsche M, Haessler M, Brandner G. Induction of nuclear accumulation of the tumour suppressor protein p 53 by DNA damaging agnets. Oncogene 1993; 8: 307-318.
51. Sullivan NF, Willis AE. Elevation of c-myc protein by DNA strand breakage. Oncogene 1989; 4:1497-1502.
52. Althaus FR, Ritcher C. ADP-ribosylation of proteins; enzymology and biological significance. Berlin Heidelberg: Springer Verlag, 1987.
53. Gradwohl G, Menissier-De M, Molinete M et al. The second zinc finger domain of poly(ADP ribose) polymerase determines specificty for single stranded breaks in DNA. Proc Natl Acad Sci 1990; 87:2990-2994.
54. Ikejima M, Noguchi S, Yamashiita R. The zinc fingers of human poly(ADP ribose) polymerase are differentially required for recognition of DNA breaks and nicks and the consequent enzyme activation. J Biol Chem 1990; 265:907-913.
55. Molinete M, Vermeulen W et al. Overproduction of the poly (ADP-ribose) polymerase DNA-binding domain blocks alkylation-induced DNA repair synthesis in mammalian cells. The EMBO Journal 1993; 2109-2117.
56. Satoh MS and Lindahl T. Role of poly (ADP ribose) formation in DNA repair. Nature 1992; 356:356-358.
57. Bhatia KG, Cherney BW, Huppi K et al. A deletion linked to the poly (ADP ribose) polymerase gene on chromsome 13q33-qter occurs frequently in the normal black population as well as in multiple tumour DNA. Cancer Res 1990; 50:5406-5413.
58. Venema J, Mullenders LHF, Natarajan AT. et al. The genetic defect in Cockaynes syndrome is associated with a defect in repair of UV-induced DNA damage in transcriptionally active DNA. Proc Natl Acad Sci 1990; 87:4707-4711.
59. Selby CP, Sancar A. Molecular Mechanism of Transcription-Repair Coupling. Science 1993; 260:53-57.
60. Madhani HD, Bohr, W and Hanawalt, P. Differential DNA Repair in Transcriptionally Active and Inactive Proto-oncogenes; c-*abl* and c-*mos*. Cell 1986; 45:417-423.
61. Schaeffer L, Roy R et al. DNA Repair Helicase: A Component of BTF2 (TFIIH) Basic Transcription Factor. Science 1993; 260:58-63.
62. Fraga GC, Shigenaga MK, Park JW et al. Oxidative damage to DNA during aging:8 hydroxy 2' deoxyguanosine in rat organ DNA and urine. Proc Natl Acad Sci 1990; 87:4533-4537.
63. Shigenaga MK, Gimeno GT, Ames BN. Urinary 8 hydroxy 2' deoxyguanosine as a biological marker of in vivo oxidative DNA damage. Proc Natl Acad Sci 1989; 86: 9697-9701.
64. Ames BN, Gold LS. Too many rodent carcinogens:mitogenesis increases mutagenesis. Science 1990; 249:970-971.
65. Cohen SM, Ellwein LB. Cell proliferation and carcinogenesis. Science 1990; 249: 1007-1101.
66. DeVita VT. In: DeVita VT, Hellman S, Rosenberg SA, eds. Cancer principles and practice of oncology. Philadelphia: Lippincott, 1989:279-300.
67. Daly A, Cholerton S, Gregory W, Idle J. Metabolic polymorphisms. Pharmac Ther 1993; 57:129-160.
68. Idle J, Armstrong M, Boddy A, 16 others. The pharmacogenetics of chemical carcinogenesis. Pharmacogenetics 1992; 2:246-258.
69. Hadidi A, Coulter C, Idle J. Phenotypically deficent urinary elimination of carboxyphosphamide after cyclophosphamide administration to cancer patients. Cancer Res 1988; 48:5167-5171.
70. Streilein JW, Taylor JR, Vincek V et al. Immune surveillance and sunlight induced skin cancer. Immunology Today 1994; 15:4-7.

CHAPTER 6

The Molecular Basis of Metastasis

1. INTRODUCTION

Metastasis is defined as the relocation of cancer from one organ to another that is not directly connected with it. This represents one of the biggest problems in cancer treatment since the widespread dissemination of disease often precludes surgical treatment. It is a highly selective process whereby only one or a few organs are the sites of growth of metastatic colonies. The invasive tumor cells must penetrate the circulatory system, survive its potentially lethal environment and lodge in particular organs in order to extravasate and proliferate. The vascular connections of the primary tumor are not, in general, sufficient to explain metastasis to some organs and other factors must be therefore be involved. Tumor cells probably progress via the acquisition of new characteristics and the final malignant cell capable of invasion and metastasis may have little relationship to the cell or tissue from which it originated. However, the order in which these changes occur are rarely clear and indeed, it is the dissection of these which is the subject of this book. In general, it appears that the alterations associated with metastasis take place relatively late in the development of the neoplasm. Moreover, studies have shown that tumor development (tumorgenicity) and subsequent metastatic behavior are under separate genetic control.[1,2] Metastasis is similar to tumorigenesis in that no single gene appears to control the overall process and thus metastasis also results from an accumulation of genetic changes. However, in contrast to tumorigenesis where there has been some insight into the mechanisms of oncogenesis[3-5] there has yet to be a molecular dissection of the pathways that lead to metastasis.

The process of metastasis requires: (a) tumor cell attachment to cells of other tissues or extracellular matrix components, (b) proteolysis of the basement membrane, the natural host barrier, (c) tumor cell locomotion and (d) relocation within the target organ. It is likely that similar biochemical processes are involved during normal angiogenesis but, that in tumor cell invasion, differences in the delicate balance between positively and negatively coordinated factors occur. At any stage of development, tumor cells must avoid host cell killing and the vast majority of the metastasizing cells are detected by the immune system. Indeed, it has been estimated that less than 0.01% of the circulating tumor cells eventually form a metastatic colony. In part, this may also be due to selection for a metastatic subpopulation in the necessarily heterogeneous primary tumor.[6]

2. TUMOR CLASSIFICATION: BENIGN OR MALIGNANT?

Tumors are usually a mixture of different cell types which show a variety of resistances to chemotherapeutics and/or radiation and often different cell morphologies, functions or growth properties. They may be divided into two classes which depend upon the degree of invasiveness: (a) benign tumors are localized to the tissue of origin and usually resemble this tissue morphologically, however, these cells may not maintain their normal spatial relationships (by definition, they do not spread to other tissues and tend to cause damage via obstruction of vital areas) and (b) malignant tumors invade and destroy the surrounding mesenchymal tissue. Continuous growth of tumor cells is limited by the oxygen supply and increases in size are often accompanied by the local production of angiogenesis factors which facilitate the formation of blood vessels. These vessels are rarely properly formed and provide a ready conduit for malignant tumor cells to enter the lymphatic system and be carried to regional lymph nodes where they can grow to form a secondary tumor. Those factors which result in this metastatic process remain one of the fundamental mysteries of cancer cell biology.

3. INITIAL CELL IMPLANTATION

The initial lodgement of the malignant cell could result from organ specific interactions or mechanical trapping, e.g., interaction with platelets. In the former case this may be due either to specific interactions with the subendothelial basement membrane, vascular endothelial cells, or to organ specific cell mobility. In this regard implantation studies of human colon carcinoma cells into nude mice have demonstrated the effect which an organ may exert on the metastatic potential of the tumor cell. Hence the transplanted human cell will only metastasize if injected into the caecum or spleen of the nude mouse.[7,8]

4. THE ROLE OF THE SUBENDOTHELIAL BASEMENT MEMBRANE

The basement membrane is a dense matrix which is normally impermeable to cells and metastasis must therefore be an active process. Indeed, tumor cell interaction with the basement membrane has been defined as the critical event of tumor invasion that signals the initiation of the metastatic cascade.[5,9] Upon adhering, malignant cells often cause a retraction of endothelial cells thus exposing the basement membrane, which in itself provides a better adhesive substrate for the tumor cells via molecules such as laminin, collagen (type IV and V), fibronectin and heparan sulphate proteoglycan. Each of these molecules have cellular receptors and changes in expression of both cell surface and extracellular matrix molecules can correlate with metastatic potential. For example, the α-6, β-1 integrin receptor for laminin can be increased as a result of chemical transformation of an osteosarcoma cell line.[10] Binding of the tumor cell to laminin can stimulate production of collagenase IV which may in itself help local invasion of the parenchyma, thus stimulating a cascade of events. Similarly, fibronectin is a prominent component of the liver extracellular matrix and some preferential binding to liver cells known to adhere to fibronectin has been demonstrated.

5. THE ROLE OF VASCULAR ENDOTHELIAL CELLS

Capillary endothelial cells express different cell surface glycoproteins depending upon the organ of origin. Malignant cells will preferentially attach to endothelial cells from the source organ and organs to which they are known to metastasize. In addition to tumor cells, lymphocytes from the blood also infiltrate, a process which is mediated by vascular addressin.[11] However, there is likely to be some redundancy in the molecules involved since two of the lymphocyte addressins (ELAM-1 and INCAM-110) can also play a role in mediating adhesins of other cell types, a colon carcinoma and melanoma cell line, respectively.[12] Similarly, other molecules such as ICAM-1 and CD44 have been implicated in tumor cell adhesion.[13]

6. DEGRADATION OF THE EXTRACELLULAR MATRIX

In order to degrade the extracellular matrix and cell adhesion molecules, tumor cells either directly secrete proteolytic enzymes or induce the host tissue to do so.[14] Lysis of the matrix occurs close to the surface of the tumor cell where the local concentration of active proteolytic enzyme exceeds that of the natural protease inhibitors, which are either secreted by surrounding normal cells, or present in the matrix and serum.[15] We must remember that proteolysis forms a normal part of maintaining tissue function, e.g., in trophoblast implantation, embryo morphogenesis and angiogenesis. In addition, the defect in tumor cells cannot be unbridled synthesis and secretion of proeolytic enzymes, since metastasis requires a balance between attachment and release. If all of the extracellular matrix components were destroyed by proteolysis, then the substratum necessary for cell traction would have been removed. The 'aggressiveness' of tumor cells has been positively correlated with several types of proteolytic enzyme: heparanases, metal dependent, serine and thiol proteases.[16,17] Proteolysis probably requires a cascade of these enzymes to act in concert, which bears similarity to the processes involved in blood coagulation. The matrix metalloproteinases have received much attention and include the interstitial collagenases which degrade type I collagen, type IV collagenases and the stromelysins, which degrade proteoylycans and the noncollagenous proteoglycans, laminins and fibronectin.[18] These enzymes are secreted as inactive zymogens and their activation represents an important step in control of their activity.

A number of natural proteinase inhibitors block either the zymogen or active forms of the metalloproteinases and include the tissue inhibitors of metalloproteinases (TIMP's) and plasminogen activator inhibitors (PAI's). These inhibitors may act to reduce tumor cell invasion and hence suppress metastasis.[19]

7. AUTOCRINE AND PARACRINE GROWTH STIMULATION AT SECONDARY SITES

The coexpression of a growth factor and its cognate receptor is unusual in normal tissues, but occurs in both benign and malignant tumor cells, more frequently in the latter. Autocrine stimulation can occur either via expression of both molecules or expression of a truncated but activated receptor (e.g. *erb*B-2). There may be two mechanisms of autocrine stimulation whereby the factor is secreted into the environment and subsequently reacts with the receptor (e.g. bombesin, GM-CSF, CSF-1, IL-2) or interaction in an intracellular compartment (e.g. PDGF, IL-3, GM-CSF, bFGF).[20] It is also common for metastatic cancer lines to have acquired apparent growth factor independence and the ability to grow independently in vitro, although this may indicate that internal autocrine loops are in operation. The use of autocrine mechanisms will most likely affect the ability of the malignant cell to grow and divide independently of the target organ although other associations may exist. However, paracrine growth stimulation may be important in determining the target organ, but in the normal course of events, important in prevention of metastasis. Indeed, the growth inhibitory and stimulatory effects of several types of liver conditioned media on various metastatic cell lines has been reported.[21] In adenocarcinoma of the prostate, which often metastasizes to the bone marrow, the growth rate of the metastasis exceeds that of the primary tumor by a considerable amount, which has been attributed to paracrine stimulation.[22] Metastatic potential also appears to correlate with heparanase cleavage of heparan sulphate which is turn may release a pool of growth factor such as FGFβ. In turn, this factor may function in angiogenesis or act directly to promote cell growth.

8. CELLULAR LOCOMOTION

Acting in concert with the action of proteolytic enzymes, tumor cells protrude pseudopodia at their migrating edge. This is generally directional and is regulated by cell surface ligand binding. This then coordinates the mobilization of those cytoskeletal elements which interact with the inner face of the cell membrane. Random tumor cell motility can be regulated by two types of cytokine, scatter factor and autocrine motility factor.[23] These latter act via a G protein dependent mechanism and

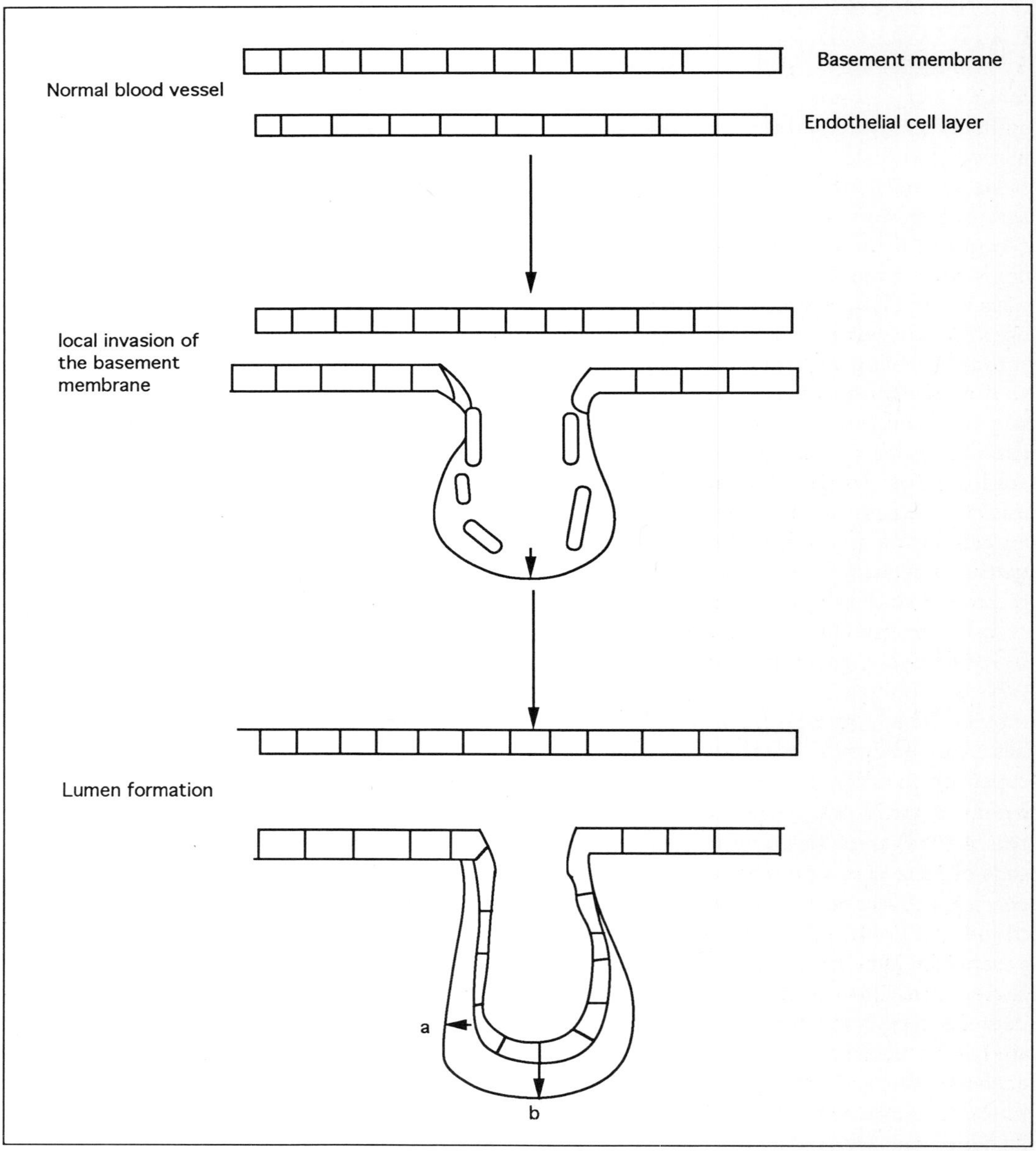

Fig. 6.1. Angiogenesis. (a) Lateral proteolysis and degradation of the ECM enables lumen formation. (b) Endothelial migration, proteolysis and cellular proliferation in response to bFGF allows vessel elongation.

are susceptible to inhibition by pertussis toxin, thus implicating a $G_{i\alpha}$ subunit. Random motility of this nature could be crucial to the dispersion and dissemination of the tumor cells. In addition to preferential adhesion and preferential cell growth due to localized growth factors, we must also consider the effects of host derived chemoattractants. Again, these may play a part in determination of directionality during tumor cell locomotion.

9. ANGIOGENESIS

The formation of new blood vessels or angiogenesis is necessary if the tumor mass is to expand in three dimensions.[24] However, angiogenesis is not a single event but a cascade of processes. In the first stage resting endothelial cells are stimulated to degrade their basement membrane and initiate a capillary sprout by invading the perivascular stroma. Migrating cells produce type IV collagenase, serine proteases and metalloproteinases, the concentration of which must exceed that of natural protease inhibitors in order for the sprout to elongate and extend the lumen in a lateral direction (Fig. 6.1).[25] Moreover, simple models have shown that the proteinase/proteinase inhibitor ratios are also important in angiogenesis.[26] Certain cytokines such as basic FGF can promote angiogenesis whilst others, e.g., TGFβ have the opposite effect.[27]

10. GENETIC INFLUENCES UPON METASTASIS

There have been few reports of genes which directly affect metastasis, although one of these is particularly interesting. This is the identification of the *nm23* gene product, expression of which is reduced up to 10-fold in cell lines of high metastatic potential.[28] The *nm23* gene has two human alleles, nm23-H1 and nm23-H2 which are 90% identical; the former has been associated with suppression of metastasis. These genes have high sequence homology to a nucleotide diphosphate kinase (NDK), the Drosophila *awd* gene product and nm23-H1 exhibits a similar enzymatic activity in vitro.[29] The latter activity has fueled speculation that nm23 may be involved in G protein mediated signal transduction, although such a function is inconsistent with the nuclear localization of the nm23 protein and the presence of a leucine zipper motif, a characteristic of a transcription factor. Indeed, NDK itself does not directly activate any GTP binding protein so far tested.[30] Perhaps a more plausible function is the demonstration that nm23-H2 may act as an in vitro transcriptional regulation of, at the very least, the c-*myc* gene.[31] To date, there is no clear association between c-*myc* expression and the extent of metastasis, so nm23-H2 may be involved in transcriptional regulation of other genes involved in this process. It is as well to note, however, that it is loss of nm23-H1 gene expression and not that of nm23-H2 that is associated with metastasis. The latter has been identified as a mouse homologue of a differentiation inhibiting factor in myeloid leukemia cells, which may explain transcriptional regulation of c-*myc*.

REFERENCES

1. Garbisa S, DeGiovanni C, Biagini G et al, Different metastatic aggressiveness by murine TS/A clones: Ultrastructure, extracellular glycoproteins and type IV collagenolytic activity. Invasion and Metastasis 1987; 8:177-192.
2. Muschel RJ, Williams JE, Lowy DR et al. H-ras induction of metastatic potential depends upon oncogene activation and the type of recipient cell. Am J Pathol 1985; 121:1-8.
3. Bishop JM. Molecular themes in oncogensis. Cell 1991; 64:235-248.
4. Fearon ER, Volgelstein B. A genetic model for colorectal tumourgenesis. Cell 1990; 61:759-767.
5. Fidler I, Radinsky R. Genetic control of cancer metastasis. J Natl Cancer Inst 1990; 82:166-168.
6. Fidler I, Hart I. Biologic diversity in metastatic neoplasms: origins and implications. Science 1982; 217:998-1001.
7. Fidler I. Orthotopic implantation of human colon carcinomas into nude mive provides a valuable model for the biology and therapy of metastasis. Cancer Metastasis Rev 1991; 10:229-243.

8. Stephenson RA, Dinney CP, Gohji K. Metastatic model for human prostate cancer using orthotopic inplantation in nude mice. J Natl Cancer Inst 1992; 84:951-957.
9. Liotta L, Steeg P, Stetler-Stevenson W. Cancer metastasis and angiogenesis: an imbalance of positive and negative regulation. Cell 1991; 64:327-336
10. Dedhar S, Saulnier R. Alterations in integrin receptor expresion on chemically transformed human cells: Specific enhancement of laminin and collagen receptor complexes. J Cell Biology 1990; 110:481-489.
11. Berg EL, Goldstein LA, Jutila MA et al. Homing receptors and vascular addressins: cell adhesion molecules that direct lymphocyte traffic. Immunological Reviews 1989; 108:5-18.
12. Rice GE, Bevilacqua MP. An inducible endothelial cell surface glycoprotein mediated melanoma adhesion. Science 1989; 246:1303-1306.
13. Gallatin WM, Rosenman SJ, Ganji A et al. Structure function relationships of the CD44 class of glycoproteins. Cell Mol Mech Inf 1991; 2:131-150.
14. Gottesman M. The role of proteases in cancer. Sem Cancer Biol 1:97-160.
15. Brown P, Levy A, Margulies I, Liotta L, Stetler-Stevenson W. Independent expression and cellular processing of the 72 kDa type IV collagenase and interstitial collagenase in human tumorigenic cell lines. Cancer Research 1990; 50:6184-6191.
16. Nakajima M, Lotan D, Baig MM et al. Inhibition of retionoic acid type IV collagenolysis and invasion through reconstituted basement membrane by metastastic rat mammary adenocarcinoma cells. Cancer Res 1989; 49:1698-1760.
17. Nakajima M, Morwikawa K, Fabra A et al. Influence of organ environment on extracellular matrix degradative activity and metastasis of human colon carcinoma cells. J Natl Cancer Inst 1991; 82:1890-1898.
18. Matrisian LM. The matrix degrading metalloproteinases. Bioessays 1992; 14: 455-462.
19. Setler-Stevenson WG, Aznavoorian S, Lioatta LA. Tumour cell interaction with the extrcellular matrix during invasion and metastasis. Annu Rev Cell Biol 1993; 9:541-573.
20. Browder TM, Dunbar CE, Nienhuis AW. Public and private autocrine loops in neoplastic cells. Cancer Cells 1989; 1:9-17.
21. Horak E, Darling DL, Tarin D. Analysis of organ specific effects on metastatic tumour formation by studies in vitro. J Natl Cancer Institute 1986; 76:913-922.
22. Chackal-Roy M, Niemeyer C, Moore M, Zetter BR. Stimuation of human prostatic carcinoma cell growth by facotrs present in the human bone marrow. J Clinical Investigation 1989; 84:43-50.
23. Gheradi E, Gray J, Stoker M et al. Purification of scatter factor, a fibroblast derived basic protein that modulates epithelial interactions and movement. Proc Natl Acad Sci 1989; 86:5844-5848.
24. Folkman J, Watson K, Ingber D et al. Induction of angiogenesis during the transition from hyperplasia to neoplasia. Nature 1989; 339:58-61.
25. Moses MA, Langer R. A metalloproteinase as inhibitor as an inhibitor of neovasculariztion. J Cell Biochem 1991; 47: 230-235.
26. Montesano R, Pepper MS, Mohle-Steinlein U et al. Increased proeotytic activity is responsible for the aberrant morphogenetic behaviour of endothelial cells expressing middle T oncogene. Cell 1990; 62:435-445.
27. Pepper MS, Belin D, Montesano R et al. Transforming growth factor beta modulates basic fibroblast growth factor induced proteolytic and angiogenic properties of endothelial cells in vitro. J Cell Biol 1990; 111:743-755.
28. Steeg PS, Bevilacqua G, Kooper L et al. Evidence for a novel gene associated with tumour metastatic potential. J Natl Cancer Inst 1988; 80:200-204.
29. Rosengard AM, Krutz HC Shearn A et al. Reduced nm 23 protein in tumour metastasis and aberrant drosphilla development. Nature 1989; 342:177-180.
30. Randazzo PA, Northup J, Kahn R. Regulatory GTP-binding proteins (ADP-Ribosylation Factor, G_t, and RAS) are not acti-

vated directly by Nucleoside Diphosphate Kinase. J Biol Chem 1992; 267: 18182-18189.

31. Postel EH, Berberich SJ et al. Human c-*myc* transcription factor PuF identified as nm23-H2 nucleoside diphosphate kinase, a candidate suppressor of tumour metastasis. Science 1993; 261:478-479.

CHAPTER 7

Acquisition of Premalignant Lesions I: Colorectal Tumor Formation

1. INTRODUCTION

Colorectal tumors are an excellent system with which to illustrate the types of genetic alterations that are involved in generation of a neoplasm, since there is not only a large volume of clinical and histological information, but several steps towards the formation of a tumor have been identified. In particular, colorectal tumors highlight the necessity for the accumulation of mutation and the role of tumor suppressor genes as dominant negative effectors. These data indicate that the majority of malignant colon carcinomas probably develop from benign adenomas and indeed, tumors at various stages of development are available for study. Both familial and environmental influences play a role in colorectal tumor formation. Whether these principles can be applied to other tumor types requires further experimentation, but they do provide a working hypothesis.

2. THE ROLE OF TUMOR SUPPRESSOR GENES AND ALLELE LOSS IN COLORECTAL TUMORS

Point mutation of one allele of the p53 tumor suppressor gene on chromosome 17p followed some later time by loss of the surviving wild type allele is a frequent occurrence in colorectal tumors. The loss of 17p is rare in adenomas, but occurs in up to 70% of colorectal carcinomas.[1] The now strong evidence for the p53 gene as a tumor suppressor is consistent with the hypotheses that this gene is normally inhibitory to tumor development and the selective growth advantage afforded by mutation of one allele may be sufficient to result in allelic loss of chromosome 17p, i.e., the other allele. Presumably, the absence of this normal allele is then insufficient to suppress further tumor progression. Thus, rather than a recessive mutation at the cellular level, p53 mutations could be considered to act as dominant negative mutations perhaps via a mechanism which involves oligomerization of the mutant and wild type forms in vivo.

A second gene, DCC (deleted in colorectal cancer), has been associated with tumor suppression in colorectal tumorigenesis[2] and may encode an adhesion molecule. The expression of this protein is either reduced or absent in many colorectal tumors and could be involved in the growth restraint mechanisms of the colonic epithelium. Since the biological efficiency of certain cell adhesion molecules is nonlinearly related to the degree of surface expression, clonal expansion could occur even if the remaining allele was normally expressed. For example, a 2-fold decrease (i.e. a heterozygote) in the surface density of cell adhesion molecules can result in almost a 30-fold reduction in adhesiveness.[3] The DCC locus represents the second most common region of chromosomal deletion in colorectal tumors and involves chromosome 18q. Deletions at this locus are found in around 50% of late adenomas and 70% of carcinomas (Table 7.1).

3. FAMILIAL CHROMOSOMAL ABNORMALITIES IN COLORECTAL CANCER

For colorectal cancer the relative contributions of hereditary and environmental influences have been subject to much debate. This is partly because of the high frequency of colon cancer in the general population, which is complicated by the difficulties in the elimination of nonhereditary factors and chance clustering from the analyses performed. It is likely that diet plays a substantial role[3] and that individual families share a common environment. As previously mentioned, studies of allelic loss in cancer prone inherited conditions (e.g. retinoblastoma and neurofibromatosis-type II) have concentrated upon the chromosome that segregates with the disease, i.e,. a linkage analysis. A similar approach has been used for colorectal neoplasia where familial adenomatous polyposis (FAP) and hereditary nonpolyposis colorectal cancer (HNPCC) have been identified.

4. FAMILIAL ADENOMATOUS POLYPOSIS

This autosomal dominant syndrome represents just 1% of colon cancer cases but does provide an insight into one of the genetic changes that may be relevant to colorectal carcinogenesis. A locus linked to FAP (APC) has been mapped to chromosome 5p21[4,5] and mutations at this locus have been observed in 30% of spontaneous colon adenomas and in between 20%

Table 7.1. Genetic changes indentified in colon cancer

Gene	Frequency	Chromosome	Comment
APC	>70%	5	Familial counterpart in FAP Tumor suppressor gene of unknown function
p53	>70%	17	Tumor suppressor gene perhaps involved in cell cycle control
DCC	>70%	18	Tumor suppressor gene. Possibly a cell adhesion molecule.
K-ras	>50%	12	Oncogene. Involved in transmembrane signaling.
FCC	>15%	2	Familial counterpart in HNPCC. Possibly involved in DNA replication/repair.
Cyclins	>4%	Various	Cell cycle regulation.
c-*myc*	>2%	8	Transcription factor.
neu/erbB2	2%	17	Growth factor receptor.

FAP, Familial adenomatous polyposis; HNPCC, Hereditary non polyposis colorectal cancer and 50% of colorectal carcinomas in patients without polyposis. Somewhat surprisingly, in FAP patients with adenomas, allelic loss of chromosome 5q21 is rare, which contrasts with the pattern of allelic loss observed in other inherited cancer prone syndromes. FAP is characterized by thousands of benign colon polyps which line the entirety of the large intestine and which usually develop in the teenage years, with complete penetrance by around the age of 40. Colorectal carcinoma in FAP patients develops in the fourth decade, a significant predisposition when compared to the development of nonfamilial colon cancer in the sixth and seventh decades. It is generally supposed that APC mutations are also an initial stage in the development of sporadic colorectal carcinomas[6,7] and predispose patients with FAP.

5. HEREDITARY NONPOLYPOSIS COLORECTAL CANCER

Hereditary nonpolyposis colorectal cancer (HNPCC) is more common than FAP and may be responsible for between 4 and 13% of colorectal cancers in the western world. In addition, HNPCC patients also suffer cancers of the stomach, endometrium, urinary tract and biliopancreatic system.[8] Via a similar linkage analysis to that used for FAP, the HNPCC gene has been localized to chromosome 2p15-16.[9] It is likely however, that other genes contribute to HNPCC, at least one of which is in the short arm of chromosome 3.[10]

Of the HNPCC associated cancers, 57% could be identified as having APC mutations, which is similar to the 49% observed in sporadic cancers.[11] This makes it unlikely that there are distinct pathways involving the development of familial and sporadic colorectal cancers.

6. HNPCC MAY REPRESENT A DNA REPLICATION DEFECT

Inheritance of the HNPCC locus appears to confer an unusual replication defect in so far as shifts in the electrophoretic mobility of $(CA)_n$ dinucleotide and $(CAG)_n$ trinucleotide repeat fragments suggest that a high frequency of replication errors have occurred during tumor development. The extent of the instability can range from either a minor change (2 bp) to a substantial heterogeneous change in repeat length. In contrast to the tumor suppressor genes, the HNPCC locus is not found to be deleted in HNPCC associated tumors and was only lost in one example out of some 46 sporadic tumors examined.[11] This argues against a role as a tumor suppressor gene and/or oncogene in the conventional sense unless loss or mutation of the second allele is a lethal event. The HNPCC gene may be acting to generally increase chromosomal instability and, if the variation in microsatellite DNA can be extrapolated to the whole genome, we would expect there to be thousands of such replication errors per cell in HNPCC patients. Microsatellite DNA is an abundant human repetitive DNA family which is characterized by stable inheritance. It is one of the more useful DNA polymorphisms used in linkage analysis. Trinucleotide repeats are a common feature of coding sequences and whilst many of these errors will be transcriptionally silent, others may have profound effects upon gene expression. One of the central themes of this book (section 3) is the role played by chromosomal instability in cancer predisposition and the value of the chromosome breakage syndromes to cancer studies. Whilst the genes involved in these syndromes are inherited in an autosomal recessive manner, there is no reason to suppose that any gene involved in maintaining chromosome fidelity and integrity is necessarily recessive. Indeed the HNPCC allele appears to act in a dominant fashion. Consistent with a general role for the HNPCC gene product in causing DNA replication errors across the whole genome, afflicted patients exhibit a wide range of tumor types, not just colorectal carcinoma. The existence of heritable unstable DNA elements occurs in a variety of other inherited disorders such as Huntington's disease, myotonic dystrophy, fragile X syndrome and Kennedy's syndrome.

Whilst it is not suggested that these elements directly cause transformation associated processes, they may be either a consequence of general genetic instability or be indirectly involved in nonspecific deregulation of gene expression, some of which will contribute to altered cell growth. Mutations in any of three yeast genes that are associated with DNA mismatch repair (PMS1, MLH1 and MSH2) lead to a 100- to 700-fold increase in instability of repeat sequences. Mutations which negate proofreading activities have no effect upon stability. If indeed such a mechanism can be translated to colorectal cancer, then mutations in the human mismatch repair genes will be implicated.[12]

These data do, however, suggest a pathway for colon cancer whereby a mutation at the HNPCC locus results in mutation generating DNA replication errors and chromosomal instability in genes associated with microsatellites. The human version of MSH2[13,14] occurs in 0.5% of the population and predisposes to colon, ovarian, kidney and uterine cancers. The strongest evidence for an association with mismatch repair in HNPCC comes from the finding that extracts derived from HNPCC tumor cells are deficient in DNA repair in vitro.[15] In heterozygotes for MSH2, the degree of mismatch repair is indistinguishable from that in normal cells, making the acquisition of a second mutation necessary for the phenotypic effect.

Some of the resultant mutations and/or instabilities may be in either oncogenes of tumor suppressor genes. The growth enhancing properties acquired therefrom would, in the former case, increase selective pressure for oncogene activation (e.g. translocations or amplifications) or in the latter case, select for loss of heterozygosity (e.g. by gene deletion). It should be noted that the deleterious effects of the mutator gene may be lost in the final tumor since there is likely to be a selective pressure for reversion of the mutator gene to prevent either lethal mutations of those which inhibit cell growth. The contribution of mismatch repair to the genesis of the final tumor may thus be underestimated.

7. THE SHERMAN PARADOX AND ITS IMPLICATIONS FOR CANCER DEVELOPMENT

Studies of fragile X mental retardation syndrome demonstrate that the risk of phenotypic effect upon any individual is dependent upon the position in the pedigree.[16] The disorder is unusual since of the carriers only 30% and 80% show mental impairment in females and males respectively. The 20% of normal transmitting males (NTMs) can pass the gene to daughters who may also not show penetrance, but grandsons may be afflicted. The brothers of NTMs show a 9% risk of phenotypic expression, but this can increase to 40% and 50% in grandsons and great grandsons respectively. This genetic phenomenon has become known as the Sherman paradox, which has until recently defied explanation. Similarly, other diseases such as myotonic dystrophy and spinocerebellar ataxia demonstrate the phenomenon of anticipation, whereby as a result of triplet repeat disorders, the illness becomes earlier in onset and more severe in successive generations. These diseases all show the unusual characterization of parental sex bias in transmission of the severe forms and increased penetrance with consecutive generations; in all cases there is a strong correlation with an increase in the number of particular trinucleotide repeats. The high copy number of the repeats in transmitting males predisposes to further amplification, but amplification occurs mostly in females, to the extent that at least one transmission via a female in a generation is required to engender a copy number that is sufficient to produce phenotypic effect.

There are 10 possible trinucleotide repeats[17] of which $p(CTG)_n$, $p(CGG)_n$ and $p(CAG)_n$ have been associated with disease states. Only polymorphic trinucleotides are tolerable in coding sequences (Table 7.2) and CGG, CAG and GAG appear to be the most frequent. CAG codes for glutamine and long stretches of this amino acid are often found in transcription factors. Similarly, tracts of polyglutamate (GAG) and polyproline (CGG) also occur in several pro-

Table 7.2. Trinucleotide repeat expansion and disease

Disease	Frequency	Repeat	Location in Gene	Size of Repeat	Predisposing Normal Alleles
Fragile X	1:2000	CGG	5' UTR	10 to 50	38 to 50
Huntingtons	1:10,000	CAG	coding sequence	11 to 34	30 to 34
Myotonic dystrophy	1:8000	CTG	3' UTR	5 to 35	20 to 35
CAG					
Spinobulbar muscular Atrophy	1:50,000	CAG	coding sequence	11 to 31	N/A
Spinocerebellar ataxia		CAG		25 to 36	

UTR, untranslated region; N/A, data not available

teins. Repeats other than trinucleotides may occur in untranslated regions although their correlation with genetic instability has yet to be demonstrated. The mechanism of dynamic mutation has not been clarified, with meiotic recombination being an unlikely scenario. However, slippage during DNA replication[18] may well be capable of generating increases in copy number, possibly by mechanisms akin to those seen in HNPCC and sporadic colon cancers.

The instability generated as a result of the increasing copy number of repeat sequences can be both meiotic and mitotic in origin. The former has been observed at medium copy number in fragile X syndrome ($n>50$) whereas the latter, which is responsible for somatic variation, appears more common if the copy number is large ($n>200$). Different sizes or multiplicities may then occur within a single tissue, again akin to that observed in some colon cancers.

The increase in susceptibility to a genetic trait over several generations may have profound implications for the way in which we view the initial stages of cancer development and may give us a clue as to the type of mutation which may initiate the process. The data in which a defect in DNA replication or repair may alter the $(CAG)_n$ repeat frequency in HNPCC patients is consistent with a model for the involvement of trinucleotide repeats in cancer development.[11] We suggest that such a mutation alters trinucleotide repeat frequencies of several genes, which may show variable phenotypic penetrance. In the HNPCC case, this can be detected within the tumor of an individual but in the case of fragile X syndrome etc., this may require either a longer period or several meiotic cycles. Many genes have been shown to exhibit trinucleotide repeat sequences in either the 5' or 3' untranslated regions or the coding sequence and some of these are proto-oncogenes. Thus increases in trinucleotide repeats over several generations could lead to small transforming changes by chromosome destabilization leading to either loss of tumor suppressor gene alleles or proto-oncogene activation via a variety of mechanisms. Alternatively, at a certain copy number, the function of the normal protein may be lost which could lead to a significant reduction in the concentration of a tumor suppressor protein. Such mechanisms if proven, could help explain familial inheritance of cancers such as breast, whereby gene penetrance is highly variable.

Of the trinucleotide repeats, $p(CGG)_n$ and $p(CGT)_n$ can be methylated and may play a role in the phenotype caused by a repeat mutation.[19] Indeed, there has been correlation of the fragile X phenotype with the extent of methylation in a CpG island adjacent to the *fmr*-1 gene, the site of the fragile X mutation. Whether such mechanisms, i.e., methylation on repeat sequences, play a role in cancer development remains to be demonstrated but will form an exciting series of experiments.

8. GENETIC ALTERATIONS IN BOTH SPORADIC AND FAMILIAL COLORECTAL CANCER: THE ROLE OF p53

Mutation of the p53 gene and loss of heterozygosity (LOH) at this locus on chromosome 17p are associated with progression of colorectal cancer. The mutated p53 may confer a selective growth advantage in the presence of the wild type gene upon cells that have already been subject to a degree of clonal selection, perhaps as a result of a mutation at the HNPCC locus and/or the APC locus. At a later stage, subsequent amplification of this growth advantage may result from loss of heterozygosity, thus compounding the effect of the first mutation. The latter is closely correlated with progression from adenoma to carcinoma. It is of interest to note that an example of a colorectal tumor exhibiting an intermediate step of mutated p53 in the presence of the wild type allele shows the two mRNA's to be equivalently expressed.[20] In other tumor types, mutations in the p53 gene tend to be associated with later stages in the transformation process. In another study, p53 mutations have not been detected in a large number of HNPCC patients, making it unlikely that inherited p53 mutations are a primary factor in the genesis of HNPCC.[21]

9. OTHER SOMATIC MUTATIONS IN COLORECTAL CANCER

We have already considered allelic loss of chromosomes 5q, 17q and 18q, but are there any other such losses, and if so, what are their relevance? In a systematic study of colorectal carcinomas, deletions in chromosomes 1q, 4q, 6p, 6q, 8p, 9p, 9q, 14q, 18p, 21q and 22q were found in over 20% of cases,[1,22] although in any given tumor, the median number of deletions was found to be between 4 and 5. These data imply two possibilities. Firstly, that the deletions are related to allelic loss of additional tumor suppressor genes, perhaps consequential upon other as yet unidentified mutations and secondly, that they are unrelated to the tumor and arise as a result of general genomic instability. Should the former be correct and a number of tumor suppressor genes remain to be identified, then the pattern of allelic loss may correspond to the observed heterogeneous biology of colorectal tumors, i.e., particular subsets of allelic loss, and hence tumor suppressor gene inactivity gives rise to a particular 'sub type' of tumor. This compounds the therapeutic problem, since inactivation of any one of the multiple pathways or biological targets will still leave a strong growth selection in place and hence also an increased probability of acquisition of a mutation at least equivalent to that treated.

Rationalization of these data is afforded by a report of somatic mutations in poly (dA.dT) repeat sequences in several sporadic cases of colon cancer.[23] 12% of colon carcinomas have been shown to carry microdeletions in these sequences which might be the result of a mutation in a factor required for DNA replication and result in a decrease in fidelity of either DNA replication or repair due to strand misalignment. These mutations are unlikely to be the result of genetic instability during tumor progression since DNA deletions occur in different sections of both adenomas and carcinomas, but not in nearby normal tissue. It is thus most likely that they occurred at an early stage of neoplastic transformation, perhaps in a colonic stem cell which then transmitted these deletions to descendant cells. The original mutation in the fidelity factor (a mutator mutation) may increase the mutation frequency in the latter cells, but a negative correlation with p53 mutations in tumors showing the deletion phenotype[23] makes p53 a less likely candidate. Simple repeat sequences are highly polymorphic in the general population and as can be inferred from their increased in vivo and in vitro mutation frequency, exhibit genetic instability. Since 88% of carcinomas do not show the hyperdeletion phenotype, colonic stem cells do not have a general inability to maintain the replication fidelity of these sequences and this mutation must be considered to be one of a class of several which are involved in the early stages of colorectal carcinogenesis. Whether this mutation is the same as the one thought to be responsible for HNPCC must await further experimentation.

In addition to tumor suppressor gene inactivity, chromosomal rearrangement, microdeletions in simple repeat sequences and mutations in the *ras* oncogene have been identified and associated with late colorectal adenoma and carcinoma. This occurs in both sporadic and familial forms of the disease. If *ras* mutation occurred in one cell of a pre-existing early adenoma, then the selective growth advantage conferred may correlate with tumor progression. In a few other cases, gene amplification (c-*myc*, c-*myb*, *neu*) and rearrangements (*trk*) have been identified, but it is not thought that these play a major role in progression of this tumor type. However, c-*myc* is often over expressed in colorectal tumors and there is often an elevation in the tyrosine kinase activity of certain proteins. The latter has been associated with particular oncogenes and is an integral part of the signal transduction machinery.

One other interesting correlation is epigenetic in nature and relates to the degree of methylation at early stages of colorectal tumor formation. In general, colorectal tumors exhibit a universal hypomethylation pattern, which is apparent even at early stages. Since a reduction in methylation has been reported to affect chromosome condensation, perhaps leading to recombination during mitosis, hypomethylation may provide a cellular mechanism which can enhance the already growth selected process of allelic loss.

10. A MODEL FOR COLORECTAL TUMORGENESIS: ARE ACCUMULATED MUTATIONS MORE IMPORTANT THAN THE ORDER IN WHICH THEY OCCUR?

The development of colorectal cancer (and probably many other types) is best regarded as a continuum whereby successive ripples of clonal expansion occur in response to successive genetic and epigenetic transforming changes (Fig. 7.1). This process occurs over many years, even in the case of familial cancer predisposition. A likely first step could be acquisition of a mutation in the HNPCC locus on chromosome 2 and/or mutation in a similar fidelity factor at another locus. As a result of DNA replication errors, this may cause an increase in the mutation frequency or destabilization of chromosome structure such that cellular hyperproliferation due to mutation or loss of the APC locus on chromosome 5 occurs. In FAP patients, the loss of one allele will be inherited. This may give rise to an adenoma which, perhaps as the result of another genetic change, has a decreased level of general DNA methylation. This may lead to aneuploidy and provide an enabling mechanism for the appearance of growth selected chromosomal rearrangements which inactivate tumor suppressor genes, perhaps in concert with the consequences of the HNPCC mutation. Mutations the c-Ki-*ras* gene in early adenomas show up at a high frequency and usually precede chromosomal deletions in chromosomes 17p and 18q, the sites of the p53 and DCC genes. If the dominant negative mutation and clonal selection theory is correct, then there must previously have been a mutation in one or both of the two (then normal) alleles of either p53 or DCC. The four most common changes in colorectal cancer (5q, 17p, 18q and K-*ras*) do not appear to have an ethnic or geographical bias, and with the exception of 5q loss, do not have any familial association. Differences in colorectal cancer frequencies, therefore, must have a basis in other genetic changes and which may be related to exposure to environmental (i.e. dietary) chemical carcinogenic influences. Further changes must be necessary (perhaps in genes such as nm23) for progression from carcinoma to a tumor with metastatic potential.

It is clear that the preferred order for the accumulation of colorectal genetic changes is 2p and/or 5p, K-*ras*, 17p and 18q, but there are several exceptions.

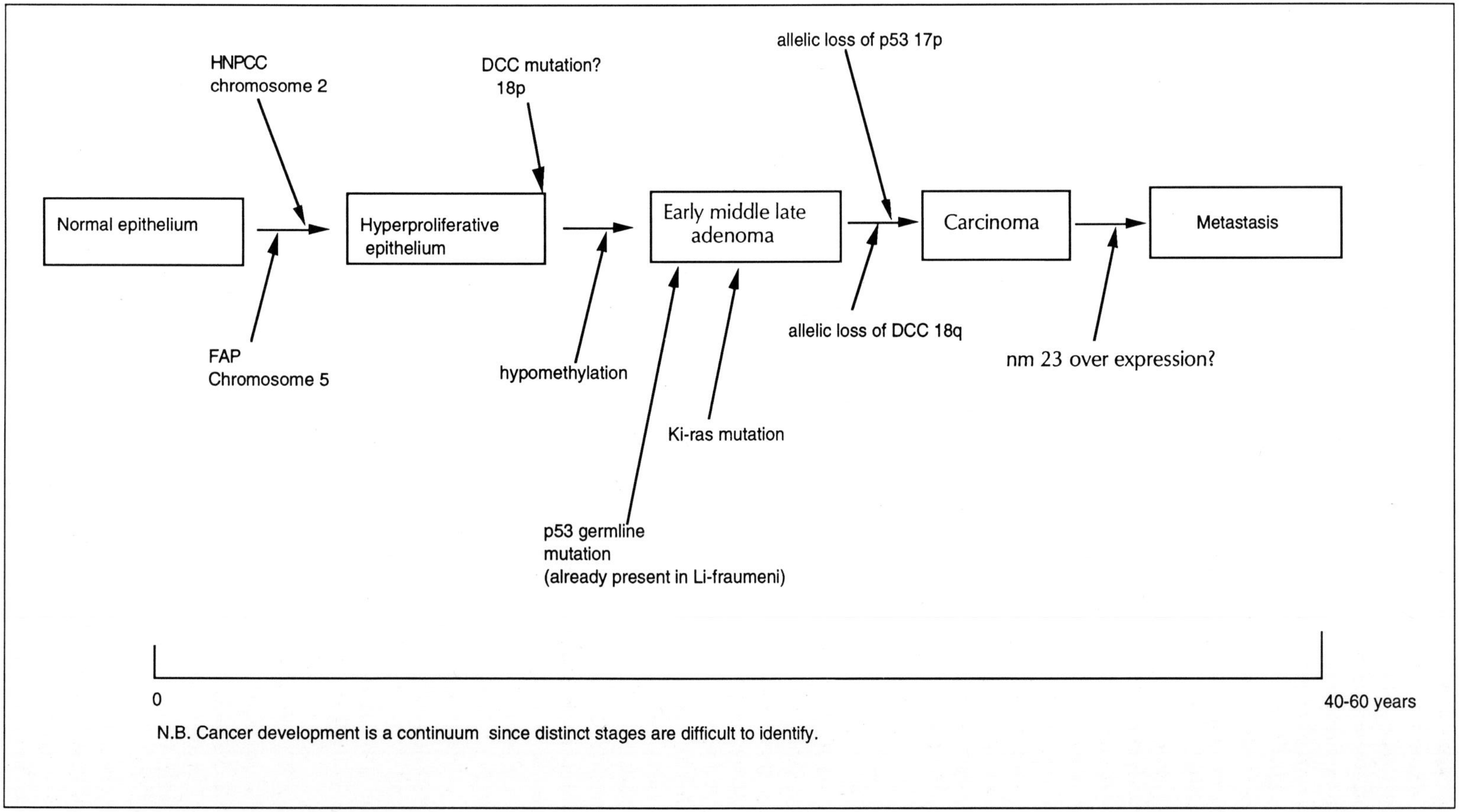

Fig. 7.1. A generalized model for colon cancer.

Whether in the cases where this occurs clonal selection is accelerated relative to those where the order is altered is not yet clear and indeed, remains a very difficult problem.

If we now consider our earlier discussion of the number of steps required for formation of a diagnosable tumor, 7% of early adenomas have more than one of the four aforementioned frequent changes, compared to 90% in the case of carcinoma.[22] It is thus likely that at least one more change is necessary for the fulfillment of metastatic potential.

Whilst many interesting questions remain unanswered, it is clear that much progress has been made in the molecular dissection of colon cancer. It is most important to investigate whether similar changes occur in other tumor types in other tissues.

References

1. Vogelstein B, Fearon ER, Hamilton SR et al. Genetic alterations during colorectal tumour development. New England Journal of Medicine 1988; 319:525-535.
2. Fearon ER, Cho KR, Nigro JM et al. Identification of a chromosome 18q gene that is altered in colorectal cancer. Science 1990; 247:49-53.
3. Hoffman S, Edelman GM. Kinetics of homophilic binding by embryonic and adult forms of the neural cell adhesion molecule. Proc Natl Acad Sci USA 1983; 80: 5762-5766.
4. Willet W. The search for the causes of breast and colon cancer. Nature 1989; 338: 389-394.
5. Kinzler KW, Nilbert MC, Su LK et al. Identification of FAP locus genes from chromosome 5q21. Science 1991; 253:661-665.
6. Nishisho I, Nakamura Y, Miyoshi Y et al. Mutations of chromosome 5q21 genes in FAP and colorectal cancer patients. Science 1991; 253:665-669.
7. Powell SM. APC mutations occur early during colorectal tumorigenesis. Nature 1992; 359:235.
8. Ichii S, Takeda S, Horii A et al. Detailed analysis of genetic alterations in colorectal tumours from patients with and without familial adenomatous polyposis (FAP). Oncogene 1993; 8:2399-2405.
9. Mecklin J-P, Jarvinen HJ. Tumour spectrum cancer family syndrome (hereditary non polyposis colorectal cancer). Cancer 1991; 68:1109.
10. Peltomaki P, Aaltonen L, Sistonen P et al. Genetic mapping of a locus predisposing to human colorectal cancer. Science 1993; 260: 810-812.
11. Lindblom A, Tannergard P, Werelius B, Nordenskojold M. Genetic mapping of a second locus predisposing to hereditary nonpolyposis colon cancer. Nature Genetics 1993; 5:279-282.
12. Aaltonen L, Peltomaki P, Leach F et al. Clues to the pathogenesis of familial colorectal cancer. Science 1993; 260: 812-816.
13. Strand M, Prolla T, Liskay RM, Petes T. Destabilisation of tracts of simple repetitive DNA in yeast by mutations affecting DNA mismatch repair. Nature 1993; 365: 274-276.
14. Leach F, Nicolaides N, Papadopoulos N et al. Mutations in a mutS homologue in hereditary non polyposis colorectal cancer. Cell 1993; 75:1215-1225.
15. Fishel R, Lescoe MK, Rao M et al. The human mutator gene homologue MSH2 and its association with hereditary non polyposis colorectal cancer. Cell 1993; 75:1027-1038.
16. Parsons R, Li G, Longley M et al. Hypermutability and mismatch repair deficiency in RER+ tumour cells. Cell 1993; 75: 1227-1236.
17. Sherman SL, Morton NE. The Marker (X) syndrome: a cytogenetic and genetic analysis. Ann Hum Genet 1984; 48:21-37.
18. Richards I, Sutherland GR. Heritable Unstable DNA Sequences. Nature (Genetics) 1992; 1:7-9.
19. Schlotterer C, Tautz D. Slippage synthesis of simple sequence DNA. Nucleic Acids Research 1992; 20:211-215.
20. Ying-Hui F, Kuhl DPA et al. Variation of the CGG repeat at the fragile x site results in genetic instability. Resolution of the Sherman Paradox. Cell 1991; 67:1047-1058.
21. Nigro JM, Baker SJ, Preisinger AC et al. Nature 1989; 342:705-708.

22. Bhaigirath T, Condie A, Dunlop MG et al. Exclusion of constitutional p53 mutations as a cause of genetic susceptibiity to colorectal cancer. Oncogene 1993; 86: 712-714.
23. Fearon E, Vogelstein B. A genetic model for colorectal carcinogenesis. Cell 1990; 61:759-767.
24. Ionov Y, Peinado M, Malkhosyan S, Shibata D, Perucho M. Ubiquitous somatic mutation in simple repeated sequences reveal a new mechanism for colonic carcinogenesis. Nature 1993; 363:558-561.

CHAPTER 8

Acquisition of Premalignant Lesions II: Myelodysplastic Syndrome and Barrett's Esophagus

1. MYELODYSPLASTIC SYNDROME

Expression of oncogenes or inactivation of tumor suppressor genes are not, in general, independently sufficient to induce transformation. The cell clearly attempts to maintain homeostasis by continuously reverting to the central 'neutral' ground. This evidence has accumulated from numerous studies on transgenic mouse models,[1] skin carcinogenesis studies and tissues which harbor preneoplastic lesions thus representing intermediate stages in the progression towards cancer. Examples of two conditions offer help in the search for intermediate stage: the myelodysplastic syndrome and Barrett's esophagus. In the future, the identification of intermediate stages for other cancers will profoundly influence our ability to diagnose, stage and treat malignancy.

Hematopoietic stem cells form the basis of the hierarchy which leads to a fully functional blood system, erythrocytes for transport of O_2 and CO_2, platelets to aid in clotting and leukocytes which form the immune system (Fig. 8.1). Stem cells undergo self renewal via a process of asymmetrical division in which one of the progeny is a replacement stem cell and the second is of a more differentiated type. More rarely, stem cells may undergo symmetrical division into two stem cells or two differentiated progeny. Humans require 5×10^{11} new terminally differentiated blood cells per day, and therefore, the stem cells must have an immense capacity for amplification. The inherent risks of amplification of a mutation by clonal selection will be apparent from our previous arguments. The controls on such proliferative cycles are of course stringent and are likely to involve regulation of: (a) proliferative rate, (b) developmental potential and (c) longevity, i.e., the apoptotic pathway that is preprogrammed in terminally differentiated cell types. Leukemias occur where there is either an uncontrolled proliferation or expansion or where

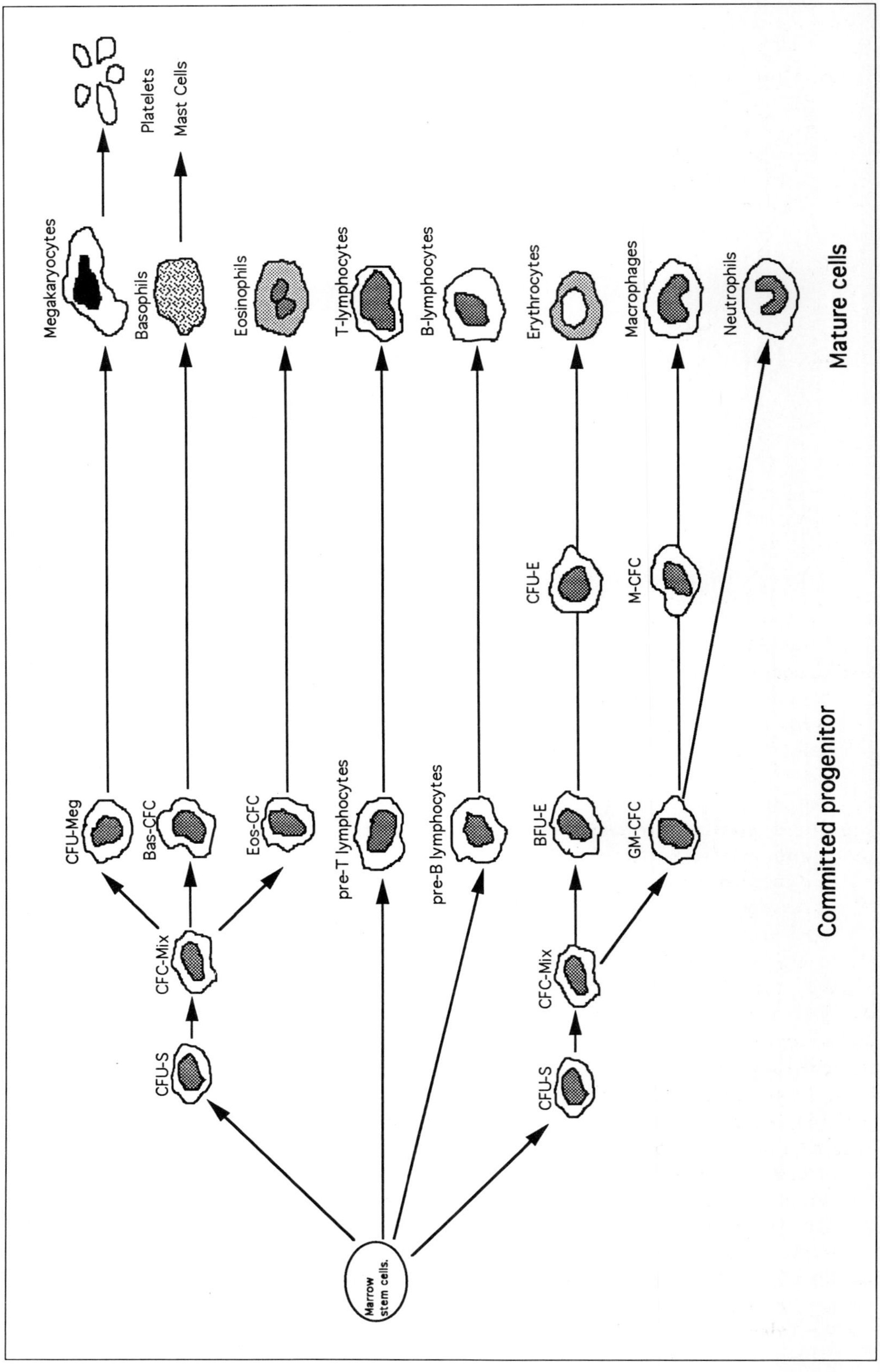

Fig. 8.1. Hematopoietic stem cell differentiation pathway. BFU-E, burst forming unit; CFC, colony forming cell; CFU, colony forming unit; CSF, colony stimulating factor; Meg, megakaryocyte; Bas, basophil; Eos, eosinophil.

the hematopoetic cells do not retain their ability to differentiate. However, some hematological disorders are not strictly leukemias since they only display a proportion of the leukemic phenotype, i.e., growth expansion (myeloproliferative syndrome) or absence of a differentiation block (myelodysplastic syndrome). Both syndromes may progress to acute leukemia and thus study of these disorders may provide an opportunity to identify the relevant oncogenic events in a stepwise manner.

Specifically, myelodysplastic syndrome (MDS) represents a failure of cells to differentiate and is characterized by a low number of circulating white blood cells. In these patients the bone marrow may show an elevated number of stem cells which do not mature normally. MDS is currently classified into five subtypes for diagnostic and operational purposes and the majority of acute leukemias after MDS fall into the acute myelocytic leukemia (AML) category. That this differs from de novo AML is firstly suggested by the differential response to chemotherapy and poorer prognosis of MDS-AML patients, and secondly, the lack of TGFβ1 inhibition of the growth of these cells. This of course suggests that MDS-AML may differ from de novo AML and sets an important precedent, i.e., that the same histological endpoint could be reached by different pathways. The cytokine TGFβ1 may inhibit growth factor dependent proliferation of both de novo AML cells and those of the normal bone marrow.

MDS may arise in progenitor cells of the B cell, T cell or both B-and T-cell lineages and is characterized by clonal dominance. The latter may also result from stem cell depletion or excess damage, e.g., as a result of chemo- and/or radiotherapy. The clonality of MDS has been indicated by X-linked restriction fragment length polymorphism analysis[2] and in some cases the abnormal clone is capable of lymphoid, monocytic and myeloid differentiation in the absence of any detectable karyotypic abnormalities. However, the stem or progenitor cell origin of MDS as a potentially multilineage disorder still remains debatable, although given the extent of amplification in the bone marrow, we can expect the effect of mutations in such cells to be profound.

i. Karyotypic Abnormalities in MDS

Around 48% of 3000 cases of primary MDS show karyotypic abnormalities in bone marrow specimens,[3] although the absolute number varies with the stage of the disease (Table 8.1). These are clustered around particular chromosomes and in some cases give clues as to which genes may be involved in the multistep pathogenesis of MDS. In MDS, which follows chemo- and radiotherapy, clonal karyotypic abnormalities occur in greater than 90% of cases. A range of abnormalities are observed although some are more common than others, e.g., deletions of 5q, 7q, 11q, 13q and 20q; monosomy of chromosomes 5 and/or 7 and trisomy of chromosome 8 (Table 8.2). Deletions of 5q predispose to cancer at a frequency of 16% with medical survival from diagnosis being approximately 5 years. The deletion has been more precisely mapped to chromosome 5q31, a region which contains two potential tumor suppressor genes, the CSF1R (*c-fms*) gene and an early growth response gene (*egr*-1).[6] Since *c-fms* mutation is common at earlier stages of MDS, the 5q31 deletion may represent a corresponding loss of heterozygosity at this locus. Also in this region is a cluster of hematopoietic growth factors and cognate receptors, one of which is GM-CSF. The latter is worthy of mention since one study of 76 patients failed to detect any structural rearrangement in the GM-CSF gene.[7] It is clear that GM-CSF may play a role in the autonomous growth properties of AML-MDS[8] and as an autocrine factor in other cases of AML. Indeed, in certain cases growth factor treatment may predispose to leukemogenesis. The positive requirement for active factor would tend to argue against loss of this locus in the pathogenesis of MDS, although the precise role of GM-CSF in MDS remains to be elucidated.

Table 8.1. Survival rate and karyotype in MDS

Karyotype	Normal	Abnormal/Normal	Abnormal
Median survival (months)*	48	11	6
% progressing to leukemia*	0	30	81
Karyotype	**Normal**	**Abnormal**	**Complex**
Median survival (months)^	36	18	8
% progressing to leukemia^	25	41	50

* Larrippa et al, 1987
^ Suciu et al, 1990

Table 8.2. Chromosomal abnormalities in primary MDS

Deletions	Frequency (%)	Chromosome loss (-)/gain(+)	Frequency (%)
5(q13-q33)	27	(+/-) 7	20
11(q14-q22)	7	(+) 8	19
12q, 20(q11-q13)	5	(-) 5	
7(q22-q34)	4	(-) 17	
13(q14)	2	(+) 21	
(-) Y			
Translocations	**Frequency (%)**	**Others**	**Frequency (%)**
t(1;7)(p11;p11)	2	i 17q	5
t(1;3)(p36;q21)	1	Inv (3) (q21;q26)	1

Chromosome 7 monosomy occurs in 15% of all MDS cases and is the most common karyotypic abnormality seen in pediatric MDS. It is associated with a poor prognosis and in two studies the median age of survival was shown to be 8 and 12 months from diagnosis. In particular, similar abnormalities have been observed in Fanconi's anemia[9] and Down's syndrome.[10] In the cases of chromosome 7 breakpoints, deletions extend from q22-34, a relatively large region which could contain several candidate MDS predisposing genes. Trisomy of chromosome 8 is also common in MDS, again with a relatively poor median survival prognosis, being 10 and 18 months in each of two studies respectively. The simplistic viewpoint would consider that this may result in excess gene dosage of an 'oncogenic' sequence. Deletion between 11q14-22 is also common and other examples include translocations at this region, albeit at a lower frequency.[3]

A number of other aberrations occur more frequently in MDS than one might expect from a random mixture of chromosome aberrations, but their biological significance is not yet clear[11] (Fig. 8.2). In most of the studies so far conducted MDS patients with ostensibly normal karyotypes have a longer median survival term than those without. Furthermore, the greater the frequency of karyotypic abnormalities, the shorter is the survival period.

ii. Oncogenic Mutations in MDS

Subkaryotypic genomic alterations may occur as an early event in MDS and may precede the appearance of cytogenetically detectable lesions. As with other examples of cancer predisposing changes, such mutations may allow clonal selection and via an increase in genomic instability, predispose to gross chromosomal rearrangement and/or LOH. It is likely that several oncogenes and tumor suppressor genes are

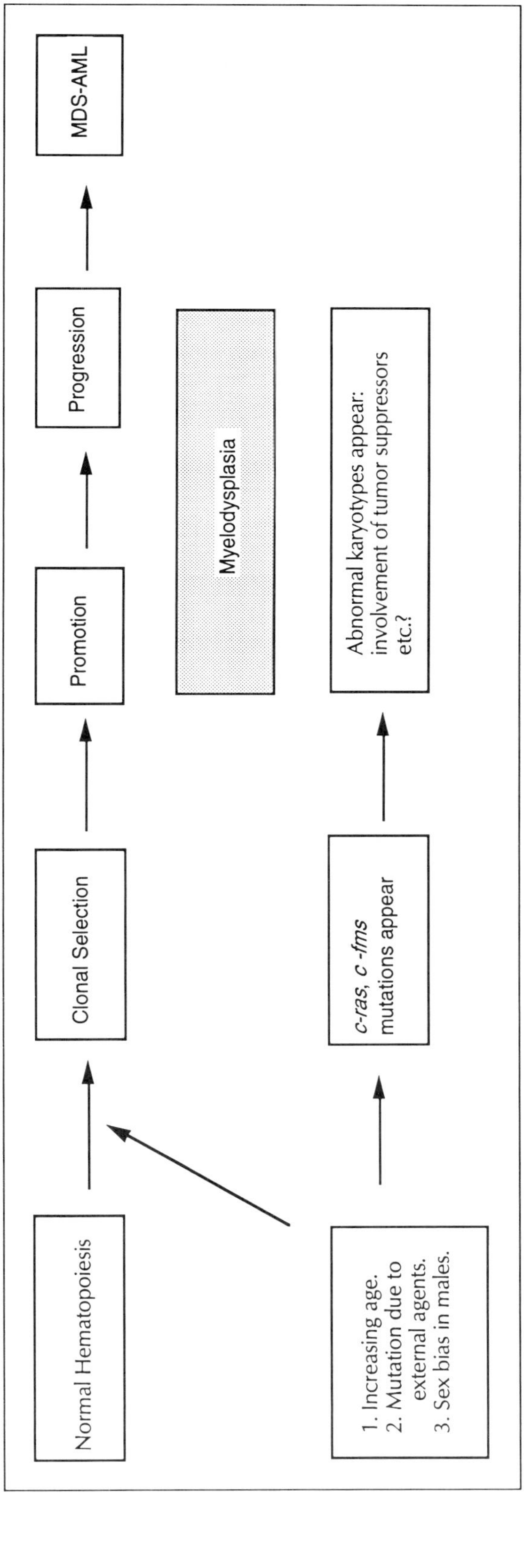

Fig. 8.2. Development of myelodysplasia.

involved in development of MDS although only a small number have been investigated to date. Three cancer associated genes have been studied in MDS c-*ras*, c-*fms* and p53. Only the former two have shown positive correlation[12,13] since only 5 out of 151 MDS patients were shown to have p53 lesions[14] of which, three showed LOH at 17p. Thus unlike with other cancers, mutations in p53 are relatively rare. Abnormalities in p53 are not excluded from participation in the hematological malignancies and occur in AML, T-cell leukemia cell lines and CML in blast crisis.

Mutations which predominantly occur at codons 13 and 61 in the N-*ras* gene are common in de novo AML (25%) and have been identified in 3 out of 8 patients in MDS.[15,16] However, point mutations in the *ras* oncogene in MDS are heterogeneous and may also involve the Ki- and Ha-*ras* alleles.[17] Several models indicate that *ras* activation may be an early or initiating event in some cancers (e.g. colon or lung cancer) but whether it performs a similar role in MDS is not yet clear. Indeed studies have not yet revealed a strong correlation between the presence of a *ras* mutation in MDS and progression to AML.[17] However, the number of cases analyzed is as yet small and given our discussion of other cancers, we realize that the multistep nature of cancer may proceed via either alternative routes and/or reassortment of the steps which constitute progression. There are at least two groups of patients with respect to the staging of *ras* mutations, being (a) a *ras* mutation in a stem cell giving mutations in bone marrow and mature peripheral blood cells and (b) later *ras* mutation resulting in evolution of a leukemic clone. During chemotherapy *ras* mutations may not completely disappear and reappear during relapse. MDS patients which exhibit a mutation in the *ras* gene have been suggested to have a higher chance of progressing to AML, with a concurrent poorer prognosis. However, *ras* may not in itself be sufficient since there are several patients with *ras* mutation and a stable disease. As with colon cancers, the most common *ras* MDS mutation is a G to A transition of the second G of codons 12 or 13, a lesion typical for alkylating agents.[18,19] Codon 12 N-*ras* mutations occur in 9% of MDS patients, but in these cases, there is a short survival period and increased probability of AML development. A separate study has revealed a higher percentage of *ras* mutations (41%) in MDS patients[13] but a similar poor prognosis in the presence of the gene.

Chromosomal alterations are frequent at 5q33 in MDS, the site of the c-*fms* gene. This codes for the receptor of the monocyte and macrophage specific growth factor known as colony stimulating factor-1 (CSF-1). The receptor demonstrates a ligand dependent tyrosine kinase activity and has two codons which are capable of activation, at positions 301 and 969. CSF-1 plays a multifarious role in myeloid hematopoiesis supporting both proliferation and differentiation of progenitor monocytes and survival of the mature differentiated derivatives. The position 301 may confer ligand independent tyrosine kinase activity, which has been shown to be disrupted in 1 out of 13 cases of MDS[6] but perhaps more significant are the 8 out of 54 cases observed with mutations at position 969, the site of a tyrosine residue which may be germane to negative regulatory activity. Subsequent studies have revealed that a significant proportion of MDS patients showed LOH at the c-*fms* locus and some of these were homozygous for gene loss.[20] This indicates the significance of deletion of c-*fms* in the development of MDS and leukemia, although we cannot yet entirely discount contributions from the IL-3, IL-4, IL-5, CSF-1 and GM-CSF genes, which also lie in the 5q region.

Other genes may be involved in MDS and an interesting example has been revealed in the NF1 gene.[21] Here a mutation in a GTPase activating protein (GAP) related domain of NF-1 results in a significant reduction in GAP activity without affecting GTP binding activity.

Thus overall, we have several candidate oncogene and tumor suppressor genes which may affect the genesis of MDS. No doubt more remain to be discovered as the genes associated with the other MDS associated chromosome breaks become clear. However, it is noteworthy that several genes could be involved and that predisposition to AML via MDS may involve acquisition of a selection of genetic changes, which vary from tumor to tumor.

iii. Therapies for MDS

A wide range of agents have been used to treat MDS patients involving differentiating agents, cytokines and alkylating agents, although with very little success to date.[22] Indeed, bone marrow allografts may be the only treatment with a reasonable chance of cure. In particular, patients with an excess of 10% of blast cells in the bone marrow have a particularly poor prognosis (median survival: 6 months). As an aside, patients with >30% immature blast cells in the bone marrow are diagnosed as AML. The poor response rate to therapy may in part be due to the acquisition of drug resistance; several studies have indicated that mdr-1 transcription is increased in MDS (25% of de novo MDS), as it is in de novo AML (21%). Recent therapies designed to circumvent this problem and make use of natural cytokines have also not proven effective. For example, GM-CSF increases the leucocyte count in MDS patients, but did not selectively stimulate normal progenitor cells and thus provide effective therapy.

2. BARRETT'S ESOPHAGUS

The condition known as Barrett's esophagus develops as a complication of stomach acid reflux and is a replacement of the normal esophageal squamous stratified epithelium by a metaplastic columnar epithelium. Barrett's esophagus predisposes to esophageal adenocarcinoma which by the time of detection is invariably incurable and mortality is in excess of 90%. It is one of the few cancer predisposing conditions in which the progress of the disease can be identified with particular morphological and histological changes and as such, provides an important model for identification of various stages of cancer development. Endoscopic examinations demonstrate progressive changes in contiguous groups of cells and provides cellular evidence of clonal evolution. As the cells progress, they increasingly express the proliferative associated antigen Ki-67, demonstrate clones with a high fraction of cells in either S or G2 phase of the cell cycle and become aneuploid. Whilst these data do not demonstrate causality in tumor development, they are suggestive of clonal changes in cell cycle control mechanisms. Many Barrett's esophageal adenocarcinomas have populations of cells that can be distinguished on the basis of increased DNA content (increased ploidy) and/or an increased G2 phase fraction by flow cytometry. Some patients with earlier stage disease also show such abnormalities. However, the central question regarding tumor cells remains: Are they intrinsically more unstable than normal cells or do they acquire abnormal karyotypes through increased proliferation rate (thus increasing the overall time in G2) and/or are subject to strong selective pressures at normal rates of chromosomal rearrangement? The columnar mucosa of Barrett's patients without cancer may show abnormal karyotypes although whether this is directly associated with the G2/aneuploid cell fraction is not yet proven.

The genetic basis of progressive development of malignancy in Barrett's esophagus may in part lie in altered expression of p53. The final Barrett's adenocarcinomas have a high frequency (53% of chromosome 17p deletions and p53 over expression.[23] This increases progressively from zero in normal epithelia[24] (Fig. 8.3) strongly implicating p53 in the development of this condition.

The correlative evidence for an increased G2/S and/or aneuploid population in Barrett's esophagus which precedes adenocarcinoma is strong. In addition, studies of many patients have revealed that this cancer is a result of the progressive accumulation of abnormalities over a several year period.[25] However, the time spent in each category (Fig. 8.2) is highly variable between subjects and is probably reflective of the rate of accumulation of both endogenous and exogenous mutations. The increased G2 phase fractions detected by flow cytometry occur over a wide region of the mucosa, thus giving a greater number of

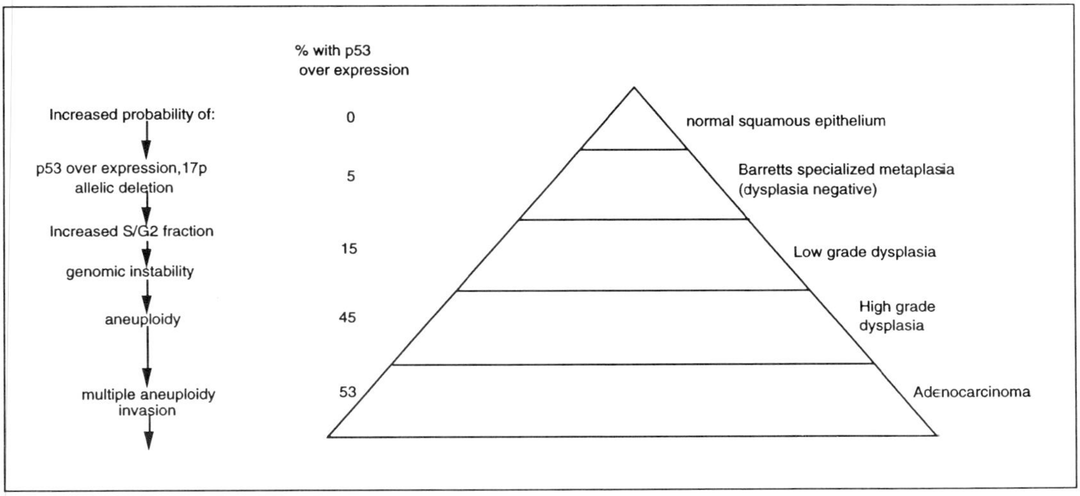

Fig. 8.3. Barrett's esophagus.

cells as possible targets for subsequent mutation. As previously discussed, the G2 phase of the cell cycle may be a time in which the cell is prone to genomic instability and development of aneuploidy. Further studies must be performed however to ascertain the prevalence of a lack of tumor suppression via p53 mutation and/or cytoplasmic localization.

References

1. Adams JM, Cory S. Transgenic models of tumor development. Science 1991; 254: 1161-1166.
2. Tefferi A. Clonal studies in the myelodysplastic syndrome using X-linked restriction fragment length polymorphisms. Blood 1990; 75:1770-1773.
3. Mufti GJ. Chromosomal deletions in the myelodysplastic syndrome. Leukaemia Res 1992; 16:35-41.
4. Larripa I, Labal de Vinuesa M, Bengiò R, Slavutsky I. Chromosome studies in human hematologic diseases: II. Myelodysplastic syndromes. Haematologica 1987; 72: 399-403.
5. Suciu S, Kuse R, Weh, HJ, Hossfield DK. Results of chromosome studies and their relation to morphology, course, and prognosis in 120 patients with de novo myelodysplastic syndrome. Cancer Genet Cytogenet 1990; 44:15-26.
6. Ridge SA, Worwood M, Oscier D, Jacobs A, Padua RA. *FMS* mutations in myelodysplastic, leukemic, and normal subjects. Proc Natl Acad Sci USA 1990; 87: 1377-1380.
7. Boultwood J, Abrahamson G, Buckle VJ, Rack K, Oscier DG, Wainscoat JS. Structure of the granulocyte macrophage colony factor gene in patients with the myelodysplastic syndromes. Am J Haemat 1990; 34:157-158.
8. Reilly AG, Kozlowski R, Russell NH. Heterogenous mechanism of autocrine growth of AML blasts. Br J Haemat 1989; 72:363-369.
9. Strivins TJ, Davis RB, Sanger W et al. Transformation of Fanconi's anaemia to acute non lymphocytic leukaemia associated with emergence of monosomy 7. Brit J Haematol 1987; 65:321-323.
10. Bunin N, Nowell PC, Belasco J et al. Chromosome 7 abnormalities in children with Down's syndrome and preleukeamia. Cancer Genet Cytogent 1991; 54:119-126.
11. Noël P, Tefferi A, Pierre RV, Jenkins RB, Dewald GW. Karyotopic analysis in primary myelodysplastic syndromes. Blood Reviews 1993; 7:10-18.
12. Paquette RL, Landaw EM, Pierre RV, Kahan J, Lübbert M, Lazcano O, Isaac G, McCormick F, Koeffler HP. N-*ras* mutations are associated with poor prognosis and increased risk of leukemia in myelodysplastic syndrome. Blood 1993; 82:590-599.
13. Yunis JJ, Boot AJM, Mayer MG, Bos JL. Mechanisms of *ras* mutation in myelodysplastic syndrome. Oncogene 1989; 4:609-614.
14. Jonveaux P, Fenaux P, Quiquandon I et al. Mutations in the p53 gene in myelodysplastic syndromes. Oncogene 1991; 6: 2243-2247.
15. Bos JL, Verlaan-de Vries M, van der Eb AJ et al. Mutations in N-*ras* predominate in acute myeloid luekaemia. Blood 1987; 69:1237-1239.
16. Hirai H, Okada M, Mizoguchi H et al. Relationship between activated N-*ras* oncogene and chromosomal abnormality during leukaemic progression from myelodysplastic syndrome. Blood 1988; 71: 256-258.
17. Lyons J, Janssen JWG, Bartram C. Mutation of Ki-*ras* and N-*ras* oncogenes in myelodysplastic syndromes. Blood 1988; 71:1707-1710.
18. Vogelstein B, Fearon ER, Hamilton SR et al. Genetic alterations during colorectal tumour development. N Eng J Med 1988; 319:525-532.
19. Bos JL. *ras* Oncogenes in Human Cancer: A Review. Cancer Res 1989; 49:4682-4689.
20. Boultwood J, Rack K, Kelly S, Madden J, Sakaguchi AY, Wang L-M, Oscier DG, Buckle VJ, Wainscoat JS. Loss of both CSF1R *(FMS)* alleles in patients with myelodysplasia and a chromosome 5 deletion. Proc Natl Acad Sci USA 1991; 88:6176-6180.
21. Li Y, Bollag G, Clark R, Stevens J, Conroy

L, Fults D, Ward K, Friedman E, Samowitz W, Robertson M, Bradley P, McCormick F, White R, Cawthon R. Somatic mutations in the neurofibromatosis 1 gene in human tumors. Cell 1992; 69:275-281.
22. Hamblin TJ. Intensive chemotherapy in myelodysplastic syndromes. Blood Reviews 1992; 6:215-219.
23. Blount PL, Ramel S, Raskind WH, Sanchez CA, Haggitt RC, Dean PJ, Rabinovitch PS, Reid BJ. 17p allelic deletions and p53 protein over expression in Barrett's adenocarcinomas. Cancer Res 1991; 51: 5482-5486.
24. Ramel S, Reid BJ, Sanchez CA et al. Evaluation of p53 protein expression in Barrett's esophagus by two-parameter flow cytometry. Gastroenerology 1992; 102:1220-1228.
25. Reid BJ, Blount PL, Rubin CE, Levine DS, Haggitt RC, Rabinovitch PS. Flow-cytometric and histological progression to malignancy in Barrett's esophagus: prospective endoscopic surveillance of a cohort. Gastroenterology 1992; 102:1212-1219.

SECTION 2

The Molecular Basis Of Cancer Predisposition-1: Environmental Carcinogens, Infective Agents and Hormonal Influences

In this section we will discuss particular examples of predisposition to cancer, both inherited and noninherited. Whilst the two categories cannot be definitely separated in the majority of cases, we hope to illustrate the roles played by particular environmental agents, infective agents and hormonal influences in the development of specific types of cancer.

CHAPTER 9

Environmental Carcinogens: Tobacco and Lung Cancer

1. THE EPIDEMIOLOGY OF LUNG CANCER

Lung cancer is the most frequently occurring cancer in UK males and is second only to breast cancer in UK females. 90% of these cancers are directly related to exposure to tobacco smoke, although we shall discuss the possible effects of exposure to ionizing radiation such as radon gas. Lung neoplasia is the overall leading cause of cancer deaths and only 13% of patients survive beyond 5 years from diagnosis. Cigarette manufacturers have responded to the evidence from the medical community by introducing filters and reducing the tar content of tobacco products. The declining social acceptance of smoking in the UK correlates with a reduction in the rate of death from lung cancer and now the highest rates are to be found in the older generation, many of whom began to smoke at an early age. One of the key epidemiological factors in lung cancer relates to the difference in age of onset of lung cancer in persons with similar smoking habits, which is perhaps suggestive of differences in the genetic susceptibility to lung cancer.

Lung tumors are divided into two classes based upon pathology and clinical characteristics; the small cell lung cancers (SCLCs) which represent 25% of those tumors observed and are probably derived from neuroendocrine cells and non-small cell lung cancers (NSCLCs). The latter include squamous cell, adenocarcinoma, large cell and undifferentiated tumor types (Table 9.1). Two of the histological types of lung cancer are definitely smoking related, small cell and squamous. The other forms, which constitute 10% of lung cancer cases (alveolar cell, carcinoma and adenocarcinoma) are not thought to be as closely related to exposure to tobacco smoke. In contrast to animal models, 90% of human lung tumors develop in the major airways as opposed to peripheral regions of the lung. Of these, 30% are squamous, 25% small cell, 10% large cell and 30% are adenomas although the spectrum may change according to the nature of the industrial or occupational exposures. Environmental and genetic factors both play a role with squamous cell carcinomas being predominant in the western world and adenocarcinoma predominant in Japan. The background level of lung tumorigenesis is difficult to assess due to the large number of chemicals that we face, together with the preponderance of respiratory infections. The identification of lung cancer predisposing genes is compounded by the low penetrance of susceptibility loci (high penetrance enables identification via the cancer prone syndromes) and the difficulties of identification of familial clustering in a population where many are (or have been) exposed to tobacco smoke, either advertently or inadvertently. However, studies have been performed that indicate enhanced susceptibility in certain families.

Besides tobacco smoke, lung cancer risk is increased in certain industrial occupations, particularly where there has been exposure to asbestos. This risk has been recognized and exposure has now been limited. In addition, industrial exposure to polycyclic aromatic hydrocarbons and to radioactive radon gas in certain mines is also of importance. In the latter case, radon may be significant in the home. For example, due to the geology of the area, the exposure of individuals in Cornwall may by 15 times the national average. The risk regarding lung cancer has yet to be quantified but if proven, radon could be an extremely important risk factor in development of all types of lung cancer.

2. GENETIC PREDISPOSITION TO LUNG CANCER

The genetic susceptibility to lung cancer is indicated by the existence of cancer prone families (e.g. in Li-Fraumeni syndrome[1]) and that some individuals who do not smoke develop lung cancer whilst not all that do smoke develop lung cancer.[2] However, one must be cautious with interpretation of these data since, (a) lung cancer can arise from proliferative effects upon any one of several cell types, each of which may be activated differently and (b) there are probable influences of passive smoking and/or genetic influences upon carcinogen metabolism. Small variations in the latter amongst individuals, e.g., via triplet repeat polymorphisms, could result in differential genetic effects. First degree relatives of lung cancer patients have a 2.4-fold excess risk factor for development of lung or other cancers, which may not be smoking related. Abnormal Ha-*ras* alleles on chromosome 11p have been found in NSCLC which suggests linkage.[3]

Familial clustering in alveolar cell carcinoma[4] has been reported in the case of siblings sharing the HLA-A28 locus and in lung adenocarcinoma associated with Li-Fraumeni syndrome. Certain in-bred mouse strains exhibit genetic susceptibility to lung carcinogenesis in response to chemical carcinogens and cancer susceptibility loci have been identified.[5] The nature and role of the homologous human genes are eagerly awaited.

Table 9.1. Lung tumor types

Tumor Type		Probable Origin
SCLC		Pulmonary neuroendocrine cells
NSCLC	adenocarcinoma	major bronchi : secretary cuboidal cells
	large cell carcinoma	undifferentiated : basal or stem cell
	squamous cell carcinoma	squamous epithelium
	peripheral airway cells	clara cells : progenitors of the bronchiolar
		Type II pneumocytes : progenitors of the alveoli

NB All bronchial carcinomas are related to cigarette smoking, except bronchial carcinoids (an SCLC with neuroendocrine features).

Overall, however, human genetic susceptibility to lung cancer has not yet been convincingly demonstrated, probably due to low gene penetrance. For the time being, exposure to environmental agents and in particular tobacco smoke, remains the most important etiological agent.

3. THE BRONCHIAL EPITHELIUM

The tracheobronchial epithelium is a pseudostratified columnar epithelium which consists of three cell types, a basal cell layer, some secretary cell types (mucous, neuroendocrine, serous and Clara cells) and ciliated cells. As with other epithelia, there is turnover of these cell types and replacement via tracheobronchial stem cells. Turnover is, however, relatively slow due to the low concentrations of positively acting growth factors and many of the tracheobronchial epithelial cells which are proliferation competent reside in the G0 phase of the cell cycle. The rate of cell turnover is probably controlled by the balance of positively and negatively acting growth and differential factors, a number of which have been identified (EGF, TGFα, TGFβ1, TGFβ2, insulin, IGF-1 keratinocyte growth factor [KGF; of the FGF family], gastrin releasing peptide [GRP] and retinoic acid derivatives). Of these EGF, TGFα, insulin, IGF-1, GRP and KGF appear to stimulate cell growth, whilst negative effects are observed with TGFβ, retinoids and indeed, factors which activate protein kinase C. Growth regulation is via both autocrine and paracrine mechanisms, for example the potential stimulatory effect of TGFα and IGF-1 released by macrophages after injury. In the transformed case, many tracheobronchial epithelial cells exhibit growth factor independence, particularly in the negative regulation of their growth. Normally, TGFβ1 and β2 inhibit the growth of these cells and cause morphological cell flattening and an increase in the levels of several enzymes such as transglutaminase type II, fibronectin and collagen IV, components of the extracellular matrix. Some lung carcinoma cells, however, remain responsive to TGFβ and acquire a differentiated phenotype upon treatment. The situation is, however, of greater complexity than this since certain lung carcinoma cell lines may show aberrant responsiveness to TGFβ, in one case resulting in enhanced ECM degradation via an excess synthesis of plasminogen activator over that of plasminogen activator inhibitor.

Important regulators of tracheobronchial epithelial cell growth are the retinoids, analogs of vitamin A. These induce a variety of effects, such as inhibition of expression of a squamous differentiated phenotype. Retinoids cause a number of changes in gene expression, such as inhibitions of the increases in transglutaminase type 1, cholesterol sulphate, keratin 13 and various other squamous cell mRNAs, which would normally accompany differentiation. Three specific high affinity retinoid receptors (RARα,β,γ) are expressed in the nuclei of these cells and bear many similarities to the steroid/thyroid hormone receptor superfamily. The RAR receptors function as ligand dependent transcription factors which act upon a set of specific genes containing a retinoic acid response element in their controlling regions. Human tracheobronchial epithelial cells are rich in the RARα, and γ mRNAs and RARβ can be induced by treatment with retinoic acid. Aberrant expression of RAR receptors in several lung carcinoma cell lines has been observed and a role for these genes as either tumor suppressor or proto-oncogenes must be considered.

Gastrin releasing peptide (GRP, often referred to as bombesin) functions as an autocrine growth factor in SCLC. GRP is produced in the fetal lung and may have a role in regulation of the normal growth and differentiation of lung tissue. It has a mitogenic effect both in vivo and in vitro and stimulates the growth of both SCLC cell lines and normal tracheobronchial epithelial cells. Reports of GRP immunoreactivity in the bronchiolavage of smokers are most interesting, since this could provide a 'promoter' for the initiation of events resulting from tobacco associated carcinogens. Stimulation of GRP activity for whatever reason would suggest a very early role for growth factor and signal transduction events in the pathogenesis of lung cancer.[6]

4. CHEMICAL CARCINOGENS IN TOBACCO SMOKE AND THEIR DETOXIFICATION

There are at least 100 chemicals which have been identified in cigarette smoke and of these, over 40 are carcinogenic in animal models. Several of these represent N-nitroso derivatives which have been shown to cause a number of different types of tumor in model systems. Besides tobacco smoke, exposure to these compounds can arise from components of the diet, atmospheric pollution and endogenous sources. N-nitroso compounds generally require metabolism and in doing so form reactive intermediates capable of alkylating DNA via the addition of methyl or ethyl moieties. Some of these show affinity for respiratory tissues, for example 4-(methyl-nitrosamino)-1-(3-pyridyl)-1-butanone (NNK) is both tobacco specific (being derived from nicotine) and highly potent in lung carcinogenicity assays (Fig. 9.1). Both NNK and the classic methylating agent N-nitrosodimethylanine (NDMA) are metabolized to the highly reactive methyl diazohydroxide via the action of the cytochrome p450 complex. This results in the formation of O^6 Me Guanine, O^4 Me Thymine and methylphosphotriesters. In addition, NNK can be hydroxylated via the p450 system on the N-methyl carbon to form a pyridyloxobutylated adduct. However, the mutation profiles observed for activation of the K-*ras* gene are identical for both NNK and NMDA, strongly suggestive of DNA methylation and not pyridyloxobutylation being the major carcinogenic pathway.[7] Also worthy of mention is the polycyclic aromatic hydrocarbon benzo[a]pyrene which can also be metabolically activated to form compounds which form adducts with DNA. It occurs as a product of incomplete combustion (e.g. tobacco smoke, engine exhausts) and its metabolic detoxification may have a genetic component. Hydrocarbons such as this are generally water insoluble and once inside the body must be made water soluble in order to be excreted in the urine. This process converts a relatively unreactive compound (e.g. benzo[a]pyrene) into an electrophilic carcinogen (Fig. 9.2).

The systems responsible for the formation of covalently binding electrophilic and nucleophilic adducts in the lung are likely to be those of the flavin mono-oxygenases, prostaglandin synthetase, xanthine oxidase and microsomal NADPH dependent cytochrome p450 reductase. Cigarette smoke induces the phase I enzyme aryl hydrocarbon hydroxylase, a mixed function cytochrome p450 dependent oxygenase and also di-methyl nitrosamine demethylase. In general, the levels of these enzymes are at higher levels in the lung tissues of smokers. In humans the enzyme system which metabolizes the antihypertensive drug debrisoquine (debrisoquine-4-hydroxylase) is coded for by the CYP2D6 allele of the p450 complex, known to metabolize at least 30 other compounds via phase I mono-oxygenation. Between 5 and 10% of the Caucasian population may be incapable of adequate debrisoquine metabolism and may also be less able to correctly metabolize the components of cigarette smoke, resulting in predisposition to cancer.[8] However, in a recent study for polymorphisms at the CYP2D6 allele in over 2000 patients statistically significant associations with lung cancer frequencies were not observed.[9] However, the relatively rare CYP1A1 allele does have a significant association with lung cancer, especially when in combination with a deletion of the glutathione-S-transferase (GST-1) locus. The latter is a phase II enzyme which decreases in response to the cigarette smoke, which is likely to have the unfortunate effect of increasing the effective concentration of carcinogens generated via phase I mono-oxygenation.

5. LOSS OF HETEROZYGOSITY IN LUNG CANCER

In fresh human tumor tissue all cases of SCLC showed loss of heterozygosity on chromosomes 3p, 13q14 (the Rb locus) and 17p.[10] In addition, up to 50% of NSCLC (including adenocarcinomas) show deletions at the 3p locus. This has led to the suggestion that a lung cancer tumor suppressor gene may exist in this region,[1] providing a restriction upon clonal expansion. Two candidate genes map to this region: c-*erb* Aβ, a thyroid hormone receptor at 3p21-25 and RARβ (3p24), a retinoic acid receptor protein. Many SCLC tumors do not show loss of the c-*erb* Aβ allele making it an unlikely contender. The preponderance of chromosome 3p deletions suggests that this may be a common step in the development of lung cancers, possibly occurring at an early stage. In NSCLCs, LOH at chromosome 17p is often associated with LOH at chromosome 11 in squamous cell carcinomas, but less so in adenocarcinomas and large cell carcinomas.

The Rb locus (13q14) has recently been the center of much attention and is worthy of further mention in the context of lung cancer. Up to 32% of primary NSCLC cancers show either absent or abnormal immunohistochemical staining for the Rb protein and in the cases where it is absent, this is often associated with LOH.[12] Similarly, LOH occurs in many examples of SCLC cell lines (76%) and primary tumors (78%).[2] Evidence suggests that survivors of hereditary retinoblastoma are predisposed to lung cancer and in addition, Rb heterozygotes have a 15-fold excess lung cancer risk.

The LOH of 17p13 correlates with loss of p53, which is also observed in other tumor types (e.g. colon, breast, brain). LOH is common to both SCLC and NSCLC and lung cancer is one of the types of neoplasms observed in Li-Fraumeni syndrome, where patients have germ line mutations in p53. The p53 gene is mutated in 45% of NSCLC tumor samples, with a different set of base changes to those observed in colon cancer. Another different spectrum of p53 mutations is observed in 73% of SCLC.[13] Benzo[a]pyrene may in part be responsible for early mutation of the p53 gene via a GC:TA transversion.[14] Either this or an *arg-pro* polymorphism in the gene may lead to clonal selection and be a prelude to LOH at this locus.

6. ONCOGENE ACTIVATION IN LUNG CANCER

Lung cancers are characterized by the extraordinary diversity of oncogenes that have been shown to be aberrantly expressed. (c-*myc*, N-*myc*, L-*myc*, c-*myb*, p53, c-*raf*-1, c-*fms*, c-*erb*B1, c-*erb*B2, c-*fos*, c-*jun*, c-Ha-*ras*, c-Ki-*ras*, c-N-*ras*). Obviously, not all of these alterations occur at the same time and perhaps these data are lacking a detailed study which correlates the precise histological type and the oncogenes which appear to be altered in expression (Fig. 9.3). Some general features can be noted and will now be discussed.

i. THE RAS FAMILY: HA-, KI- AND N-RAS

In lung tumors and cell lines, the Ki-*ras* gene is frequently mutated, usually at position 12. Reports of mutations in c-Ha-*ras* and c-N-*ras* have been sporadic, although LOH of the c-Ha-*ras* locus has been reported for aggressive NSCLC tumors. Nearly all adenocarcinomas show mutation of the c-Ki-*ras* gene with a wide variety (codons 12, 13, 18 and 61) of mutations having been observed. Activation of the c-Ki-*ras* gene has been suggested as an early event in lung carcinogenesis which is directly related to exposure to tobacco smoke. NNK induces c-Ki-*ras* codon 12 mutations in 76% (13 out of 17) of hamster lung tumors,[15] as does benzo[a]pyrene in 93% of mouse tumors examined.[16] Thus there appears to be a direct correlation between exposure to known tobacco carcinogens and activation of Ki-*ras*. However, this does not prove that smoking helped cause the tumor in any individual case and given the time scales involved, this is likely to be difficult.

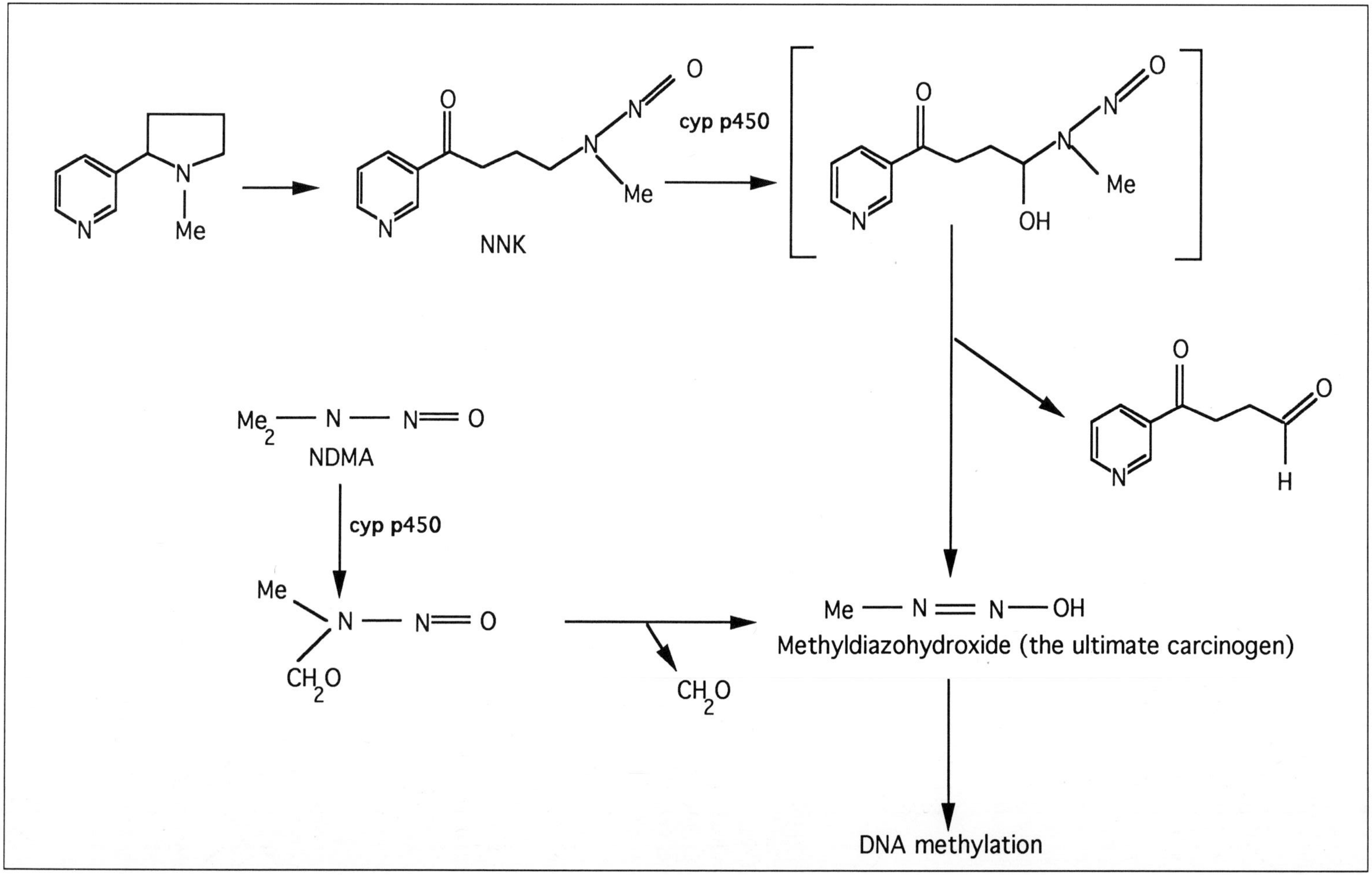

Fig. 9.1. Chemical carcinogens in tobacco smoke. 4-(methyl nitrosoamino)-1-(3-pyridyl)-1-butane arises as a consequence of burning nicotine. It is metabolized to methyldiazohydroxide, a methylating agent (it produces O6Me Guanine and O6 Me Thymine) and the ultimate carcinogen. For comparison we include the pathway to metabolism for NDMA (N-nitrosodimethylamine) a compound often used in lung carcinogenesis and alkylation studies. This may also be metabolized by the CYP P450 complex to methyldiazohydroxide.

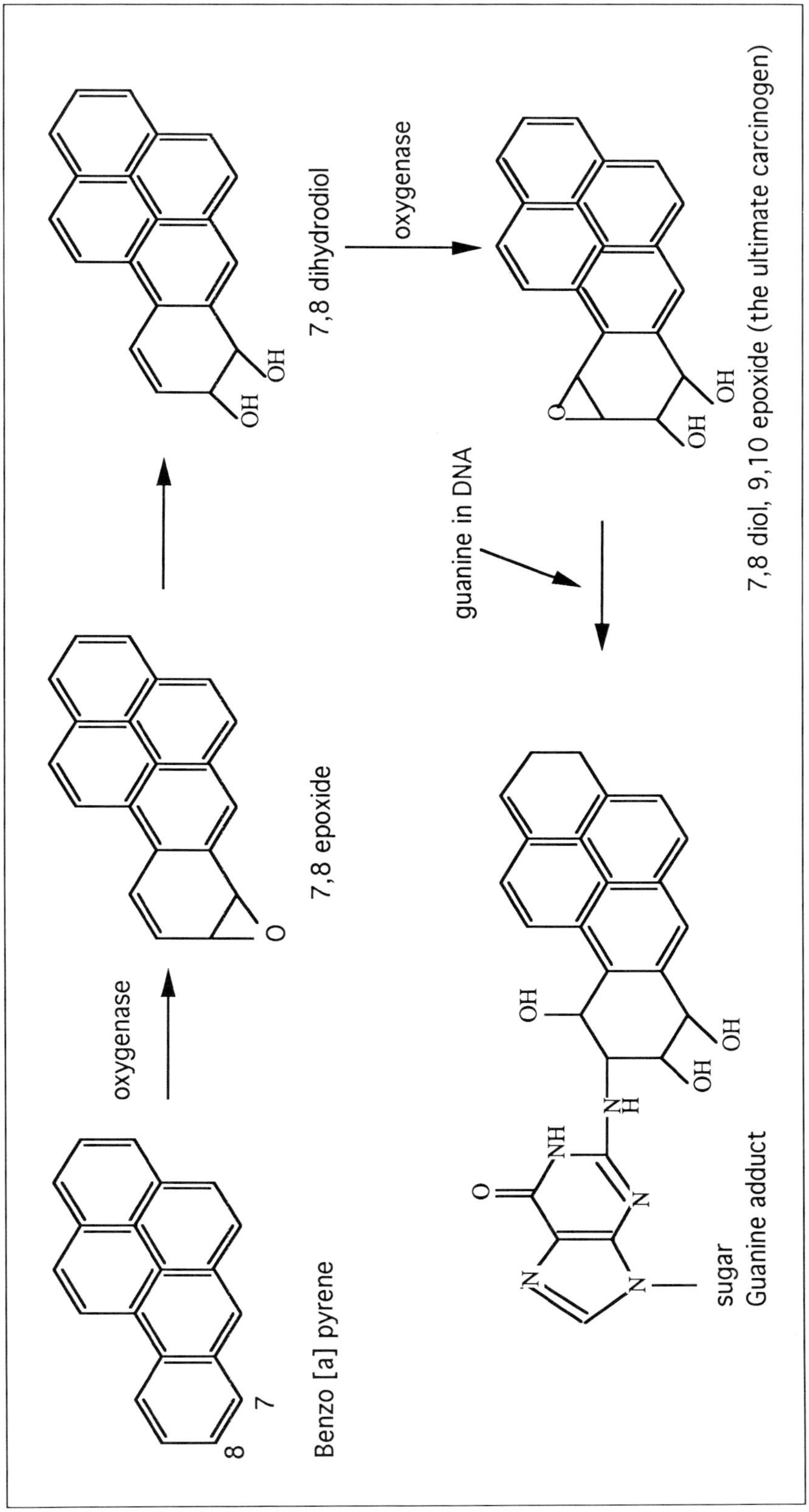

Fig. 9.2. Chemical carcinogens in tobacco smoke.-2. Benzo [a] pyrene can be converted into several products only one of which is shown here. The ultimate carcinogen (7,8, diol 9,10, epoxide) is capable of forming adducts with guanine residues in DNA, eventually resulting in GC to AT transversions.

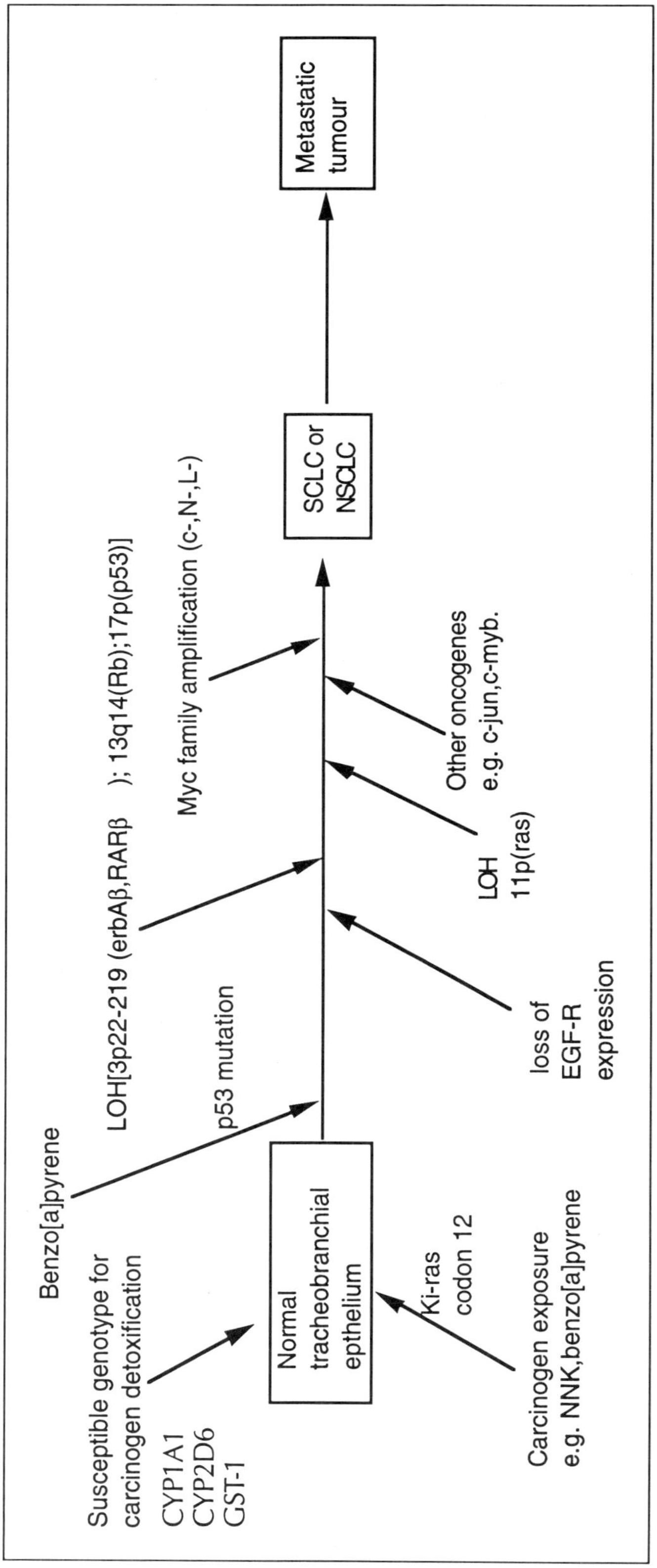

Fig. 9.3. A generalized model for lung cancer.

ii. C-*RAF*-1

LOH of the c-*raf*-1 allele (chromosome 3p25) occurs in up to 80% of SCLC cell lines and in many SCLC (100%) and NSCLC (42%) tumors. Of the SCLC cell lines, 100% express higher levels of the c-*myc* mRNA and transcriptional activation of c-*raf*-1 in NSCLC cell lines is common. It is of interest to note that the c-*raf*-1 locus is often retained if there is LOH at the more proximal c-*erb*Aβ locus (3p21-25), which may perhaps indicate a relationship between them at the level of signal transduction.

iii. THE *MYC* FAMILY

The expression of the c-*myc* and N-*myc* oncogenes is altered in SCLC cell lines and tumor tissues by gene amplification, in contrast to the chromosomal translocation events observed in B cells. The mRNAs are, however, often transcriptionally upregulated even without gene amplification by a mechanism which involves enhanced transcription rates, rather than an increase in mRNA stability. This alteration in c-*myc* expression is associated with aggressive clinical progression of the disease. There are also examples of the over expression of c-*myc* in NSCLC, but this has not yet been reported for N-*myc*. The L-*myc* gene was identified as a cross hybridizing band in studies of SCLC using a c-*myc* probe. As for c-*myc*, it is frequently amplified and over expressed in both SCLC and NSCLC and in particular, L-*myc* expression may be of prognostic significance to cancer.[17]

iv. Other Oncogenes Associated with Lung Cancer

Besides the *ras* and *myc* family, certain other oncogenes are expressed in lung cancer tumors and cell lines, albeit with low frequencies. Some reports indicate that both SCLC and NSCLC express EGF receptors (c-*erb*B1), whilst others report a lack of EGF binding activity and c-*erb*B1 gene expression at both the mRNA and protein levels. This may reflect a loss of growth factor dependence as the transformation state of the cells increases. The c-*erb*B2 (*neu*) oncogene has been detected as an amplified product in adenocarcinoma, but is an infrequent event. The c-*myb* and c-*fms* oncogenes are often over expressed in SCLC. The nuclear oncogene and transcription factor c-*jun* is strongly expressed in lung tissue and may produce chronic tumor promoting effects similar to the phorbol esters, which of course induce its expression.

v. The Link Between Chemical Carcinogenesis in the Lung and Oncogene Activation

There is clearly a correlation between exposure to tobacco smoke and the incidence of lung cancer, but to what extent does the evidence indicate causality? A few of the components in tobacco smoke have been identified and shown to be mutagenic via DNA damage. Some are also carcinogenic. Some of these compounds activate known oncogenes in vivo and in vitro in ways which are consistent with the types of changes seen in oncogenes in the final tumor. However, these data, although strong, are not sufficient to build up a cause and effect model for lung carcinogenesis. We do not know exactly which chemicals are most important in cell transformation and hence which lesions they cause. Thus we cannot decide which oncogene(s) and tumor suppressor genes (and remember that some may remain to be identified) are activated in response to a given chemical or indeed, if this hypothesis is correct in the first place. Perhaps most importantly we cannot yet build up as complete a picture of the series of events which may lead to lung cancer, in the way that it is possible to do so for colon cancer. This is vital to our understanding of the disease and derivation of strategies for intervention. Furthermore, once in remission, lung cancer patients have a significant risk of developing a second malignancy such as acute leukemia or cancers of the lung, liver, breast, pancreas and several other organs. Conversely, patients with other malignancies, e.g., lymphoma are at increased risk from developing lung cancer. Whether this relates to the increased metastatic capability of lung cells or the increased capacity of the lung as a recipient for other cell types remains an interesting problem.

References

1. Hartley AL, Birch JM, Marsden HB et al. Malignant melanoma in families of children with osteosarcoma, chondrosarcoma and adrenocortical carcinoma. J Med Genet 1987; 24:664-668.
2. Buchhagen DL. Molecular mechanisms in lung pathogenesis. Biochimica et Biophysica Acta 1991; 1072:159-176.
3. Heighway J, Thatcher N, Cerny T et al. Genetic predisposition to human lung cancer. Br J Cancer 1986; 53:453-457
4. Paul SM, Bahrach B, Geopp C. A genetic influence on aveolar cell carcinoma. J Surgical Oncology 1987; 36:249-256.
5. Garibaldi M, Manenti G, Canzian F. A major susceptibility locus to murine lung carcinogenesis on chromosome 6. Nature Genet 1993; 3:132-136.
6. Jetten AM, Vollberg TM, Nervi C et al. Positive and negative regulation of proliferation and differentiation in tracheobronchial epithelial cells. Am Rev Respir Dis 1990; 142:S36-S39.
7. Belinsky SA, Devereux TR, Foley JF et al. Relationship between the formation of promutagenic adducts and the activation of the K-ras protooncogene in lung tumours

from A/J mice treated with nitrosamines. Cancer Research 1989; 49:5305-5311.
8. Caparaso NE, Tucker MA, Hoover RN. Lung cancer and the desbrisoquine metabolic phenotype. J Natl Cancer Inst 1990; 82:1264-1271.
9. Wolf CR, Smith CA, Gough AC et al. Relationship between the desbrinoquine hydroxlase polymorphism and cancer susceptibility. Carcinogenesis 1992; 13: 1035-1058.
10. Yokota J, Wada M, Shimsato Y et al. Loss of heterozygosity on chromosomes 3, 13 and 17 in small-cell carcinoma and on chromosome 3 in adenocarcinoma of the lung. Proc Natl Acad Sci USA 1987; 84:9252-9256.
11. Daly MC, Xiang RH, Buchhagen D et al. A homozygous deletion on chromosome 3 in a small cell lung cancer cell line correlates with a region of tumor suppressor activity. Oncogene 1993; 8:1721-1729.
12. Reissmann PT, Koga H. Inactivation of the retinoblastoma susceptibility gene in non-small-cell lung cancer. Oncogene 1993; 8: 1913-1919.
13. Takahashi T, Takahashi T, Suzuki H et al. The p53 gene is very frequently mutated in small-cell lung cancer with a distinct nucleotide substitution pattern. Oncogene 1991; 6:1775-1778.
14. Puisieux A, Lim S, Groopman J et al. Selective targeting of p53 gene mutational hotspots in human cancers by etiologically defined carcinogens. Cancer Research 1991; 51:6185-6189.
15. Oreffo V, Lin H-W, Padmanabhan R et al. K-ras and p53 point mutations in 4-(methylnitrosamino)-1-(3-pyridyl)-1-butanone-induced hamster lung tumors. Carcinogenesis 1993; 14:451-455.
16. You M, Candrian U, Maronpot RR et al. Activation of the Ki-*ras* protooncogene in spontaneously occuring and chemically induced lung tumours of the strain A mouse. Proc Natl Acad Sci USA 1989; 86: 3070-3074.
17. Kawashima K, Shikama H, Imoto K et al. Close correlation between restriction fragment length polymorphism of the L-*MYC* gene and metastasis of human lung cancer to the lymph nodes and other organs. Proc Natl Acad Sci USA 1988; 85:2353-2356.

CHAPTER 10

Infective Agents in the Cancer Process

1. INTRODUCTION

The role of the infective agent in triggering cancer has long been suspected and indeed demonstrated with the transmission of an infective agent (Rous's sarcoma virus) between chickens in 1911 and induction of rabbit skin tumors by papilloma viruses in 1932. After a period in the wilderness, the importance of infective agents to the cancer process is again beginning to be realized as evidence accumulates for their involvement in several tumor types (Table 10.1). Indeed, on a worldwide basis viral infections may be associated with up to 20% of all human cancers. Epstein Barr virus (EBV) has been associated with Burkitt's lymphoma and nasopharyngeal carcinoma and more recently Hodgkin's disease and non-Hodgkin's lymphoma. Some bladder, oral and skin cancers may have infectious causes and indeed, specific agents have been identified as being associated with cervical, hepatocellular and gastric cancers.

2. HUMAN PAPILLOMA VIRUS AND CERVICAL CANCER

Studies in the 1960s showed that women who were more sexually active had an increased risk of cervical cancer, which was attributed to infection by human papilloma virus (HPV) in the 1970s. Certain types of HPV (16, 18, 31, 33, 35) have now been detected in 90% of cervical cancers and women with cervical cancer are thirty times more likely to be infected than control women. This contrasts with an increased likelihood of infection of 2-fold for herpes virus (type II) and 3-fold for *chlamydia trachomatis*. However, this is still not compelling evidence since the epidemiology can only suggest a correlative association and more studies need to be performed in order to prove causality. The same HPV strains may be associated with vaginal, anal and vulval cancers and in particular, HPV's 16 and 18 have been found in both oral and bladder cancers.[1] The HPV E6 protein has a profound role in inhibiting transcriptional activation by the p53 gene product, though it remains to be proven if this has direct relevance to the development of cervical carcinoma.

Table 10.1. Infective agents in human cancers

	Linkage to Tumor Type
Viral	
Epstein Barr	Burkitts Lymphoma
	Nasopharyngeal carcinoma
Hepatitis B	Liver cancer
HTLV II (a human retrovirus)	T cell lymphoma
Papilloma	Carcinoma of uterine cervix
Bacterial	
Helicobacter pylori	Stomach cancer
Parasitic	
Schistosoma hematobium	Bladder cancer

3. HEPATITIS B VIRUS AND HEPATOCELLULAR CARCINOMA

In the developing countries, carcinogenesis due to infective agents such as hepatitis B virus is of great concern. Since the 1970s, there have been reports that patients with hepatocellular cancer are more likely to be hepatitis B virus (HBV) carriers than the overall population. However, in a more definitive study in Taiwan whereby 22,707 males were screened for HBV and subsequently monitored for liver cancer, HBV carriers were shown to be two hundred times more likely to contract hepatocellular carcinoma.[2] In addition, certain dietary toxins such as the fungal aflatoxin found in moldy peanuts and maize tend to enhance the effect of HBV by damaging DNA[3] and might do so in other cancers. Being viral in origin, there are good opportunities for developing anti-HBV vaccines and indeed, clinical trials are now in progress.

HBV is likely to be an early event in hepatocellular carcinogenesis (HCC) perhaps contributing to the transformation process by random integration into the genome and causing either gene activation or inactivation. HBV infected normal or cirrhotic liver reveals the HBV sequences to be randomly distributed in the genome, revealed as a smear by DNA hybridization techniques. In contrast, liver tumor material reveals discrete HBV hybridizing bands, which indicates both clonal selection processes are in operation and that the tumor is monoclonal. An additional level of complexity is observed with histopathological evidence which often reveals a 'tumor within a tumor'. Indicative of further clonal selection, the more malignant tissues show p53 mutations, whilst the surrounding 'tumor' tissues exhibit a normal p53 gene.[4] In geographical regions where HBV is a risk factor, most p53 mutations are in a single nucleotide pair (codon 299) contrasting significantly with the spectrum seen in other tumor types (chapter 2).

A further late stage in HCC is LOH on chromosome 16q 22-23, since these deletions are observed in the larger, poorly differentiated and often metastatic tumors, but not in early stage HCC.[5] In human HCCs, LOH has also been associated with chromosome 4, 11p and 13q, but whether or not these correlate with any particular stage of HCC development is as yet unknown. LOH on chromosome 16 frequently coexists with the LOH on chromosome 4.[5]

4. STOMACH CANCER

Our second example illustrates the possible role of diet and bacterial infection as cancer predisposing factors. Stomach cancers are perhaps the second most important type of cancer in terms of frequency of occurrence, although the incidence is declining. Whilst there is as yet no clear etiological agent, a great deal of research has focused upon the diet. However, from an epidemiological viewpoint, such studies are obviously difficult to control, but there are indeed protective effects due to a high intake of fresh fruit and vegetables and an increased disease risk due to excessive preserved food products and a high salt intake. In particular, the protective effects of antioxidant compounds such as beta carotene or vitamin C may be important, together with compounds found in the onion and brassica families of vegetables. In certain preserved foods, carcinogenic N-nitroso derivatives may play a role. These may arise from reduction of nitrate to nitrite which is then available for nitrosation of proteins. Clearly, this process could be prevented by antioxidants present within the diet.[6]

An additional predisposing factor to stomach cancer is "chronic atrophic gastritis," a loss of the acid secreting cells. This may be due to irritation and chronic inflammation of the stomach lining, perhaps due to a high salt intake, certain drugs such as aspirin or the action of the *helicobacter pylori* bacterium. The mechanism of transmission of this bacterium is not clear, but it appears to attach to the stomach lumen beneath the mucous layer and its uncontrolled proliferation, perhaps as a result in a change in stomach pH, may result in a chronic inflammatory response. The association between chronic infection with this bacterium and stomach cancer has yet to be definitively demonstrated, but it is a frequent pathogen of the noninvolved gastric mucosa of patients with gastric cancer and has been suggested as a causal agent.[7] Seropositivity to *helicobacter pylori* correlates with the geographical distribution of gastric cancer in China,[8] the UK[9] and the US.[10] The 3-fold increased risk resulting from *helicobacter pylori* infection is much lower than the 200x increased risk associated with HBV infection, but this may reflect the importance of other factors in the development of gastric cancer. Recent experiments have identified the Lewis blood group antigen as the receptor for *helicobacter pylori* in the human gastric mucosa. This antigen is reduced in blood group A and B individuals relative to group O and it will be interesting to see if this correlates with the occurrence of gastric adenocarcinoma in group O individuals.[11]

Unlike with lung cancer, there are several instances of familial stomach cancer inheritance, which are usually transmitted with an autosomal dominant mode of inheritance, although susceptibility genes have not yet been identified. In particular, the stomach cancer incidence appears to increase in certain inherited syndromes, for example, Lynch type II, familial adenomatous polyposis coli (FAP, chapter 7), Li-Fraumeni and ataxia telangiectasia. A number of chromosomal abnormalities have been associated with stomach cancer and mutations in the p53 tumor suppressor gene may occur in stomach cancer metastasis.

5. ACQUIRED IMMUNE DEFICIENCY SYNDROME RELATED CANCERS

The most common cancer observed in Acquired Immune Deficiency Syndrome (AIDS) patients is Kaposi's sarcoma, an extremely rare tumor of the general population. It has been suggested that this may be due to transmission of an as yet unidentified agent which opportunistically infects as a result of AIDS related immunosuppression.[12] It is also noteworthy that non-Hodgkin's lymphoma is found with a 60-fold increased frequency in AIDS patients and many of these are Epstein Barr virus (EBV) related B-cell malignancies. EBV has also recently been associated with non-Hodgkin's lymphoma in patients with immunosuppression,[13] and also in Hodgkin's disease.[14]

6. EPSTEIN BARR VIRUS AND BURKITT'S LYMPHOMA

Burkitt's lymphoma is a particularly interesting and relatively rare tumor which occurs in two forms, one of which has a direct pathogenic association with the

Epstein Barr virus. However, in all cases there is activation of the same oncogene (c-*myc*), albeit via slightly different mechanisms. In human B cells several types of chromosomal translocations have been identified and usually involve translocation of the c-*myc* locus on human chromosome 8 to any one of the immunoglobulin loci on chromosomes 2, 22 or 14. Two distinct classes of translocation associated with Burkitt's lymphoma (BL) have been identified: (a) EBV associated endemic BL, in which translocation involves the region 5' to the c-*myc* gene and (b) sporadic BL, which is not universally associated with EBV, but where translocations occur within the c-*myc* gene itself, specifically in the vicinity of exon 1.[15,16] The linkage with EBV is dependent upon geography and is almost always found in the endemic form prevalent in equatorial Africa and Papua New Guinea, where malaria is holoendemic, at a rate of 5-10 cases per 100,000 children below the age of 16.[17] The exact role of EBV in the development of BL is still unclear. It is postulated that EBV-induced B-cell proliferation results in the expansion of the number of cells in which a translocation can occur, or provide the final step in the transformation of a B cell in which a translocation has already occurred.[18] However, it has also been shown that the EBNA 1 protein, the only EBV latent protein expressed in BL, is also capable of increasing the immunoglobulin enhancer activity and would thus upregulate a c-*myc* gene coupled to such an enhancer.[19] EBV could therefore elevate the incidence of BL by providing a mechanism for the complete deregulation of the c-*myc* gene. As has been discussed previously, high levels of the c-*myc* protein can result in apoptosis. This does not occur in EBV infected cells thus suggesting that this virus has mechanisms for overriding this cellular control. Indeed it has been shown that activation of the EBV latent genes protect human B cells from death by apoptosis, and moreover, it appears that this may in part be achieved by the upregulation of *bcl*-2 by the latent membrane protein LMP1.[20,21]

References

1. Shibutani YF, Schoenberg MP, Carpiniello VL, et al. Human papillomavirus associated with bladder cancer. Urology 1992; 40:15-17.
2. Beasley RP, Hwagn l-Y, Lin C-C et al. Hepatocellular carcinoma and hepatitis B virus. A prospective study of 22,707 men in Taiwan. Lancet 1981; 2:1129-1133.
3. Ross RK, Yuan J-M, Yu MC et al. Urinary aflatoxin biomarkers and risk of hepatocellular carcinoma. Lancet 1992; 339:943-946.
4. Sugimura T. Multistep carcinogenesis: a perspective. Science 1992; 258:603-607.
5. Tsuda H, Zhang W, Shimosato Y et al. Allele loss on chromosome 16 associated with progression of human hepatocellular carcinoma. Proc Natl Acad Sci USA 1990; 87:6791-6794.
6. Ames B, Shigenaga M, Hagen T. Oxidants, antioxidants and the degenerative diseases of aging. Proc Natl Acad Sci USA 1993; 90:7915-7922.
7. Correa P, Ruiz B. Campylobacter pylori and Gastric Cancer. In: Rathbone BJ, Heatly RV, eds. Campylobacter pylori and Gastroduodenal disease. Oxford: Blackwell, 1989:139-145.
8. Forman D, Sitas F, Newell DG et al. Geographic association of Helicobacter pylori antibody prevalence and gastric cancer mortality in rural China. Int J Cancer 1990; 46:608-611.
9. Forman D, Newell DG, Fullerton F, et al. Association between infection with Helicobacter pylori and risk of gastric cancer: Evidence from a prospective investigation. Br J Med 1991; 302:1302-1305.
10. Correa P. Is gastric carcinoma an infectious disease? N Eng J Med 1991; 325:1170-1171.
11. Boren T, Falk P, Rothe K et al. Attachment of helicobacter pylori to human gastric epithelium mediated by blood group antogens. Science 1993; 262:1892-1895.
12. Beral V, Bill D, Darby S et al. Risk of Kaposi's sarcoma and sexual practices associated with faecal contact in homosexual or bi-sexual men with AIDS. Lancet 1992; 339:632-635.
13. Loxton JC, Thomas JA, Crawford DH. Aetiology and pathogenesis of non-Hodgkin

lymphona in AIDS. Cancer Surveys 1991; 10:103-119.

14. Jarrett R, Onions D. Viruses and Hodgkins disease. Leukaemia 1992; 6:14-17.
15. Pelici PG, Knowles D, Magrath IT et al. Chromosomal break points and structural alterations of the c-myc locus differ in endemic and sporadic forms of Burkitt's lymphoma. Proc Natl Acad Sci 1986; 83:2984-2988.
16. Neri A, Barriga F, Knowles DM et al. Different regions of immunoglobulin heavy cahin locus are involved in chromosomal translocations in distinct pathogeneic forms of Burkitt's lymphoma. Proc Natl Acad Sci 1988; 85:2746-2752.
18. Magrath IT. African Burkitt's lymphoma. History, biology, clinical features and treatment. Am J Ped Oncol 1991; 13:222-246.
19. Magrath IT, Jain V, Bhatia K. Epstein-Barr virus and Burkitt's Lymphoma. Sem Cancer Biol 1992; 3:285-295.
20. Gregory CD, Dive C, Henderson S et al. Activation of EBV latent genes protects human B cells from death by apoptosis. Nature 1991; 349:612-614.
21. Henderson S, Rowe M, Gregory C et al. Induction of bcl-2 expression by EBV latent membrane protein 1 protects infected B cells from programmed cell death. Cell 1991; 65:1107-1115.

CHAPTER 11

Hormonal Influences upon Cancer Development

1. INTRODUCTION

In this chapter the role played by hormonal influences in the development of breast cancer will be discussed. The etiology of several types of cancer is probably under hormonal influence,[1] particularly breast, endometrial, ovarian and prostate. In newly diagnosed cancers in the US, hormonal influences are thought to account for 40% of newly diagnosed female and 20% of newly diagnosed male cancers.[2] Thus, chemoprevention via administration of antihormone therapeutics in order to reduce the rate of cell division in the apposite epithelium has become a major focus in cancer research.

2. MOLECULAR PREDISPOSITION TO BREAST CANCER

Mortality from breast cancer has held relatively constant over the past few years although there is an apparent increase in overall risk, probably as a result of improved detection methods of both in situ tumors, i.e., those that have not invaded surrounding tissue and smaller tumors, (those less than 2 cm in diameter).

A great deal of effort has been expended in the identification of potential environmental risk factors which may be associated with breast cancer, with no clear correlate emerging. Some researchers believe that alcohol taken around the ovulation period and the late luteal phase causes an increase in estrogen levels, which may in turn provide an increased risk factor in breast cancer. However, this link must be regarded as tenuous, since alcohol could be carcinogenic by other means. Attention is now shifting back towards hormonal exposure, as the declining age of first menarche and tendency for both later childbirth (after 35 years of age) and late menopause increases the temporal span of exposure to two natural hormones, estrogen and progesterone. During the productive reproductive lifespan, women have a four weekly ovulation cycle which subjects them to cyclical exposure to estrogen and progesterone, which stops during pregnancy as both hormones reach a steady state level. A mitogenic effect of estrogen upon breast tissue may in part be involved, particularly if we consider amplification of mutations which may already be in residence in the stem cell population. You will note, however, that the latter presupposes either previous exposure to an environmental carcinogen or inheritance of a cancer predisposing lesion.

There are a number of lines of evidence supporting the case for a role for estrogen in breast cancer: (a) patients who have had ovarectomy in early life rarely succumb to breast cancer, (b) women who ovulate less frequently than average (e.g. are both young and obese) have a lower risk of breast cancer, however, in obese women, postmenopausal estrogen production from body fat may become an important risk factor. In contrast to the data obtained for colon cancer, an association between a fatty diet and increased risk of breast cancer has not been convincingly demonstrated, despite the wide acceptance of this theory in the 1980s,[3] (c) women using estrogen replacement therapies and combination oral contraceptives have a higher relative risk at contracting breast cancer, but in both cases this reduces when the treatment ceases. Indeed, oral contraceptives appear to reduce the incidence of cancer in the endometrium and ovary, (d) in contrast to the other types of tumor, the age incidence of breast, ovarian and endometrial cancer does not follow a straight line and the rate of increase slows at menopause[4] indicating involvement of premenopausal etiologies.

Several proteins have been shown to contribute to the altered growth of breast cancer cells. This includes growth factors and their receptors and the tumor and metastasis suppressor genes, p53 and nm23. Indeed 40% of sporadic breast cancers contain p54 mutations.[5] Additional prognostic indicators include those enzymes which degrade the basement membranes (e.g. collagenases and cathepsins) and those involved in angiogenesis and interactions between the epithelial and stromal layers.

3. FAMILIAL BREAST CANCER

Early epidemiological evidence showed that the risk of contracting breast cancer was increased if either a mother or sister died of breast cancer before the age of 50. Subsequent refinements indicated dominant mutations in an autosomal gene, perhaps suggesting the involvement of a tumor suppressor gene. A locus responsible for about 5% of all breast cancers, BRCA 1 has been mapped to a 2-3 x 10^6 base pair region of chromosome 17q21.[6,7] Tumors from patients who have inherited a mutant form of BRCA1 often exhibit LOH of the normal allele at 17q.[8] The rationale, of course, is that identification of the breast cancer susceptibility gene may identify a factor that plays a role in the development of sporadic, i.e., noninherited breast cancer. At the very least, it could add a valuable reagent for the early diagnosis of this disease in familial cases. It is, however, unlikely that this is the only gene involved and several others with less conspicuous but equally profound biological effects probably remain to be identified. Acquired (i.e. somatic) mutations are responsible for 95% of breast cancers, but the high frequency of this disease (10% of all women) means that the remaining 5% of breast cancers associated with inherited mutation are a highly significant proportion and indeed, breast cancer is an extremely common genetic disease.

One candidate for a breast cancer predisposing gene is the tumor suppressor gene p53 which may account for up to 10% of hereditary breast cancers. Up to 1% of women with breast cancer that are diagnosed before the age of 30 have inherited p53 mutations[9] and there is a high frequency of breast cancer in Li-Fraumeni syndrome. Mutation of p53 results in loss of cell cycle control, but may also be responsible for gene amplification by unknown mechanisms. Indeed, as we shall discuss later, this may be related to the amplification of the c-*erb*B2 gene, a prognostic marker for breast cancer. In addition to Li-Fraumeni syndrome, a number of genetic disorders have been associated with predisposition to breast cancer (Table 11.1). The multifarious nature of these syndromes probably points to the existence of more than one genetic susceptibility locus for breast cancer.

4. THE METASTATIC PROCESS IN BREAST CANCER

To date, five factors are associated with poor prognosis (i.e. possible metastasis) in breast cancer: (a and b) loss of the estrogen and progesterone receptors, (c) production of angiogenic proteins by the tumor cells (e.g. basic fibroblast growth factor and vascular-endothelial growth factor, (d) amplification of the *neu*/*erb*B2/HER2 genes and (e) decreased expression of the nm23 gene. The relative contributions of each of these remains to be elucidated.

5. LOSS OF HORMONE RECEPTORS

The absence of the estrogen and progesterone receptors is an indicator of poor prognosis, usually resulting in prescription of chemotherapy subsequent to radiotherapy. Given our previous discussion where estrogen and progesterone have a growth stimulatory effect on normal breast cells and prolonged lifetime exposure may be a risk factor, the loss of these receptors may seem beneficial. However, this loss appears to allow the cells to grow in the absence of hormones and makes them refractive to conventional therapies, which are based on receptor antagonism. This includes both the antiestrogen drug tamoxifen and antiprogesterone drug RU-486. In these cases, the receptor is mutated such that the extracellular binding domain is lost and the inner portion remains functional and continuously stimulated. Again we are left with the question as to how and why receptor mutation has occurred. Is there a mutational hot spot, a reduced ability to repair lesions in these genes or a particular class of environmental carcinogen which targets this region of DNA?

Table 11.1. Inherited breast cancer predisposing syndromes

Breast/ovarian cancer
Cowden disease
Klinefelter syndrome
Li-Fraumeni
Lynch type II
Peutz-Jegher syndrome
Rivalcabu-Myre-Smith Syndrome

6. AMPLIFICATION OF c-*erb*B2

The *erb*B2 gene (also known as the HER2 or *neu* oncogene) is probably the receptor for a growth factor. If amplified in breast cancer cells, the prognosis is poor, and indeed, in vitro studies whereby *erb*B2 is transfected into breast cancer cells cause an increase in both their growth rate and ability to form tumors in nude mice.[10] Therapies which involve humanized antibodies against the overexpressed and thus overexposed *erb*B2 protein are currently being devised.[11]

7. A METASTASIS SUPPRESSOR GENE

A gene (*nm23*-H1) which suppresses the metastatic capabilities of melanoma cells has been isolated and shown to be under expressed in breast cancers that have poor prognosis.[12] It has been subsequently demonstrated that reduced survival of breast cancer patients correlates with underproduction of the nm23-H1 protein and that restoration of nm23-H1 expression by transfection into metastatic melanoma cell lines in vitro results in a reduction of metastasis.[13] The nm23-H1 gene product appears to prevent migration of cells towards different chemoattractants.

8. BREAST CANCER IN MALES

In males, breast cancer is approximately 100-fold less common than in females, which may be associated with the lower levels of estrogen and higher levels of androgens. Risk factors for males include a family history of the disease and clinical conditions which result from androgen insufficiency. A family has been identified whereby breast cancer in two brothers was associated with a clinical and endocrinological resistance to androgens; a germ line mutation in the DNA binding domain of the X-linked androgen receptor gene was identified in these patients.[14] The androgen receptor mediates the action of both testosterone and dihydrotestosterone and germ line mutations in this gene are responsible for testicular feminization. Variation in the degree of androgenization as a result of altered receptor function may in part be due to differences in the number of $(CAG)_n$ repeat units in the first exon of the gene, which have also been associated with X-linked spinal and bulbar muscular atrophy. As has been discussed, the variation in such trinucleotide repeats may be associated with neoplasia.

9. TESTOSTERONE IN PROSTATE CANCER

Prostatic adenocarcinoma is a slow growing tumor that affects 50% of the male population over the age of 70. Although only a small number of these tumors reach a sufficient size to escape from the primary site, metastatic prostate tumors correlate with a high mortality rate. The precise complement of androgens which are associated with this disorder have yet to be defined, although as might be expected, the malignant prostate produces a large quantity of 5-α dihydrotestosterone. This compound is a much more powerful mitogen than testosterone and it is likely that it is required for growth of the tumor. Cultured cells from prostate tumors confirm this clinical observation since they show increased growth in the presence of testosterone and 5-α dihydrotestosterone, yet are inhibited by antiandrogens such as flutamide.

References

1. Henderson BE, Ross RK, Pike MC. Endogenous hormomes as a major factor in human cancer. Cancer Res 1982; 42:3232-3239.
2. Henderson BE, Ross RK, Pike M. Towards the primary prevention of cancer. Science 1991; 254:1131-1134.
3. Prentice RL, Pepe M, Self SG. Dietary fat and breast cancer: A quantitative assessment of the epidemiological literature and a disscussion of methodological issues. Cancer Res 1989; 49:3147-3156.
4. Henderson BE, Ross RK, Pike MC. Hormonal chemoprevention of cancer in women. Science 1993; 259:633-638.
5. Coles C, Candie A, Chetty U et al. p53 mutations in breast cancer. Cancer Resaerch 1992; 52:5291-5298.
6. Hall JM, Lee MK, Newman B et al. Linkage of early onset familial breast cancer to chromosome 17q21p. Science 1990; 250: 1684-1692.
7. Narod SA. Familial breast and ovarian cancer locus on chrosome 17q12-q23. Lancet 1991; 338:82-87.
8. Smith SA, Easton DF et al. Allele losses in the region 17q12-21 in familial breast and ovarian cancer involve the wild-type chromosome. Nature Genetics 1992; 2:128-131.
9. Malkin D. Germline p53 mutations in a familial syndrome of breast cancer, sarcomas and other neoplasms. Science 1990; 250:1233-1238.
10. Varley JM, Swallow JE, Brammer WJ et al. Alterations to either c-erb B-2 or c-myc proto-oncogenes in breast carcinomas correlate with poor short term prognosis. Oncogene 1987; 1:423-430.
11. DeSantes K, Slamon D, Anderson S et al. Radiolabeled antibody targeting of the HER-2/neu oncoprotein. Cancer Res 1992; 52:1916-1923.
12. Barnes R, Masood S, Barker E et al. Low nm23 protein expression in infiltrating ductal breats carcinomas correlated with reduced pateint survival. Am J Path 1992; 139:245-248.
13. Postel EH, Berberich SJ, Flint CA et al. Human c-myc transcription tractor PuF identifird as nm23-H2 nucleotide diphosphate kinase, a candidate suppressor of tumour metastasis. Science 1993; 261: 478-480.
14. Wooster R, Mangion J et al. A germline mutation in the androgen receptor gene in two brothers with breast cancer and Reifenstein syndrome. Nature Genetics 1992; 2:132-134.

SECTION 3

The Molecular Basis of Cancer Predisposition-2: The Inherited Syndromes

As should now be apparent, cancer research is beset by the problem of having tumor tissue and normal tissue, but a dearth of material which represents intermediate stages. The cancer prone inherited syndromes afford a possibility to dissect the molecular mechanisms which lead to neoplasia, and hopefully, these familial examples will reveal genes and interactions that can be applied to their sporadic counterparts. These syndromes already help delineate the plethora of molecular mechanisms that could lead to growth defects. In this chapter we will illustrate some of these pathways with specific examples of tumor suppressor gene inheritance (Li-Fraumeni syndrome), genomic imprinting (Beckwith-Wiedemann syndrome) and DNA repair deficiency syndromes.

The latter include syndromes whereby an inability to repair radiation damage may result in altered control at the G1/S checkpoint (ataxia telengiectasia) and others showing a DNA repair deficiency in DNA ligase I (Bloom's syndrome), an inability to repair DNA strand cross links (Fanconi's anemia) and an inability to repair DNA damage due to ultraviolet light (xeroderma pigmentosum and Cockayne's syndrome). We will also consider the molecular implications arising from two syndromes, van Hippel-Lindau and Bloom's, whereby patients succumb to an unusually wide range of tumor types. We will suggest that the defects manifested in these diseases represent an alteration in a fundamental and universal cellular process.

CHAPTER 12

Ataxia Telangiectasia

1. CLINICAL AND CELLULAR CHARACTERISTICS

One of the most important examples of the cancer prone phenotype lies in the autosomal recessive chromosome breakage syndrome known as ataxia telangiectasia (AT). This disease is noteworthy for the high frequency of occurrence of cancer and the extreme radiosensitivity of both patients and cell lines derived therefrom.[1] AT was first noticed as a syndrome due to the abnormal sensitivity of certain patients undergoing radiotherapy. It occurs at a frequency of about 1 in 40,000 in the general population with a heterozygote frequency which is estimated to be about 1%. The occurrence of AT as a syndrome does not reveal any ethnic bias.[2] The AT patients have a mean age of survival of 25 with the most frequent cases of death being due to neoplasia and pulmonary infections. Patients homozygous for the mutant gene (located on chromosome 11q23) develop cancer at an astonishingly high rate of 30% to 40%, and of these, 80% are cancers of the lymphoid system. Heterozygotes also show an increased frequency of cancer and in particular, up to a 15-fold increase in breast cancer in females.[3,4] Other cancers which may be increased in frequency are those of the pancreas, stomach, bladder and ovary. As such, AT may provide a model for a number of different tumor types. Also relevant to the increased cancer frequency may be the immune deficiency observed in AT, whereby there are disorders in both B-cell and T helper cell function, often together with reduced levels of IgA (to 70%) and IgE (to 80%). As a result of the T helper cell dysfunction, AT patients have reduced cell mediated immunity. They also show hyperpigmentation in sun exposed regions, often accompanied by a progressive cutaneous atrophy. Also common is a progressive cerebellar ataxia which leads to neuronal loss in the cerebellar cortex and thus mental retardation.

Cell lines derived from AT patients show abnormal sensitivity to DNA strand breakage induced in response to both direct γ-irradiation and γ-mimetic agents such as bleomycin, neocarzinostatin and calicheamycin γ^1_1. They are also sensitive to the tumor promoting agent phorbol 12-myristate 13-acetate, which activates protein kinase C. These data, together with evidence demonstrating that the G1/S checkpoint is abolished in AT cells,[5] have led to the suggestion that these AT mutation(s) lead to a deficiency in the repair of DNA damage, perhaps via altered cell cycle control.

Cytogenetically, in AT there are increases in random chromosome aberrations such as breaks, translocations and gaps in cultured cell lines, which are significantly increased by both X-irradiation and radiomimetic agents. Patient lymphocytes show increased breaks and rearrangements at the sites of the T-cell receptor and immunoglobulin genes. Clonal populations of cells may arise, which often involve chromosome 14q32 and which are generally associated with malignancy. Both fibroblasts and lymphocytes derived from AT patients show an increased number of spontaneous DNA chain breaks, in addition to a greater than expected increase in response to clastogenic agents. In fibroblasts, these breaks tend to be randomly distributed, but less so in lymphocytes, where rearrangements at the immunoglobulin and T-cell receptor loci are more common. Such breaks have been reported to be 40 times more frequent than in a normal cell.[6] The most common T-cell rearrangements in AT involve 14q32 and the IgH locus, the site of the *tcl*-1 proto-oncogene.

Thus there are a number of apparently unrelated clinical and cellular characteristics of AT, which all appear to be a consequence of a mutation in a single autosomal recessive gene. There are at least five different complementation groups of AT (A to E) all of which show the same phenotypic characteristics, suggesting that up to four related proteins could contribute to the biochemical defect in AT perhaps as part of a multienzyme complex. These groups have been defined on the basis of showing resistance to ionizing radiation induced inhibition of DNA synthesis.[7-9]

2. THE GENE WHICH CORRESPONDS TO AT GROUP A COSEGREGATES WITH THE THY-1 LOCUS

An Amish family (AT complementation group A) has been screened for restriction fragment length polymorphisms and a *Thy*-1 polymorphism on chromosome 11q 22-23 was found to cosegregate with the condition.[10] The results of several groups have now more precisely linked the gene to chromosome 11q23 and shown it to be distinct from the c-*ets*-1 oncogene, which is also in this region.

Of the four AT complementation groups, three of the relevant genes are thought to map in a similar chromosomal region with the fourth (group E), being as yet unmapped due to a dearth of patients. As yet, it cannot be ascertained that there are five different genes clustered into this chromosomal region or mutational hot spots within a smaller number of genes which are responsible for the different properties of each of the complementation groups.

3. THE DEFECTIVE BIOCHEMICAL FUNCTION IN AT

Several possibilities have been suggested for the function of the AT gene product although unfortunately none have satisfactorily explained all of the clinical and cellular characteristics of this disease. The 11p23 region contains several genes associated with the assembly of T-cell receptor and immunoglobulin genes; *Thy*-1, γ-CD3, δ-CD3, ε-CD3 and N-CAM, none of which are suitable candidates for the AT gene. This has led to the suggestion that the AT gene product(s) may be involved in the regulation of gene expression within this family.[1] The increased sensitivity to oxygen free radical associated DNA damage provides the most likely explanation for the characteristics of AT, that is, there may be a defect in a step(s) which relates to the efficiency of repair of oxygen free radical induced DNA strand breakage. The latter generates both single and double strand DNA chain interruptions. Such DNA damage is constantly occurring within the cell and repair requires the action of base specific DNA glycosylases, a DNA polymerase and a DNA ligase at the very least. There is also a requirement for the action of DNA gyrases and topoisomerases and in addition, it is known that poly ADP-ribose polymerase plays an adjunct role in the repair of DNA strand breakage. A single recombinase is responsible for the rearrangement of the T-cell receptor and immunoglobulin genes[11] and a defect in such a recombinase may also be a candidate for the AT gene.

It is likely that several other enzymatic activities will be required and that a defect in any one of these could seriously impair the cell's ability to repair DNA damage, thus leading to enhanced cytotoxicity. Let us consider then, the evidence for the AT gene being in one of these enzymes.

AT cell lines are able to repair double strand DNA chain breaks as efficiently as control cell lines and there have not been reports of deficiencies in either DNA polymerases, DNA ligase I, DNA ligase II or poly ADP-ribose polymerase. However, there is an elevation in the synthesis of poly ADP-ribose which suggests a higher endogenous level of DNA strand breakage and an enhanced rate (10-fold) of misrepair. Cell lines derived from AT patients are sensitive to killing by agents which generate oxygen free radicals, but not to those that require the use of the excision repair pathways, such as methylation and ethylation associated damage.

4. DOES THE AT GENE(S) AFFECT THE G1/S CELL CYCLE CHECKPOINT?

Cell lines derived from AT patients continue to initiate DNA replication after γ-irradiation, in contrast to heterozygous AT and normal cells,[5] thus implicating an aberration in a checkpoint at the G1/S boundary (Fig. 12.1). A similar phenomenon is associated with inactivation of p53 in that after γ-irradiation the G1/S delay is abrogated[12] and the p53 gene product can be induced by γ-irradiation in normal cells but not in AT cell lines.[13] These and other data imply that the AT gene(s) may lie upstream of p53 in a pathway that is in some way related to control of the G1/S checkpoint. However, the system increases in complexity since exit from the G1 phase of the cell cycle is not necessary for AT cell lines to exhibit an increased frequency of DNA strand breakage[14] which thus implies a role for the AT gene(s) in DNA repair, independent of the p53 gene product. Similarly, whilst γ-irradiated cells which are already in S phase and contain a mutant p53 will continue replication and complete S phase, AT cells do not and arrest both new replicon initiation and elongation of ongoing replicative DNA synthesis. This implies a role for the AT gene(s) in higher order control, whereby it is associated with repair of DNA damage both in the G1 and S phases and has a controlling influence upon the transcriptional regulator p53. Amongst other functions the AT gene(s) controls expression of the γ-irradiation inducible GADD45 gene and the genomic surveillance mechanisms at the G1/S transition. These data also imply that S phase may be regulated at positions other than at the very beginning.

5. A MOLECULAR PATHWAY FOR AT REGULATED G1/S ARREST

To reiterate, at least one of the genes which are defective in AT are required for the radiation inducible increase in the levels of the p53 gene product. The radiation dependent induction of the GADD45 gene product is dependent upon a functional p53 gene product and wild type (but not mutant) p53 binds to a conserved intron within the GADD45 gene sequence, thus implicating a direct role for p53 in control of GADD45 transcription. Cell lines from at least two AT complementation groups (A and C) are also deficient in the induction of the GADD45 transcript. However, GADD45 can also be induced by a number of p53 independent mechanisms and as yet, there is no evidence to suggest that it is directly involved in control at the G1-S checkpoint. The GADD45 and the GADD135 genes are inducible by both methylmethane sulphonate and UV light, which implicates a role for other transcriptional mechanisms.

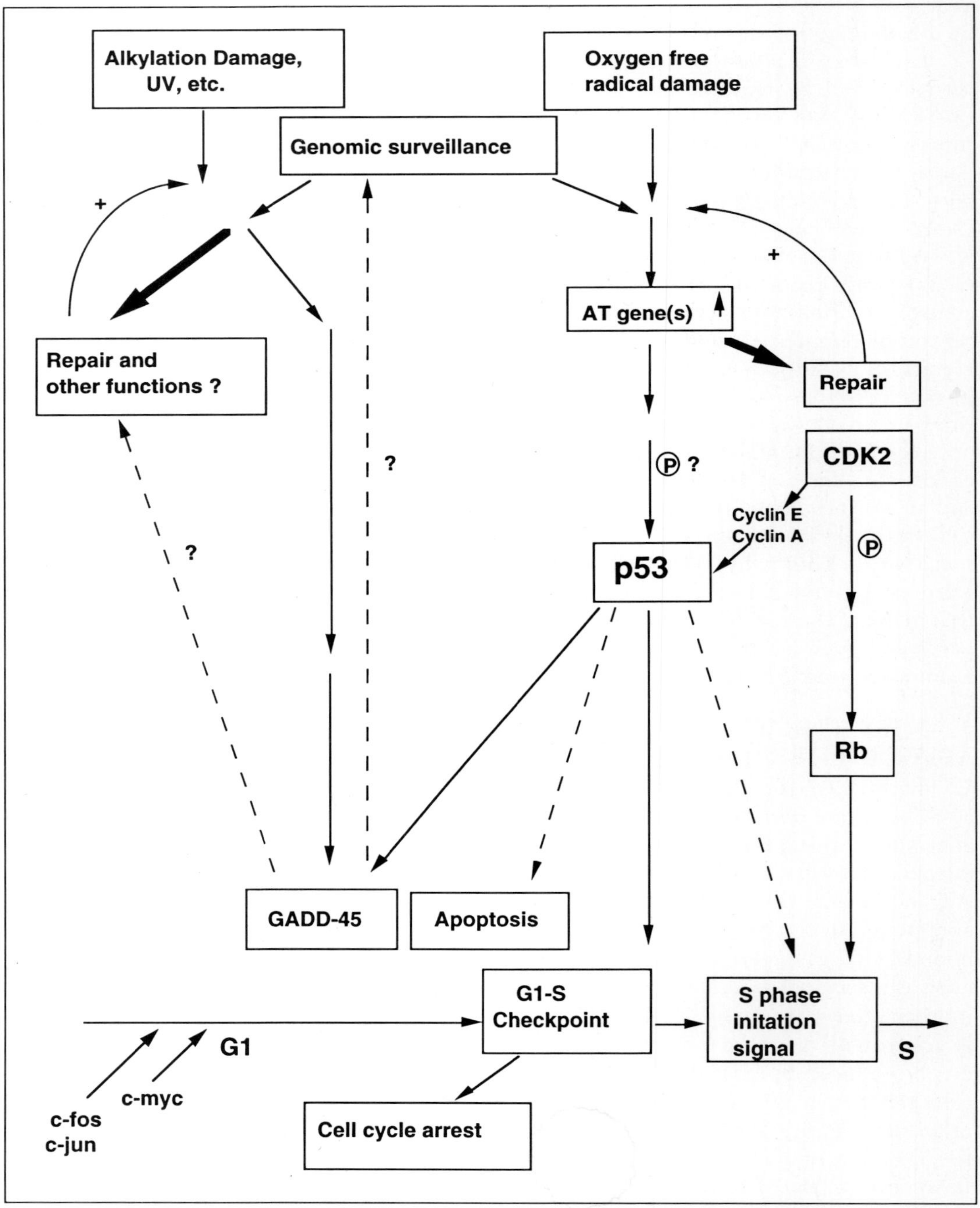

Fig. 12.1. The role of the ataxia telangiectasia gene product(s) in checkpoint control.

References

1. Peterson R, Funkhouser JD et al. Cancer susceptibility in Ataxia-Telangiectasia. Leukemia 1992; 6:8-13.
2. Swift M. Genetic aspects of ataxia telangiectasia. Immunodefiency Reviews 1990; 2:67-81.
3. Swift M, Reitnauer P, Morrell D, Chase CL. Breast and others cancers in families with ataxia telangiectasia. N Eng J Med 1987; 316:1389-1836.
4. Morrell D, Chase CL, Swift M. Cancers in 44 families with ataxia telangiectasia. Cancer Cell Cytogenetics 1990; 50:119-123.
5. Painter RB. Structural changes inchromatin as the basis for radiosensitivity in ataxia telangiectasia. Cancer Cell Cytogenetics 1982; 33:139-144.
6. Fiorilli M, Carbonari M, Crescenzi M et al. Nature 1985; 313:186-190.
7. Bates PR, Lavin MF. Comparison of gamma irradiation induced accumulation of ataxia telangiectasia and control cells in the G2 phase. Mutation Research 1989; 49: 259-263.
8. Houldsworth J, Lavin MF. Effect of ionizing radiation on DNA synthesis in ataxia telangietasia cells. Nucleic Acids Research 1980; 77:7315-7317.
9. Painter RB, Young BR. Radiosensitivity in ataxia telangiectasia: a new explanation. Proc Natl Acad Sci USA 1980; 8:7315-7317.
10. Gatti RA, Berkel I, Boder E et al. Localisation of an ataxia telangiectasia gene to chomosome 11q22-23. Nature 1988; 336:577-580.
11. Yancopoulos GD, Alt FW. Ann Rev Immunol 1986; 4:339-368.
12. Kastan MB, Onyekwere O, Sidransky D et al. Participation of p53 protein in the cellular response to DNA damage. Cancer Res 1991; 51:6304-6311.
13. Kastan MB, Zhan Q et al. A mammalian cell cycle checkpoint pathway utilizing p53 and GADD45 is defective in ataxia-telangiextasia. Cell 1992; 71:587-597.
14. Cornforth MN, Bedford JS. On the nature of a defect in cells from individuals with ataxia-telangiectasia. Science 1985; 227: 1589-1591.

CHAPTER 13

Bloom's Syndrome

1. INTRODUCTION

When considering cancer predisposing syndromes, one of the most important and informative is that of Bloom's syndrome (BS). This is largely due to the predisposition to a wide variety of tumor types in a number of different tissues, which may indicate an alteration in a fundamental molecular process. Around 20% of all BS patients develop cancer, usually before the age of 20. Leukemias and lymphomas predominate although there is a high frequency of carcinomas in a number of regions (larynx, esophagus, stomach, colon and cervix). The latter tumors may be multiple in nature and patients rarely survive to become adults. Three patients have succumbed to Wilms' tumor.

Besides cancer predisposition, there are a number of other potentially relevant clinical symptoms, notably a growth deficiency, telangiectasia, hypo- and hyperskin pigmentation and sensitivity to sunlight. Compared to certain ataxia telangiectasia patients, those with BS have a normal range of intelligence. However, it is interesting to note that BS patients often present with immune deficiency. This can lead to gastrointestinal and respiratory infections and we cannot discount the contribution of inflammatory responses to the cancer predisposing phenotype. In particular, there is often a reduction in the levels of specific immunoglobulins, notably IgA and IgM. There are also several cellular characteristics which are worthy of note, being: (a) a high frequency of sister chromatid exchange, unique to BS, (b) an abnormal profile of the intermediates of DNA replication and (c) demonstration of defects in several key cellular enzymes such as DNA ligase I, uracil DNA glycosylase, DNase I etc.

We will be examining all of these clinical and cellular points in some detail but before we do so, a critical point must be illuminated. Any suggestion for a candidate mutation for BS must include reference to *all* of these points. It is crucial to be able to explain, or at the very least rationalize, these characteristics in molecular terms, including the autosomal mode of inheritance.

2. CLINICAL CHARACTERISTICS OF BS PATIENTS

One of the first noticeable features of Bloom's syndrome (BS) is that patients with this disorder have a low birth weight and show growth retardation. Hence, the average birth weight after a normal 40 week gestation period is 1960-2620 gm for males and 1880 gm for females and the birth length is reduced to about 40-55 cm. Throughout childhood the growth rate is comparable to that of normal children; however, an increase in growth rate which normally occurs before puberty is either lacking or minimal in BS individuals, thus contributing to an average adult height of about 150 cm for males and 145 for females. The body proportions in BS patients are normal in contrast to those seen in achronoplastasia (dwarfism).

BS individuals also show dolicholcephaly (a long narrow head) and they have a marked sun sensitivity resulting in telangiectasia on the butterfly regions of the face (nose, cheekbones and tips of the ears). Immunodeficiency is another important feature of this syndrome and immunological examination has revealed decreased serum levels of the immunoglobulin classes IgG, IgM or IgA, a reduction which varies markedly from one patient to another.[1] From an assessment of two patients with an IgM deficiency it is apparent that this could result from a B-cell dysfunction, since whilst there is a reduction in the numbers of IgM secreting cells, an alteration in the percentage of IgM bearing cells was not observed.[2,3]

The most important clinical characteristic of BS syndrome is the high incidence of neoplasia. Solid tumors (the carcinomata) are the predominate type of neoplasm in BS occurring in skin, breast, large intestine, tongue, esophagus, cervix, uteri and lung. These manifest at an average age of 35 in BS patients compared to 65 years of age in the general population. Acute leukemia, lymphoma and Hodgkin's disease are also represented in BS and again the incidence of occurrence is much earlier than is normally observed, with an average age of onset of 22 in the affected which contrasts with 55 years of age in the general population. Skin cancers are also found in BS patients, but at unusual locations such as the scalp, iliac crest and at the base of the penis.[4]

3. INHERITANCE OF THE BS MUTATION

BS is an autosomal recessive disorder. Its incidence is elevated in the Ashkenazi Jewish population and studies on this sector of the Jewish population in Israel show a disease incidence of 1:57,000 (i.e. in homozygotes) which suggests the gene frequency in this population to be 1:120 (heterozygotes). Analysis of the patients' ancestors shows the gene to be concentrated in the Ukraine and neighboring eastern European regions. In the rest of the population the incidence of BS is much lower and generally only occurs where there has been consanguinous mating. Only one complementation group has been observed for BS which suggests that the defect probably arises from a single gene.

Cell lines derived from patients with BS have been studied with regard to their: (a) cytogenetics (b) sensitivity to chemical carcinogens and (c) tumorigenicity. Each has given particular insights into the biology of BS, which we will now consider.

4. THE CHARACTERISTICS OF CELL LINES DERIVED FROM BS PATIENTS

i. Cytogenetic Studies

BS is a member of the family of chromosome breakage disorders, since cell lines derived from BS patients display chromosomal instability although they have a normal chromosome complement. Hence, BS cell lines show isochromatid breaks with acrocentric fragments[4] and a high level of sister chromatid exchange (SCE). SCEs occur at apparently random homologous sites between a chromosome pair and BS cell lines contain between 45 and 62 SCEs per cell compared to controls which exhibit between 1 and 14 per cell.

The extent of SCE in BS can be reduced to by lowering the temperature to between 30 and 32°C.[5,6] Since cells grown at low temperature have a lengthened cell cycle, relatively speaking they may have a longer period of time in which to repair replication defects such as SCEs and indeed, it has been proposed that DNA replication factors may be involved in the formation of SCEs.[7] This model does not of course account for the reduced rate of DNA repair enzyme activity at the lower temperature. In addition, increasing the concentration of thymidine in the BS cell culture media also results in a reduction in SCE levels[8] suggesting that a perturbation in the thymidine pool may be relevant. It is possible to decrease SCE in BS cells by cell-cell fusion with control cell lines. Euploid somatic cell hybrids between BS and normal fibroblasts reduce the level of SCE from an average of 75 per cell to 3.5 per cell.[9] In hybrids formed between BS cell lines and those derived from acute lymphoblastic leukemia or chronic lymphocytic leukemia the elevated numbers of SCEs are still maintained.[10] Taken together, these data suggest that the high numbers of SCEs observed in BS are a consequence of a specific abnormal function,[11] but there is as yet no molecular explanation.

It is possible to isolate cells with differing numbers of SCE from BS patients, i.e., some cells with a high level of SCE and others with near normal levels of SCE.[12] It is rather difficult to explain how this could occur in cellular terms since BS is inherited as an autosomal recessive disease and one would expect that the same defect would manifest in each cell, although there is the possibility that some cells have reverted to a "normal" phenotype. Three classes of BS lymphoblastoid cell lines (BSLCL) have been isolated from BS patients; a normal karyotype and normal SCE, high SCE but normal karyotype and finally high SCE and abnormal karyotype.[13] It has been proposed that variations in SCEs may result from the transformation process of BS cells with EBV. The number of SCEs in BSLCLs can be decreased to 10% of the initial value by EBV transformation, and moreover, infection of T-cell lines with EBV causes a reduction in the number of SCE's to between 70% and 30% of the original value.[14] In addition, it appears that BS cells are abnormally sensitive to bromodeoxyuridine (BrdU) and it has been proposed that the difference in SCEs observed are in part due to differing sensitivities to this compound. For example, in an SCE assay which utilized a reduced amount of BrdU, the numbers of SCE fell from 130-140 per cell to 38-60 per cell.[15]

However, despite this confusion in the literature, it is likely that chromosomal aberrations are an important feature in BS, and indeed, chromosomal abnormalities have been shown to occur in exfoliated cells from the urinary tract and the oral cavity of BS patients. In these cells there was an elevation in the frequency of cells with micronuclei, hence demonstrating that chromosomal instability probably occurs in vivo.

Other cytogenetic studies have suggested that the chromosome breaks and subsequent crossingover events found in BS occur at nonrandom sites, e.g., a particular nonrandom banded chiasma has been observed.[16] It has been proposed that crossing over at specific sites could lead to homozygosity of transformation associated loci, or alternatively, if the crossing over were not precise, it could lead to rearrangements or amplification of such genes. Abnormalities at chromosome positions 5q31, 3p14 and 16q22 occur at a higher frequency in BS families compared to normal controls. Deletions in 5q are associated with a variety of hematological malignancies which include refractory anemia, acute myeloid anemia and nonlympholytic leukemia. Since 30% of all BS patients develop hematological malignancies, these observations may have relevance to tumorigenesis in BS.[17]

From a study of single chromosome breaks, it has been suggested that any abnormality in BS must occur exclusively in S/G2, since a much greater number of dicentric chromosomes were observed in diploid rather than tetraploid cells.[18]

ii. Mutation Rates in BS Cell Lines and Their Sensitivity to Mutagens

Cell lines derived from BS patients have a rate of mutation that is greater than that found in cells from healthy individuals. Utilizing a 6-thioguanine resistance as a marker, a mutation rate of 17 times above normal has been found in BS[19] and furthermore, herpes simplex virus I mutants have a significantly higher reversion frequency to a nontemperature dependent sensitive phenotype in BS cells when compared with control fibroblasts.[20] In addition, a glycophorin A assay has been used to estimate the frequency of mutations that accumulate in vivo in somatic cells of patients with BS.[21] This assay indirectly measures mutational or recombinational events in erythroid precursor cells since it detects the lack of an allelic form of glycophorin A in red blood cells. In this study the BS patients show a 50- to 100-fold increase in the frequency of mutational and recombinational events. These elevated mutation rates are likely to be a consequence of a biochemical defect in BS cells and could arise one of at least two ways: (a) the defect in BS could be located in a DNA repair enzyme which may indirectly increase the mutation rate via a lack of repair or (b) the defect in BS could be due to an effect upon chromosomal stability and the increase in the mutation rate could arise from unequal crossing over events etc.. The high mutation rate could accelerate the process by which cancer predisposing mutations are acquired and hence shift the spectrum of cancer causality to younger ages, whilst still maintaining the variety of tumor types that are observed.

In contrast to the other members of the family of chromosome breakage syndromes, which are generally only hypersensitive to one type of DNA damage, BS cells are sensitive to the cytotoxic effects of a wide range of different DNA damaging agents. This implies either that: (a) a number of different repair enzymes are defective in BS or (b) the defect is in a protein that is central to the repair process.

a. Sensitivity to UV irradiation

BS cell lines are abnormally sensitive to all wavelengths of UV radiation but this sensitivity is slight when compared to that observed in cell lines derived from patients with xeroderma pigmentosum. BS cell lines which have been treated with UV light (313-365 nm) show an increase in the number of DNA strand breaks when compared to control cells.[7] The BS cell survival curves of some lines were found to be biphasic.[22] A number of specific enzymes are involved in the repair of DNA damage induced by UV, yet there is no evidence for a defect in any one of these in BS. Moreover, BS cells are able to repair thymine dimers to the same extent as control cells.[23] This perhaps suggests that BS cells are more sensitive to the lethal effects brought about by nondimer damage which could include, for example, 6-4 photoproducts or DNA strand breaks caused by UV induced oxygen free radicals.

b. Sensitivity to alkylating agents

Cell lines derived from patients with BS are sensitive to the cytotoxic effects of a range of different alkylating agents and are four times more sensitive than control cells to the lethal effects of ethylnitrosourea (ENU). They are also hypersensitive to the induction of SCE by this agent[24] and it is interesting to note that if BS cells are left to recover after ENU treatment, a reduction in SCE frequency is not observed, thus contrasting with control cells. This may reflect the efficiency of the repair process in the G2-S phase when SCEs are more likely to occur. BS cell lines are more sensitive to cytotoxic effects and hyper-SCE induction by ethyl methane sulphonate (EMS).[25] However only those BS cell lines with a high frequency of SCE show EMS sensitivity and low SCE BS cell lines exhibit the same degree of sensitivity as normal cells. BS cell lines are more sensitive than control cell lines to the cytotoxic effects of dimethyl sulphate, although the number of DNA strand breaks induced by this treatment is comparable to that observed in corresponding normal lines.[26]

As all these types of damage are repaired by different enzymes, the possibility again arises that either BS is deficient in a number of different DNA repair enzymes or that a particular protein is common to all of these processes.

c. DNA crosslinking agents

Interstrand crosslinks represent an important class of chemical damage to DNA since they prevent DNA strand separation and could result in blocks to DNA replication and gene transcription. These compounds include mitomycin C, nitrogen mustard and some anticancer drugs such as cis-platin and 5-flurouracil (5FU). BS cells are more sensitive to the cytotoxic effects of mitomycin C than control cells,[27] yet the amount of unscheduled DNA synthesis is the same as for control cells, suggesting that the defect in BS must involve a repair pathway for mitomycin C induced DNA damage. BS cells lines are also hypersensitive to 5FU, resulting in an increase in DNA fragmentation. This is presumably due to an inability to repair the lesions induced by 5FU.[28]

iii. The Tumorgenicity of BS Cell Lines

BS patients are predisposed to cancer and therefore, one of the key questions to ask of cell lines derived from BS patients is whether they are already tumorigenic in nude mice or whether some other transforming change is required. It is possible to obtain tumors in nude mice and cells which are capable of growing in soft agar from BS lymphoblastoid cell lines, but this only occurs after prior exposure of these cells to the carcinogens 4-nitro quinoline oxide (4-NQO) and methyl N-nitrosoguanidine (MNNG).[29] However, this effect is only observed in the BS cell lines with a high SCE (in excess of 70 per cell) and which had been previously transformed by EBV. Subsequent studies using a different series of EBV transformed BS cell lines have not demonstrated tumorigenicity, perhaps indicating that other mutations may be required for the full transformation of these cell lines.[30] Perhaps only BS cell lines with an elevated level of SCEs are highly susceptible to the transforming action of carcinogens, and whilst BS patients are clearly predisposed to cancer, some other alterations may be necessary in order to give a malignant phenotype. This could include EBV infection for B and T cells and/or the action of other viruses or particular carcinogen action.

5. THE BIOCHEMICAL BASIS OF BS

There have been several hypotheses as to the biochemical defect in BS but which at first analysis appear to be inconsistent with one another. Since there is only one complimentation group and hence one defective gene, the expectation is that there is a primary biochemical defect in BS which may affect the activity of a wide variety of enzymes.

i. Alterations in the Detoxication of Active Oxygen Species

Addition of conditioned media from BS cell lines to control cells induces chromosomal aberrations. Hence there are probably epigenetic factors produced by BS cells into the culture media which have clastogenic activity. It has been proposed that abnormal oxygen metabolism is occurring in BS since addition of super oxide dismutase (SOD) to BS conditioned media can affect its clastogenic action.[31] BS cells exhibit elevated levels of superoxide dismutase activity which suggests that they have a high intracellular superoxide content. Treatment of control lymphoblastoid cells with compounds that increase the steady state concentration of superoxide results in elevated numbers of SCE, hence indicating that the SCE in BS cells could result from oxidative stress.[32] However, as high levels of SOD cannot reasonably explain the other cellular characteristics of BS it is unlikely that oxidative stress plays a causative role, being a consequence of some other perturbation of cellular metabolism.

ii. Possible Alterations in DNA Repair Enzymes

DNA repair enzyme defects have been reported in BS cell lines which could in part explain the cellular sensitivities and some of the clinical characteristics of the syndrome.

a. Uracil DNA glycosylase

There are various mechanisms whereby uracil can arise in DNA, for example the deamination of cytosine. This would result in the formation of a UG mispair and can eventually lead to a GC to AT transition. Uracil DNA glycosylase catalyzes the hydrolysis of the N-glycoylic bond which links uracil to the deoxyribose-phosphate backbone and thus is capable of removing the defective base. Enzymatic assays do not show differences in the activity of uracil DNA glycosylase as a function of cellular protein concentration between normal and BS cell lines, with an average of 42 units of uracil DNA glycosylase activity per mg cell lysate between the two cell types.[33] However, examination of synchronous cultures shows a number of alterations. In control cells which have been synchronized by serum depletion, a peak of uracil DNA glycosylase activity occurs after 21 hours, which is followed (after 26 hours) by a peak of DNA polymerase α activity and simultaneous DNA synthesis. In BS cell lines the increase in the DNA glycosylase activity occurs at a delayed time of 32 hours, which presumably reflects the slower growth rates of these cells, but the DNA polymerase activity and DNA synthesis *also* occurs at the same time, i.e., 32 hours. Therefore in BS, these cells are likely to be entering DNA synthesis with an increased probability of maintaining errors in the DNA. Whilst control cells show an enhanced amount of DNA glycosylase enzyme after DNA damage, in BS cells an overall increase in the amount of this enzyme is not observed.[34,35] Immunological differences have been reported in human uracil DNA glycosylase from BS. Hence, the enzyme which was obtained from control cell lines was able to react with a monoclonal antibody in enzyme linked immunosorbent assays, but the enzyme from BS cells did not show reactivity. However, denatured uracil DNA glycosylase derived from BS cells was able to react with this antibody which suggested that there may be structural differences between the control and BS enzymes.[36]

b. Hypoxanthine DNA glycosylase

Hypoxanthine is produced in DNA by the deamination of adenine and is excised by the action of hypoxanthine DNA glycosylase (chapter 5) and the inability to remove such altered bases can result in DNA mutations. Whilst BS cells contain normal amounts of hypoxanthine DNA glycosylase, it appears to be aberrantly regulated; in normal human fibroblasts which are synchronized in either the G1 or G0 phase of the cell cycle, maximal enzyme levels are reached prior to DNA synthesis yet in BS fibroblasts these two activities are coincident. Cells that have been synchronized at the G1-S checkpoint using hydroxyurea normally enter DNA synthesis after removal of the drug; this is followed by another round of DNA synthesis after 18-21 hours. In normal human fibroblasts there is a peak of hypoxanthine DNA glycosylase activity 9 hours before the second round of DNA synthesis, yet in BS fibroblasts these activities occur simultaneously.[36] Hence in BS there appear to be alterations in the coordination of the processes of DNA repair and DNA replication.

c. O^6 methylguanine DNA methyl transferase

The O^6 alkylguanine lesion is implicated in the mutagenesis; this is due to alkylating agents since it can mispair with cytosine during semiconservative DNA synthesis. The enzyme O^6 methylguanine DNA methyl transferase (O^6 MG) is able to remove this lesion from DNA by transferring it to a specific amino acid within the protein. There is considerable evidence which indicates that O^6 alkylguanine is involved in the production of tumors in experimental animals[37] and hence a deficiency in this enzyme could aid in the acquisition of cancer predisposing mutations. The regulation of O^6 MG is altered in BS cells when synchronous cell populations of both BS and control cells are compared. In the control cell lines the level of enzyme activity is increased 2.4-fold prior to the induction of DNA replication, yet in the BS cells this does not occur.[38,39]

The alterations observed in the control of uracil DNA glycosylase, hypoxanthine DNA glycosylase and O^6 MG in BS suggests a deficiency in proliferation dependent regulation of base excision repair genes. Presumably the levels of these enzymes normally increase before S phase to enable lesions which would result in the insertion of mutations in DNA to be removed. If DNA repair is stimulated concomitantly with DNA replication as appears to occur in BS, then the damaged bases might not be repaired until after replication has taken place. This may contribute towards the elevated mutation rate which is observed in BS.

iii. A Defect in DNA Replication in BS?

a. Examination of replication intermediates

When the propagation of newly forming DNA chains in individual replication units is examined in BS cells (using the technique of DNA fiber radiography) the rates are slower than in control cells. These data demonstrate that in S phase, most if not all of the replication units exhibit a reduced rate of chain growth.[40] However, when the replication behavior was examined in BS cells grown in in vitro culture at high density, no differences were observed in the rate of DNA chain growth. If grown at low density there is a lower rate of chain growth.[41] In another study, the maturation of newly synthesized DNA was also found to be delayed in BS cells when compared to normal cells, and moreover, when a bromo-deoxyurdine substituted template was used, the DNA replication in normal cells was delayed by an additional 12 hours. In BS cell lines replication is not complete even after 30 hours. However, it should be noted that BS cell lines do not exhibit a strong delay in the joining of Okazaki fragments.[26] Taken together, these data indicate that in BS there could be a defect which occurs at some stage of the DNA replication processes.

b. Enzymes that are associated DNA replication

As cells derived from BS patients appear to be less efficient than control cells in some stages of DNA replication, the activities of enzymes that are normally associated with this process will now be examined.

DNA polymerases

In mammalian cells the polymerases that are necessary for DNA synthesis during replication are DNA polymerase α and DNA polymerase δ, whilst it has been proposed that DNA polymerase β is utilized mainly in repair situations. When the amount of DNA polymerase α and β activities were determined in cell extracts derived from BS and control cells differences in their abilities to promote the incorporation of labeled nucleotides were not observed. Additionally, the enzymes isolated from both sources had equal mobilities on SDS PAGE, thus helping to preclude an effect of post translational modification.[42,43]

DNA ligases

DNA ligases are required in both DNA replication where they are responsible for joining Okazaki fragments and in DNA repair to ligate short patches formed as a result of the excision repair. DNA ligases form 3'-5' phophodiester bonds in DNA in a two step reaction which involves an enzyme AMP intermediate. To date three DNA ligases have been isolated from mammalian cells and have been termed DNA ligase I, II and III repectively.[44] DNA ligase I is the major DNA ligase in mammalian cells and is induced upon cell proliferation,[45] but it also appears to be involved in the repair of DNA damage.[46] It has been proposed that DNA ligase II plays a role in both DNA repair and DNA recombination,[47] but as yet no specific role has been proposed for the more recently discovered DNA ligase III.

Partially purified cell extracts made from cell lines derived from patients with BS have up to 70% less DNA ligase I activity than control cell lines, although there appears to be an equivalent amount of protein present.[48-50] The partially purified BS enzyme is less efficient at forming enzyme AMP intermediates.[51] Moreover, when the DNA joining ability of cells from BS patients was measured in vivo, using a shuttle vector, it was found that these cells had a 1.4- to 3-fold reduction in the ability to ligate the plasmid, again suggesting a defect in a DNA ligase.[52] However, the DNA ligase I gene cloned from normal cells was unable to rescue the BS phenotype.[53] Moreover, the BS DNA ligase I gene was able to complement *S. cervisiae* DNA ligase I mutants. The sequence of the DNA ligase I gene from BS cell lines was determined and compared to that from wild type cells; no coding mutations have been identified.[45] The levels of DNA ligase II activity were found to be equivalent to those in control cells[48] and hence other factors must be involved which could explain the reduced DNA ligase I activity in BS cells. The DNA ligase I activity in the BS was determined, before the discovery of DNA ligase III, on extracts that had been partially purified by size fractionation. It was proposed, therefore, as DNA ligase I and III are of similar molecular weights, that the alteration in ligase activity in BS could be due to a reduction in DNA ligase III activity. However, DNA ligase III activity has been measured in both control and SV40 transformed BS fibroblasts and the enzyme appears to be equally active.[54] A specific inhibitor of DNA ligase I has been discovered which copurifies with the enzyme through several chromatographic steps.[55] The over expression of such an inhibitor in cells from BS patients would be expected to cause an apparent reduction in DNA ligase I activity, although this has yet to be determined. It is also possible that DNA ligase I in BS requires some type of post translational modification for full activity. For example, this enzyme is a phosphoprotein, therefore aberrant phosphorylation of this enzyme would result in a reduction in activity. A series of precise biochemical experiments are now required to elucidate this interesting problem.

A reduction in the enzymic activity of a DNA ligase I alone is insufficient to explain the other biochemical alterations that have been found in BS. One possible explanation for the disparity/confusion as to the nature of the defect in BS has come from studies on the CHO cell lines DNA repair mutant EM9. These cells have cellular characteristics that are similar to those observed in cell lines of BS origin. Hence, they exhibit cellular sensitivities to alkylating agents and ionizing radiation and they have an elevated number of SCE per cell. However, a defect in either the activities of DNA ligase I or II has not been observed in EM9 cells.[56] The human gene that corrects the EM9 defect has been cloned and codes for XRCC 1.[57] This particular repair protein is involved in the rejoining of DNA single strand breaks that arise following the treatment of cells with either alkylating agents or ionizing radiation. When a cDNA encoding an XRCC 1 mini-gene was inserted into EM9 cells and the resulting protein product purified, it was found to copurify with DNA ligase III. This provides some evidence that these two proteins physically interact within the cell, perhaps as part of a repair complex.[58] Moreover, the XRCC 1 protein is able to stimulate DNA ligase III activity and consistent with this, the EM9 cells have a reduced activity of DNA ligase III.[59] In mammalian cells, DNA damage is probably repaired by large protein complexes which are analogous to replication complexes and indeed, a mammalian protein complex of 550-600 KDa has been identified which repairs both double strand breaks and deletions, using homologous recombination.[60]

6. A MODEL FOR THE BIOCHEMICAL DEFECT IN BS

In BS one could envisage a lack of, or reduced levels of, a protein (X) that is able to stimulate the activity of DNA ligase I. In BS there is no delay in the joining of Okasaki fragments suggesting that there is a sufficient amount of enzymic activity present to join together pieces of DNA on the lagging strand. There is a delay in the movement of replication forks and in the accumulation of higher molecular weight fragments in BS, so perhaps there is an insufficient amount of DNA ligase I activity present to carry out this reaction at high growth rates. The aberrant regulation of the DNA glycosylase activity observed in BS could also result from the lack of the stimulatory action of such a protein, which would suggest that the levels of this protein X are regulated coordinately with DNA synthesis and that it is present in both replication units and in repair units. This protein would most likely be a DNA binding protein which would either physically interact with or is of the same molecular weight as DNA ligase I, hence resulting in its copurification in the normal lymphoblastoid cells. There are a number of candidate proteins from those that have already been identified which are capable of stimulating the activity of DNA ligase I. This protein is unlikely to be XRCC 1,[61] but a candidate could be the human equivalent of bovine single stranded binding protein (SSBP) which is able to stimulate the activities of both DNA ligase I and DNA polymerases 4-fold.[58] This protein may also be required for effective polymerization and ligation of the leading strand replication complex.[59]

7. A MODEL FOR CANCER PREDISPOSITION IN BS

As mentioned above, it is possible to malignantly transform some EBV immortalized BS cell lines that have high SCE with carcinogens such that they give rise to tumors in nude mice.[29] EBV immortalized B-cell lines derived from BS patients have an elevated amount of the c-*myc* protein and it has been previously suggested that over expression of the c-*myc* gene and infection with EBV alone are sufficient for the acquisition of tumorgenicity in nude mice. However, this is clearly not the case.[30] In addition, studies performed on B cells over expressing c-*myc* protein have demonstrated that additional oncogenes are required for tumorgenicity[62,63] and several reports have also shown that c-*myc* gene and EBV immortalization will not support tumorgenicity in nude mice.[64,65] Hence, whilst over expression of the c-*myc* gene and immortalization by EBV may play a predisposing role, it is likely that other cellular changes, e.g., activation of other oncogenes are necessary for LCLs derived from BS patients to progress toward malignancy. However, in vivo and in vitro cells from these patients (perhaps due to the biochemical defects, e.g. defects in DNA repair capacity and DNA ligase activity) have elevated mutation rates, so the likelihood of additional transforming changes will be much greater.[19,20]

The next key question to ask is how could one of the biochemical defects in BS, e.g., in DNA ligase activity result in the elevation of c-*myc* protein and a predisposition to cancer. A clue to the mechanism by which this was occurring came from the observation that the elevated levels of c-*myc* protein were directly proportional to the reduced activity in DNA ligase I (Fig. 13.1).[66] The reduced ligase activity results in increased number of DNA strand breaks[52] and further work demonstrated that the level of c-*myc* protein can be increased by agents that cause breaks in DNA.[67] This suggests a novel route to tumor formation in BS. The decrease in DNA ligase I activity due to the lack of some stimulatory protein causes an increase in the levels of DNA strand breakage and thus results in an elevation in the amount of the c-*myc* protein. The high incidence of chromosome breakage and recombination events including

SCEs in BS may eventually result in tumor suppressor gene inactivation, chromosomal rearrangement and amplification of other oncogenes. The mutator phenotype in BS perhaps due to the defects in the repair ability of these cell could also result in other transforming changes. These could conceivably lead to the greatly increased frequency of cancer in BS patients by an acceleration of the process by which mutations are required (Fig. 13.1).

8. THE 46BR ENIGMA

46BR is a human fibroblast cell line derived from a young female who had clinical symptoms similar to those of BS. Hence the patient had stunted growth, cutaneous photosensitivity, elf-like features and eventually died from lymphoma at 19 years of age.[68] Cells derived from this patient are hypersensitive to a wide variety of different DNA damaging agents and in particular to methylating agents, but differ from BS cell lines as they do not have an elevated level of SCE.[69] These cells additionally also show a dramatic hypersensitivity to the cytotoxic effects of 3-amino benzamide, a potent inhibitor of poly (ADP-ribose) polymerase, which is required for the efficient ligation of DNA strand breaks in damaged chromatin. Biochemical studies revealed a reduced capacity to ligate DNA strand breaks following excision repair processes and an accumulation of Okasaki fragments during DNA replication. Missense mutations in both alleles of the DNA ligase I gene have been identified and cell lines from this patient contain a reduced amount of DNA ligase I activity.[45,71]

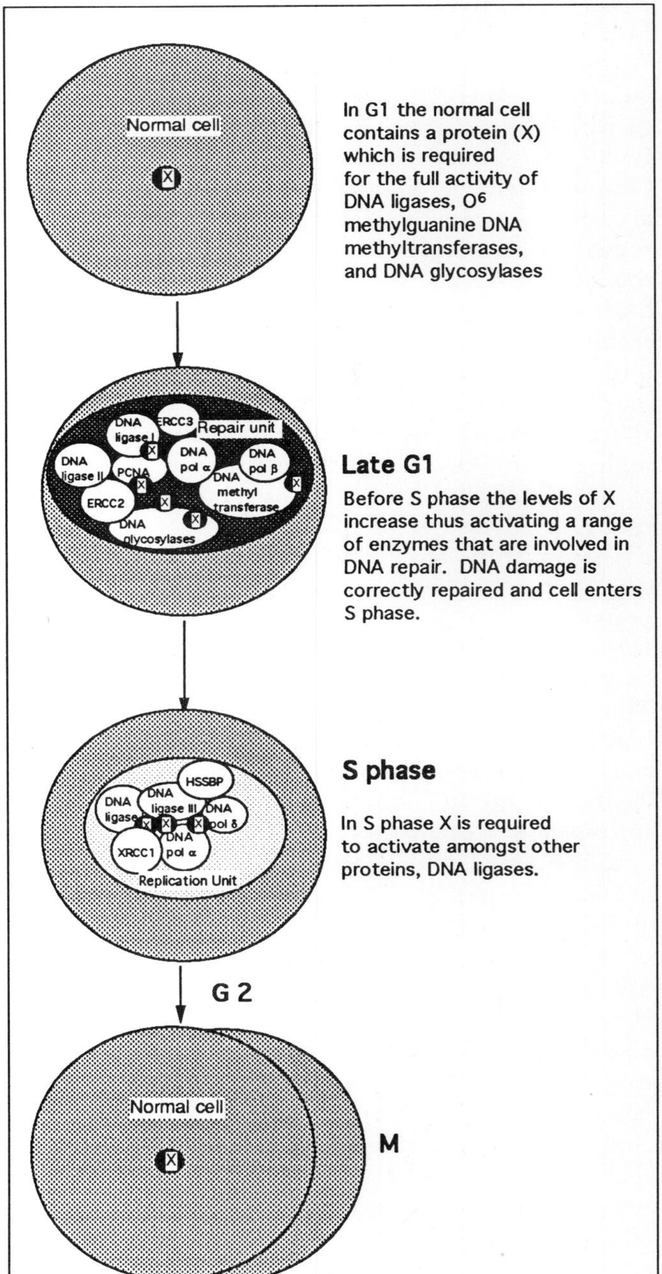

Fig. 13.1. (left half) *A model for cancer predisposition in Bloom's syndrome.*

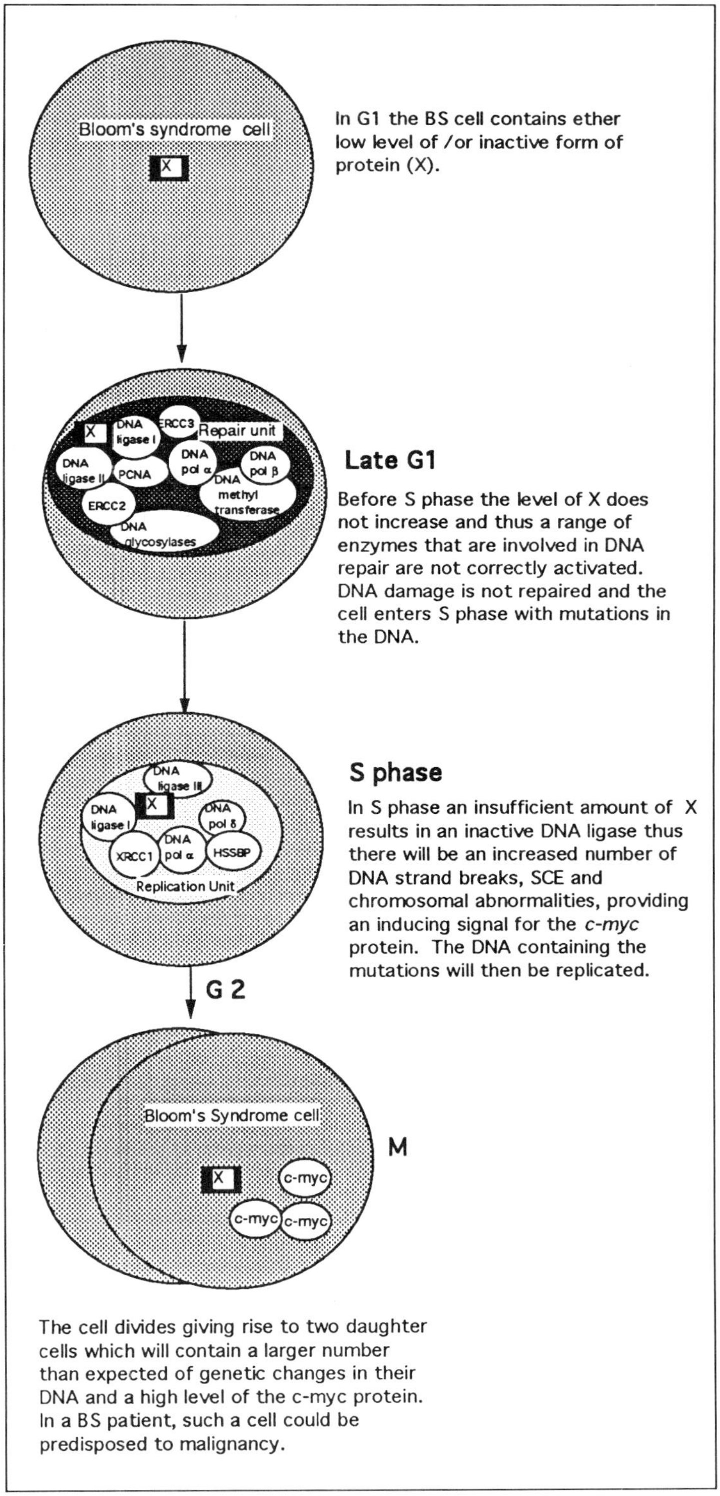

Fig. 13.1. (right half) *A model for cancer predisposition in Bloom's syndrome.*

References

1. Taniguchi N, Mukai M, Nagaoki T. Impaired B-cell differentiation and T-cell regulatory function in four patients with Bloom's Syndrome. Clin Imm and Immunopath 1982; 22:247-258.
2. Kondo N, Ozawa T, Kato Y. Reduced secreted μ mRNA synthesis in selective IgM deficiency of Bloom's Syndrome. Clin Exp Immunol 1992; 88:35-40.
3. Kondo N, Motoyoshi F, Mori S. Long term study of the immunodeficiency of Bloom's Syndrome. Acta Paediatr 1992; 81:86-90.
4. German J, Passarge E. Bloom's syndrome XII. Report from the registary for 1987. Clin Genet 1989; 35:57-69.
5. West J, Lyttleton MJ, Giannelli F. Effect of incubation temperature on the frequency of sister chromatid exchange in Bloom's Syndrome lymphocytes. Human Genet 1981; 59:204-207.
6. Shiraishi Y, Miyagi T, Miwa M. Effects of temperature on sister chromatid exchange in Bloom's Syndrome cells. Gann 1982; 73:514-516.
7. Giannelli F, Pawsey SA, Botcherby PK. Tendency to high levels of UV induced unscheduled DNA synthesis in Bloom's Syndrome. Mut Res 1981; 81:229-241.
8. Shirashi Y. Effects of cell fusion and deoxynucleosides on sister chromatid exchange in B-lymphoblastoid cell lines from 5 Bloom's Syndrome patients. Mut Res 1988; 199:75-83.
9. Bryant EM, Hoehn H, Martin GM. Normalization of sister chromatid exchange frequencies in Bloom's Syndrome by euploid cell hybridisation. Nature 1989; 279: 795-796.
10. Shiraishi Y, Koduchi H, Utsumi K. Levels of sister chromatid exchange in hybrids between BS B-cells and various cell lines with lymphoid malignancy. Mut Res 1990; 243:13-20.
11. Alhadeff B, Velivasakis I, Charry WC et al. High rates of sister chromatid exchange in Bloom's Syndrome chromosome is corrected in rodent human somatic hybrids. Cytogenet Cell Genet 1980; 27:8-23.
12. Gianelli F, Benson PF, Pawsey SA et al. uv light sensitivity and delay DNA-chain maturation in BS fibroblasts. Nature 1977; 265:466-469.
13. Shirashi Y, Kubonishi I, Sandberg A. Establishment of B-lymphoblastoid cell lines retainig cytogenetic characteristics of Bloom Syndrome. Canc Genet Cytogenet 1983; 9:129-131.
14. Shirashi Y, Yoshimoto S, Miyoshi I et al. Dimorphism of sister chromatid exchange in BS B-and T-cell lines transformed with EBV and adult T-cell leukaemia virus. Cancer Res 1983; 43:3836-3840.
15. Shirashi Y, Ohtsuki Y. Sister chromatid exchange levels in BS cells at very low concentrations of BrdU. Mut Res 1987; 176:157-164.
16. Kuhn E, Therman E, Denniston C. Mitotic chiasmata, gene density and oncogenes. Hum Genet 1985; 70:1-5.
17. Fundia AF, Gorla NB, Bounduel M et al. Increased expression of 5q31 fragile site in a BS family. Hum Genet 1992; 89:569-572.
18. Therman E, Kuhn E. Incidence and origin of symmetric and asymmetric dicentrics in Bloom's syndrome. Cancer Genet Cytogenet 1985; 13:293-301.
19. Warren S, Scultz R, Chan C et al. Elevated spontaneous mutation rate in Bloom's Syndrome fibroblasts. Proc Natl Acad Sci 1981; 78:3133-3137.
20. Bubley GJ, Schnipper LE. Effects of Bloom's Syndrome fibroblasts on genetic recombination and mutagenesis of herpes simplex virus type 1. Somatic Cell and Mol Genet 1987; 13:111-117.
21. Langlois RG, Bigbee WK, Jensen RH et al. Evidence for increased in vivo mutation and somatic recombination in Bloom's syndrome. Proc Natl Acad Sci 1989; 36: 670-674.
22. Zbinden I, Cerutti P. Near-ultra violet sensitivity of skin fibroblasts of patients with Bloom's syndrome. Biochem Biophys Res Comm 1981; 98:579-587.
23. Smith PJ, Paterson MC. Lethality and the induction and repair of DNA damage in far, mid or near UV-irradiated human fibroblasts: Comparison of effects in normal, XP and Bloom's syndrome cells. Photochem Photobiol 1982; 36:333-343.
24. Kurihara T, Inoue M, Tatsumi K. Hypersensitive of Bloom's syndrome fibroblasts

to N-ethyl-N-nitrosourea. Mut Res 1987; 184:147-151.
25. Krepinsky AB, Heddle JA, German J. Sensitivity of Bloom's syndrome lymphocytes to ethyl methansulfonate. Hum Genet 1979; 50:151-156.
26. Lehmann AR, Willis AE, Broughton BC et al. Relation between the human fibroblast strain 46BR and cell lines representitive of Bloom's syndrome. Cancer Res 1988; 48:6343-6347.
27. Ishizaki K, Yagi T, Inoue M et al. DNA reapair in Bloom's syndrome fibroblasts after UV irradiation or treatment with mitomycin C. Mut Res 1981; 80:213-219.
28. Lonn U, Lonn S, Nylen U et al. Increased levels of 5-flurouracil induced DNA lesion in Bloom's syndrome. Int J Cancer 1990; 45:494-499.
29. Shirashi Y. Bloom syndrome B-cells are hypersensitive towards carcinogen and tumour promoter-induced chromosomal alterations and growth in agar. EMBO J 1985; 4:2553-2560.
30. Sullivan NF. Nontumorigenicity in Bloom's syndrome lymphoblastoid cell lines in immunodeficient mice. Eur J Cancer 1990; 26:930-931.
31. Emerit I, Cerutti P. Clastogenic activity from Bloom's syndrome cultures. Proc Natl Aca Sc 1981; 78:1868-1871.
32. Nicotera TM, Notaro J, Notaro S et al. Elvevated supreoxide dismtuase in Bloom's syndrome: a genetic condition of oxidative stress. Cancer Res 1989; 49:5239-5243.
33. Vilpo JA, Vilpo LM. Normal uracil-DNA glycosylase activity In Bloom's syndrome cells. Mut Res 1989; 210:59-62.
34. Gupta PK, Sirover MA. Altered temporal expression of DNA repair in hypermutable Bloom's Syndrome cells. Proc Natl Acad Sci USA 1984; 81:757-761.
35. Yamamoto Y, Fujiwara Y. Abnormal regulation of uracil-DNA glycosylase induction during cell cycle and cell passage in Bloom's Syndrome fibroblasts. Carcinogenesis 1986; 7:305-310.
36. Seal G, Brech K, Karp SJ et al. Immunological lesions in human uracil DNA glycosylase: association with Bloom syndrome. Proc Natl Acad Sci USA 1988; 85: 2339-2343.
37. Dehazya P, Sirover MA. Regulation of hypoxanthine DNA glycosylase in normal human and Bloom's Syndrome fibroblasts. Cancer Res 1986; 46:3756-3761.
38. Willis AE. DNA ligases their biochemical characterisation and a defect in Bloom's Syndrome. PhD thesis University of London 1987.
39. Kim S, Vollberg TM, RoJ-Y et al. O^6-Methylguanine methyltransferase increases before S phase in normal human cells but does not increase in hypermutable Bloom's Syndrome cells. Mutation Res 1986; 173: 141-145.
40. Hand R, German J. A retarded rate of DNA chain growth in Bloom's Syndrome Proc Natl Acad Sci 1975; 72:758-762.
41. Ockey CH. Quantitative replicon analysis of DNA synthesis in cancer prone conditions and the defects in Bloom's Syndrome. J Cell Sci 1979; 40:124-144.
42. Spanos A, Holliday R, German J. Bloom's Syndrome XIII. DNA polymerase activity of cultures lymphoblastoid cells. Hum Genet 1986; 73:119-122.
43. Parker VP, Leiberman M. The levels of DNA polymerases α and β in control and repair deficient human diploid fibroblasts. Nucleic Acids Res 1977; 4:6-10.
44. Tomkinson AE, Lasko DD, Daly G et al. Mammalian DNA ligases. J Biol Chem 1990; 265:1-7.
45. Barnes DE, Tomkinson AE, Lehman AR et al. Mutations in the DNA ligase I gene of an individual with immunodeficiences and cellular hypersensitivity to DNA -damaging agents. Cell 1992; 69:495-503.
46. Soderhall S, Lindahl T. Mammalian DNA ligases sereological evidence for two separate enzymes. J Biol Chem 1975; 250: 8438-8444.
47. Tomkinson AE, Roberts E, Daly G et al. Three distinct DNA ligases in mammalian cells. J Biol Chem 1991; 266: 21728-21735.
48. Willis AE, Lindahl T. DNA ligase I deficiency in Bloom's Syndrome cells. Nature 1987; 325:357-359.
49. Willis AE, Tomlinson S, Weksberg R et al. Structural alterations of DNA ligase in Bloom syndrome. Proc Natl Acad Sci 1987;

84:8016-8020.

50. Chan JYH, Becker FF, German J. Altered DNA ligase I activity in Bloom's Syndrome cells. Nature 1987; 325:357-359.
51. Chan JYH, Becker FF. Defective DNA ligase I in Bloom's Syndrome. J Biol Chem 1988; 263:18233-18234.
52. Runger TM, Kraemer KH. Joining of linear plasmid DNA is reduced in error-prone Bloom's Syndrome cells. EMBO J 1989; 8:1419-1425.
53. Petrini JHJ, Huwiler KG, Weaver DT. A wild-type DNA ligase I gene is expressed in Bloom's Syndrome cells. Proc Natl Acad Sci 1991; 88:7615-7619.
54. Tomkinson AE, Starr R, Schultz RA. DNA ligase III is the major high molecular weight DNA joining activity in SV40 transformed human fibroblasts: Normal levels of DNA ligase III activity in Bloom's Syndrome fibroblasts. Nucleic Acids Res 1993; 21: 5425-5430.
55. Yang SW, Becker FF, Chan JYH. Indentification of a specific inhibitor of DNA ligase I in human cells. Proc Natl Acad Sci 1992; 89:2227-2231.
56. Chan JYH, Thompson LH, Becker FF. DNA ligase activites appear normal in CHO mutant EM9. Mut Res 1984; 131:209-214.
57. Thompson LH, Brookman LW, Jones NJ et al. Molecular cloning of the human XRCC 1 gene which corrects defective DNA strand break repair and sister chromatid exchange. Mol Cell Biol 1990; 10: 6160-6171.
58. Caldecott KW, McKeown CK, Tucker JD et al. An interaction between the mammalian DNA repair protein XRCC 1 and DNA ligase III. Mol Cell Biol 1994; 14:68-76.
59. Jessberger R, Podust V, Hüblsecher U et al. A mammalian protein complex that repairs double-strand breaks and deletions by recombination. J Biol Chem 1993; 268: 15070-15079.
60. Waga S, Stillman B. Anatomy of a DNA replication fork revealed by reconstitution of SV40 DNA replication in vitro. Nature 1994; 369:207-212.
61. McDaniel LD, Scultz RA. Elevated sister chromatid exchange phenotype of Bloom syndrome cells is complemented by human chromosome 15, Proc. Natl Acad Sci 1992; 89:7968-7962.
62. Alexander WS, Bernard O, Cory S et al. Lymphogenesis in Eμ-*myc* transgenic mice can involve *ras* mutations. Oncogene 1989; 4:575-581.
63. Vaux DL, Cory S, Adams JM. Bcl-2 gene promotes haemopoietic cell survival and cooperates with *c-myc* to immortalise pre-B-cells. Nature 1988; 335:440-442.
64. Hotchin NA, Allday MJ, Crawford DH. Deregulation of *c-myc* expression in EBV immortilised B-cells induces altered growth properties and surface phenotypes but not tumourigenesis. Int J Cancer 1990; 45: 566-571.
65. Wolf J, Pawlita M, Bullerdiek J. et al. Suppression of the malignant phenotype in somatic cell hybrids between Burkitts' lymphoma cells and EBV immortalised lymphoblastoid cells despite deregulated c-myc expression. Cancer Res 1990; 50: 3095-3100.
66. Sullivan NF, Willis AE, Moore JP et al. High levels of the c-myc protein in cell lines of Bloom's syndrome origin. Oncogene 1989; 4:1509-1511.
67. Sullivan NF, Willis AE. Elevation of *c-myc* by DNA strand breakage. Oncogene 1989; 4:1497-1502.
68. Webster D, Arlett CF, Harcourt SA et al. A new syndrome of immunodeficiency and increased cellular sensitivity to DNA damaging agents. In: Bridges BA, Harden D, Eds. Ataxia Telangiectasia, A cellular and Molecular link between cancer, neuropathology and immune deficiency. New York: Wiley 1982:378-386.
69. Henderson LM, Arlett CF, Harcourt SA et al. Cells from an immunodeficient patient (46 BR) are hypomutable but hypersensitive to the induction of sister chromatid exchanges. Proc Natl Acad Sci 1985; 82: 2044-2048.
70. Teo IA, Broughton BC, Day RS et al. A biochemical defect in the repair of alkylated DNA in cells fdrom an immunoedeficient patient (46BR). Carcinogenesis 1983; 5:559-564.
71. Prigent C, Satoh MS, Daly G et al. Aberrant DNA repair and DNA replication due to an inherited enzymatic defect in human DNA ligase I. Mol Cell Biol 1994; 14: 310-317.

CHAPTER 14

Fanconi's Anemia

1. INTRODUCTION

Patients with Fanconi's Anemia (FA) are predisposed to acute myelogenous leukemia (AML). The cellular defect is manifested in chromosomal instability, hypermutability for allele loss mutations and hypensitivity to peculiar forms of DNA damage, especially repair of DNA strand cross links. However, patients do not show consistent karyotypic abnormalities and either oncogene associated chromosomal translocations or consistent tumor suppressor gene LOH events have not been identified. However, a gene for one of the complementation groups has recently been cloned so a biochemical analysis of its function will provide an interesting clue to an early stage event in AML.

2. CLINICAL CHARACTERISTICS

FA is an autosomal recessive disorder with a homozygote frequency of about 1:360,000. The heterozygote (carrier) occurs at about 1:200 of the population. All affected individuals are at risk of developing leukemias, particularly AML or carcinomas and of the latter, hepatocellular carcinoma is common. Approximately 15% of patients develop either AML or preleukemia[1] and nearly all show clonal karyotype abnormalities in bone marrow specimens. This represents a 15,000 fold excess cancer incidence over children in the normal population; the average age of death is at only 15 years. FA associated leukemias showed a high frequency of chromosome 7 loss and duplications of chromosome 1q. Chromosomal abnormalities were observed in patients who ultimately died from complications which resulted from aplastic anemia. In these cases hematopiesis was shown to be clonal via cytogenetic studies and were similar to the types of changes observed in preleukemic patients. However, the marked increase in AML in FA patients suggests that this disease may present a significant opportunity to study the etiology of this tumor.

FA heterozygotes have a relative excess cancer risk of 3-fold, but this has not reached statistically significant proportions. Other disorders of the disease include various congenital abnormalities (thumb/radius, skin hyperpigmentation, kidney and urinary tract, micropthalmia, microcephaly and growth retardation). Hematologically, there is often a low platelet count.[2] Variant examples (Estren-Dameshek) show hypoplastic anemia and may be the result of different level of phenotypic expression of FA.

Indeed, diagnosis is complicated by the extreme variability in symptoms although there have been improvements in detection via induced chromosome breakage in response to DNA cross linking agents (e.g. diepoxybutane and mitomycin C). However the variety of clinical manifestations is difficult to attribute solely to a deficiency in the ability to repair DNA cross links.

3. CELLULAR CHARACTERISTICS

Hypersensitivity to the clastogenic effects of DNA cross linking agents is a unique marker for FA, which can be used to identify either preleukemia or aplastic anemia cases who do not present with the characteristic physical symptoms. The baseline expression of chromosomal instability is in some cases low and probably could not be diagnosed in the absence of treatment. Using the DNA cross linking agent diepoxybutane, treated FA cells show an increase in frequency of chromosome breakages compared to that observed for non-FA cells.[2] However, the variability in metabolic activation mechanisms, the extent of mono adduct formation (requiring simple excision repair) and the multiplicity of cellular sensitivities preclude this as a reliable test for FA carriers, since there is significant overlap between the relevant heterozygote and normal populations. At the cellular level FA cell lines are characterized by sensitivity to DNA cross linking (mitomycin C) and alkylating agents which result in chromosome damage. Subsequently, sensitivity to the cross linking agents diepoxybutane (DEB), photo activated psoralens and cis-diamine dichloroplatinum (II) (cis-DPP) has been demonstrated and becomes accepted as a key diagnostic criteria of the disease. Thus it has been suggested that FA cells may exhibit a defect in the processing of DNA cross links. However, reports have been conflicting and range from a partial to complete incision defect, to a normal efficiency of repair. Also FA-A and FA-non-A groups differ in sensitivity to DNA strand cross linking agents,[3] although these sensitivities to MMC have been corrected by transfection with normal DNA.[4] These experiments paved the way towards cloning of the FA-C gene.

4. HYPOMUTABILITY OF FA CELL LINES FOLLOWING PHOTOADDITION OF PSORALEN

In FA-B cells there is a decrease in mutation frequency at a marker locus (hypoxanthine phosphoribosyl transferase, HPRT) following photoaddition of psoralens and an increase in the deletion frequency at this locus.[5] Similarly, FA-A cells show hypomutability at two loci, HPRT and a Na^+/K^+ ATPase.[6] Photoactivated 4,5'-8 trimethylpsoralen (Me_3Pso) gives both monoadducts and cross links post-365 nm irradiation and monoadducts post-405 nm irradiation. These data contrast with normal cells where point mutations predominate and suggests that the chromosomal instability in Fanconi's anemia is more likely to be associated with the cancer predisposition than any general change in mutation frequency.

5. G2 ARREST AND OXIDATIVE STRESS IN FA

In in vitro culture FA cells often permanently arrest in G2 and show a prolongation of G2 phase. This may be an attempt to repair residual DNA damage retained after S phase due to unrepaired or partially repaired endogenous cross linking or adduct formation, prior to entering M phase. Such damage could of course trigger the chromosomal abnormalities seen in FA. The FA defect may be related to the generation of oxygen free radicals since the G2 arrest is greater if the cells are cultured in a high oxygen concentration (35% vs 5%)[7] and the degree of chromosome breakage can be reduced by reducing the oxygen concentration in which the FA cells are cultured. Antioxidants such as superoxide dismutase and catalase appear to have a protective effect upon cultured lymphocytes, although it is not clear whether FA cells are hypersensitive to oxidative damage per se. Mitomycin C (MMC) may generate cytotoxicity via the generation of free radicals and causes a disproportionate increase in 8-hydroxy deoxyguanosine (8-OH dG) in FA cells. 8-OH dG is a sensitive marker for oxidative damage and is both mutagenic and carcinogenic in vivo. However, this only occurs at very high doses of MMC and this drug is effective as a cytotoxic agent at doses which do not reveal any detectable increase in 8-OH dG. Thus additional factors must be responsible for the differential sensitivity of FA cells to MMC.[8]

6. THE COMPLEMENTATION GROUPS OF FA AND IDENTIFICATION OF THE FA(C) GENE

The phenotypic heterogeneity in FA patients is accompanied by genetic heterogeneity, as illustrated by somatic cell fusion analysis. Subsequent complementation studies using gene transfer to circumvent the hypomutability of FA cells has revealed a minimum of four complementation groups: FA-A, B, C and D.[9] The locus heterogeneity complicates strategies for gene identification which are based on positional cloning via linkage analysis. In this case, cloning via functional complementation, thus exploiting the sensitivity to cross linking agents is likely to be a viable approach. This has been used to clone the FA-C gene, designated FACC (Fanconi's anemia group C complementing) via transfection of a cDNA library into a FA-C cell line showing sensitivity to diepoxybutane and MMC.[10] The FACC gene is ubiquitously expressed in many replicating and nonreplicating tissues although extensive searches of the databases have not revealed sequence homology with any other known genes. The FACC gene which was cloned from a confirmed FA-C cell line, was shown to exhibit a single base mutation which converts a leucine to a proline in the coding sequence. Similar analyses may help unequivocally identify FA-C cell lines. A subsequent study of FA cell lines has demonstrated FACC type mutations in 24% of cases and it was noted that in two of these samples of Ashkenazi Jewish origin an identical splice site mutation was observed. Due to founder effects, several autosomal recessive disorders cluster in this ethnic group (Tay-Sachs, Gauchers, Bloom's syndrome) and indeed, upon screening 21 new families, three new patients were discovered, all of which carried the same splice site mutation.[11] The FACC gene has been localized to chromosome 9q22.3 by in situ hybridization, which contrasts with earlier provisional reports of the gene being on chromosome 2. The cloning of this gene makes a most important step towards a reliable diagnosis for FA-C and it is important to obtain genes for the other complementation groups. In particular, given that bone marrow transplantation is an option for FA treatment, the current success with ex vivo manipulation of hematopoietic stem cells for adenosine deaminase deficiency suggests that gene therapy may be an alternative option.

In conclusion then, FA shows pronounced predisposition to AML and may provide a model for this disorder. Progress is being made at identification of the genetic causes and a gene which represents one of the four complementation groups had been identified. This has no known homologues and we may only guess at its function. It may be ancillary to the repair of DNA strand cross links, but it is difficult to reconcile the variety of cellular and clinical characteristics by this fact alone. For leukemia development in FA, we may envisage clonal selection as a result of either the intrinsic cellular defect or of damage to a stem cell as a result of environmental exposure. The latter mechanisms may be more common than is generally realized, especially since in patients treated with alkylating agents as a chemotherapeutic, the subsequent frequency of AML is dramatically increased.

References

1. Auerbach. Fanconi anaemia and leukemia: tracing the genes. Leukemia 1992; 6:1-4.
2. Auerbach AD et al. International Fanconi anemia registry:relation of clinical symptoms to diepoxybutane sensitivity. Blood 1989;

73:391-396.

3. Poll EHA et al. Fanconi anaemia cells are not uniformly deficient in unhooking of DNA interstrand crosslinks, induced by mitomycin C or 9-methoxypsoralen plus UVA. Hum Genet 1984; 68:228-234.
4. Diatloff-Zito C et al. Abnormal response to DNA crosslinking agents of Fanconi anemia fibroblasts can be corrected by transfection with normal human DNA. Proc Natl Acad Sci USA 1986; 83:7034-7038.
5. Papadopoulo D et al. Mutagenic response of Fanconi's anemia cells from a defined complementation group after treatment with photoactivated bifunctional psoralens. Cancer Res 1990a; 3289-3294.
6. Papadopoulo P et al. Hypermutability in Fanconi anemia cells is assoicated with increased deletion frequency at the HPRT locus. Proc Natl Acad Sci USA 1990b; 87:8383-8387.
7. Schindler D, Hoehn H. Fanconi Anemia Mutation Causes Cellular Susceptibility to Ambient Oxygen. Am J Hum Genet 1988; 43:429-435.
8. Takeuchi T, Morimoto K. Increased formation of 8-hydoxydeoxyguanosine, an oxidative DNA damage, in lymphoblasts from Fanconi's anemia patients due to possible catalase deficiency. Carcinogenesis 1993; 14:1115-1120.
9. Strathdee CA, Duncan A, Buchwald M. Evidence for at least four Fanconi anaemia genes including FACC on chromosome 9. Nature Genetics 1992; 1:196-198.
10. Strathdee CA, Gavish H, Shannon W, Buchwald M. Cloning of cDNAs for Fanconi's anaemia by functional complementation. Nature 1992; 356:763-767.
11. Whitney AW et al. A common mutation in the FACC gene causes Fanconi anaemia in Ashkenazi Jews. Nature 1993; 4:202-205.

CHAPTER 15

Xeroderma Pigmentosum and Cockayne's Syndrome

1. XERODERMA PIGMENTOSUM: A LINK BETWEEN INEFFICIENT DNA REPAIR AND CANCER

Xeroderma pigmentosum (XP) represents one of the key cancer predisposing disorders since it not only provides a unique model for skin cancer, but also a logical molecular basis for the union of DNA repair mechanisms and cancer. The homozygote frequency in XP is 1 in 250,000 in the US and Europe,[1] yet this relatively low incidence should not belie the importance of this syndrome as a cancer model, since it is the first to clearly implicate defective DNA repair in the cancer process. The syndrome has been identified as a hereditary cancer predisposing disease since 1882 when it was first identified by Kaposi.[2] It is heterogenous in nature with 7 complementation groups and one 'variant' form. Patients usually die from multiple disseminated tumors by their 20s or 30s.[3] A related disorder, Cockayne's syndrome has many features in common with XP and these will be discussed towards the end of this chapter. Patients with XP show hypersensitivity to ultraviolet (UV) light and demonstrate a high frequency of UV induced skin cancers.[4,5] They are karyotypically normal, but cells derived from XP patients show considerable chromosomal damage after exposure to UV light. Over 50% of patients show clinical onset of XP before 1.5 years of age with freckling of sun exposed regions and a telangiectatic stage, followed by numerous varieties of benign tumors such as keratoacanthoma, keratoma and cutaneous horns. There is a 2000-fold increased frequency of malignant skin cancers at an early median age (8 years) when compared to the general population (60 years).[6] In particular, sun exposed areas show malignant melanoma and multiple malignant basal and squamous cell carcinomata. A number of other tumor types may develop in the eyes, tongue, oropharynx and mucous membranes at a 10,000-fold elevated risk. In addition, an increased frequency of internal cancers (10- to 20-fold) has been suggested to occur, which involves a wide variety of tissues such as lung, brain, breast and testicle. The latter point suggests that there may be more to the etiology of xeroderma pigmentosum related tumors than is apparent from solely repair of sunlight associated damage. Indeed, this suggests that either the mechanisms used to repair DNA damage are applicable to other types (i.e. non-UV associated) of DNA damage or, that these mechanisms are used in other fundamental cellular processes. Each of the complementation groups so far described has a variable capacity for the UV associated excision repair of DNA lesions, which in turn are associated with variations in clinical severity. There are a number of XP related conditions, being: (a) an XP variant where the neurological defects common in XP do not develop, (b) Cockayne's syndrome (CS), (c) long wave UVA sensitivity, (d) De Sanctis-Caccione syndrome, which is similar to XP complementation group D and which usually includes neurological complications and (e) trichothiodystrophy.[7] Both XP and CS show a wide range of neurological defects, which together with the diversity of other clinical syndromes, makes reconciliation with a defect in nucleotide excision repair an interesting conceptual problem. For example, why should the central nervous system be a particularly sensitive target for aberrant DNA repair? Whilst we cannot expect reconciliation of these issues in the near future, progress has been rapid and these data will now be discussed.

2. UV DAMAGE TO DNA IN XP

To briefly reiterate our previous discussions, both UV light and ionizing radiation generate different lesions in DNA, which are repaired by different DNA repair pathways. In the case of UV, the predominant pyrimidine dimer lesions are repaired by a nucleotide excision repair pathway. On the other hand, the single and double strand breaks, oxidized bases, ring saturated and fragmented lesions generated by ionizing radiation are repaired by base excision repair utilizing a variety of glycosylase enzymes.

In XP, there is a defect in incision at cyclobutane pyrimidine dimers and 6-4 pyrimidine-pyrimidones, providing a rationalization for the multiple skin cancers and skin eye lesions which result from exposure to sunlight. It is, however, a little more difficult to explain the 10- to 20-fold increase in internal cancers in XP patients and the neurological deterioration which is observed in some of the complementation groups.

We have already discussed how mutations are perpetuated in the genome, i.e., via the action of replicative polymerases on incorrectly repaired or unrepaired DNA. The p53 gene clearly plays a central role in blocking S phase progression in the presence of DNA damage. What is also becoming clear, is that the genes responsible for at least some of the XP complementation groups have much more general cellular functions, outside the processes of nucleotide excision repair. This realization has in part arisen from study of a series of repair mutants of somatic rodent cell lines, the excision repair cross complementing (ERCC) mutants of which there are now at least eleven examples. Of these ERCC 2,

Table 15.1. Complementation of XP defects by genes of heterologous species

Phenotype	Mutation Complementing Genes		
	Human	Rodent	*S. cerevisiae*
XP	XPA		RAD14
XPCS	XPB	ERCC 3	RAD25
XP	XPC		
XP, CS, TTD	XDD	ERCC 2	RAD3
XP	XPE		
XP	XPF	ERCC 4	
XP, CS	XPG	ERCC 5	RAD2
CS	CS-A		
CS	CS-B	ERCC 6	

3, 4, 5 and 6 appear to have relevance to XP and/or CS.

3. RODENT AND YEAST MUTANTS HELP IDENTIFY THE FUNCTION OF THE XP GENES

Recent progress has been made via exploitation of the genetic diversity of the yeasts *Saccharomyces cerevisiae, Schizosaccharomyces pombe*, the fruit fly *Drosophila menalongaster* and a number of in vitro derived mutant rodent cell lines which have been selected on the basis of their hypersensitivity to DNA damaging agents (Table 15.1).

The ERCC 2 gene is involved in nucleotide excision repair,[8] has high homology to the *S. cerevisiae* gene RAD3 and complements the XPD mutation.[8,9] Functionally, the RAD3 gene encodes an ATP dependent 5'-3' DNA helicase which can be inhibited by damaging the strand to which it binds. This suggests that it is involved in the detection of damage during excision repair.[10] Subsequent studies have shown the purified XP-D protein to have a single stranded DNA dependent ATPase and DNA helicase activity[11] and that this protein can complement RAD3.

Similarly, the ERCC 3 gene also has characteristics of a helicase and corrects a defect in an early step in rodent excision repair. Extraordinarily, the conjunction of the XP-B and CS disorders can be corrected by ERCC 3 and a single mutation in the human gene is responsible for the defect.[12] There is only one patient which has been identified to date as representing the XP-B phenotype. Remarkably, this female patient manifests the clinical symptoms of both XP and CS. The cells derived from this girl have virtually no excision repair as measured by UV induced unscheduled DNA synthesis, which would otherwise be unusual in CS and furthermore, show hypersensitivity to UV light. Since both XP and CS are extremely rare, then it is highly improbable that this patient has a double mutation which affects both XP and CS loci, especially since the family does not otherwise have anyone suffering from either disease.

Microinjection experiments utilizing the whole ERCC 3 gene fully correct the repair defect in XP-B and demonstrate that the effect is not due either to large scale deletions or gene rearrangements. The ERCC 3 gene must therefore participate in one of two pathways: firstly, it may be involved in two excision repair pathways predominantly associated with either disorder or secondly, that there could be a common step in the route to both disorders. The XP-B patient shows a C to A transversion in the final intron, thus creating a new splice site 4 bp upstream of that normally used. The phenotypes of some *Drosophila haywire* mutants may also give insight with the function of ERCC 3,[13] if one can give credence to 66% identity between the two proteins. *Haywire* mutations confer hypersensitivity to UV irradiation but not to methane methyl sulphonate, which is repaired via a different pathway. Furthermore, *haywire* mutants show motor defects, reduced fertility in males or females depending upon the allele and a reduced life span. Since XP and CS patients often show neurological defects and CS males show reduced fertility (undescended testes), there is a reasonable correlation between *haywire* and these genetic disorders. In particular, the progeny of females which carry a mutated allele derived from maternal sources show defects in the central nervous system.[13] This is consistent with the inability to detect transcripts without the 4 bp insertion which is characteristic of the mutation. For an as yet unexplained reason the paternal allele does not appear to be expressed.[12]

Comparison of the sequence of the ERCC 3 protein with other proteins reveals that it may have functional domains indicative of a helicase and the high mobility group 1 protein family which associate with the basic histones of chromatin.[14] The ERCC 3 gene product is identical to a subunit of the basal transcription factor BTF2 (TFII-H),[15] and is directly implicated in excision repair by antibody depletion of ERCC 3 in cell free extracts.[16] This abrogates the possibility that ERCC 3 was indirectly affecting the transcription of excision repair genes. Both ERCC 2 and ERCC 3 may fulfill similar or complementary functions, which is consistent with the consequence of phenotype: sensitivity to UV but not X-rays or DNA cross linking agents, a similar degree of UV associated mutagenesis and a defect in an early step of excision repair, probably at the preincision stage. It is possible that these two proteins work in concert to unwind DNA either side of a lesion, where one protein works in the 5' to 3' direction (ERCC 2) and the other unwinds from the 3' to 5' direction (ERCC 3). In this way the two proteins could "trap" a lesion in a single stranded region, in preparation for the incision of excision repair. Both proteins may cooperate in scanning for distortions or for local cleaving of nucleosomes which could otherwise sterically prevent access to the incision enzymes. Microinjection of a dominant negative mutant ERCC 3 protein which has lost helicase activity has shown that there is abrogation of excision repair and transcriptional activity with a concomitant collapse of chromatin.[16] Clearly then, there is a convergence of repair and transcription, at least via ERCC 3, thus raising the possibility that a component of the cancer predisposition in XP-B could be due to aberrant transcriptional effects.

The ERCC 4 protein may complex with the ERCC 1 protein to complement XP-F mutations,[17,18] but final proof must await purification of the ERCC 4 and XP-F proteins. The XP-F phenotype is apparently a milder form of XP where patients show sensitivity but are not as susceptible to cancer, as for example, XP-A patients. However, there is the possibility that the existing symptomatically mild forms of XP are the result of a 'leaky' or less profound mutation and that there is another class of XP-F mutation that leads to nonviable offspring. This hypothesis is supported by the isolation of a neurologically compromised severely affected XP-F patient.[19] This patient eventually died of bile duct cancer at the relatively late age of 50 years when compared to other XP patients. CT scanning of the brain demonstrated a severe cerebral atrophy, in addition to the mild photosensitivity which had been noted for 30 years.

A further rodent mutation, that of ERCC 5, has been shown to complement XP-G[20] as has the human homologue of the yeast RAD2 protein.[21] The ERCC 6 mutation completes the picture to date by rescuing CS-B cells[22] which represents a form of CS that is not further complicated by symptoms of XP. The biology of this gene will be discussed in the CS section which follows.

One gene homology to note is that of the protein encoded by the human XP-AC gene that complements XP-A cell lines and that of the yeast RAD14 gene. The latter functions in the excision repair pathway probably at the point of incision of the damaged DNA.[23]

Thus the ERCC and yeast mutants have firmly demonstrated that the mutations which represent the various XP complementation groups are associated with the enzymes responsible for excision repair of damaged bases. Whilst this is a significant step forward, it is important to consider exactly why a deficiency in a DNA repair enzyme could be a cancer predisposing factor. Simplistically, one might assume that DNA damage potentiated by UV light in sun exposed regions of the body and due to UV mimetic agents/bulky adduct formation in nonexposed regions, is ultimately responsible for mutagenesis. Failure to repair damaged bases may lead to errors of transcription during replication. The mutagenic effects are likely to be due to the incorrect repair of 6-4 pyrimidine-pyrimidones, rather than cyclobutane pyrimidine dimers, which result in a block DNA replication but not mutagenesis.

4. NEUROLOGICAL DETERIORATION IN XP

What then, is the basis for internal cancers and neurological defects in XP patients, where UV exposure is not a factor? This problem has in part been addressed with a unique biochemical assay, which involves sequential removal of characterized lesions from irradiated plasmids and examination of ATP dependent repair synthesis.[24] By use of pyrimidine hydrate DNA glycosylase (Nth protein) and formamido pyrimidine DNA glycosylase (Fpg protein) these authors were able to remove purines with an oxidized or fragmented imidazole ring or pyrimidines without a 5-6 double bond, leaving closed circular DNA containing another as yet unidentified lesion(s). The latter was repaired by normal, but not XP cell extracts prepared from complementation groups A, B, C, D and G. The evidence is consistent with a rate limiting excision repair pathway. Furthermore, mixing the cell extracts derived from XP-A, B and C restored a significant fraction of repair activity, indicating complementation and thus augmenting the argument for a nucleotide excision repair pathway. The nature of the lesion which cannot be removed by the XP extracts is unclear, although a number of possibilities have been eliminated.[24] The key point, however, is that there is probably an oxygen free radical induced lesion which requires the same nucleotide excision repair system as used for UV induced pyrimidine dimers and cannot be removed in XP. These data could explain the increase in internal cancers in XP. The neurological abnormalities seen in both XP and Cockayne's syndrome might conceivably result from the accumulation of these lesions over the lifetime of the individual although how this may subsequently affect cellular behavior is at present unclear.

5. XP VARIANTS

There is an additional class of XP patients, whereby in contrast to the classical XP, UV induced photoproducts are excised at a near normal rate. However, these patients show the same clinical characteristics of classical XP and have the same predisposition to skin cancer. Fibroblasts from XP variant cells are only slightly more sensitive to the cytotoxic effects of UV but are significantly more susceptible to its mutagenic action. Clearly, this hypermutability in response to UV irradiation may contribute to skin cancer predisposition in XP variant patients, although as with XP, the mechanisms are still unclear. Unlike with XP, this mutability cannot be attributed to a defect in excision repair mechanisms since irradiation of synchronized variant cells at different time periods prior to S phase shows a decrease in mutation frequency in proportion to the increase in the length of time which is available for repair. However, there is no difference between non-XP cells and XP variant cells in the rate of excision of cyclobutane pyrimidine dimers and 6-4 pyrimidine-pyrimidones, but the two differed significantly in the spectrum of mutations that are induced.[25,26] In particular, this may be associated with the reduced probability of XP variants to incorporate dAMP and dGMP opposite photoproducts during replication, when compared to normal cells. The most likely mechanism for the increased mutation frequency in XP variants is that of a defective (error prone) replication complex, whereby unexcised lesions are bypassed and are less likely to incorporate the correct nucleotide opposite the lesion during S phase.

6. CLONING OF THE XP-A AND XP-C GENES AND ISOLATION OF THEIR PROTEINS

The XP complementation group A includes cases with many degrees of clinical severity manifesting both with and without neurological symptoms. However complementation group C is the most commonly described form of the disease and most patients in this class do not express neurological abnormality. The XP-A gene has been cloned and shown to confer resistance to ultraviolet light in cells derived from XP-A but not other complementation groups.[27,28] In particular, the gene reveals a zinc finger motif which indicates that it may encode a protein which has a DNA binding activity.[28,29] In the latter study, a missense mutation and two deletions in the zinc finger consensus region disrupt the putative zinc finger domain of the XP-A protein. The identity of a protein involved in

XP-A was first suggested by microinjection of partially purified cell fractions into XP-A cells, resulting in the restoration of unscheduled DNA synthesis in the defective cells. Subsequently, the XP-A protein has been purified[30-32] and shown to preferentially bind to damaged DNA.[33]

Similarly, the XP-C gene has been cloned via a selective procedure which involves restoration of unscheduled DNA synthesis and ultraviolet radiation resistance to XP-C cells to normal levels,[34,35] a study which revealed significant homology to the yeast RAD4 gene.[34] Subsequent studies have shown that XP-C complementing activity probably resides in a complex of two proteins, each with homology to yeast RAD4 and RAD23 respectively.[36]

Progress towards the cloning of the XP-E gene is being made with the identification of a lack of a DNA damage binding protein (DDB) in two consanguinous XP-E patients.[37] This protein recognizes UV irradiated DNA and has been purified[37,38] but its role in nucleotide excision repair, if indeed it has any, has not yet been elucidated. However, only some XP-E patients show a reduction in DDB activity and in a similar study indeed, twelve cell lines from ten XP-E families did not show this defect: microinjection of purified DDB protein into XP-E cells lacking this protein specifically corrected the defect by restoration of repair synthesis but had no effect on XP-E cells which did not lack the protein or cell lines derived from other XP complementation groups.[39] Thus DDB participates in excision repair but its precise role has yet to be ascertained. These data suggest the possibility of two subclasses of XP-E complementation, only one of which is due to a defect in DDB.

7. REMOVAL OF UV INDUCED LESIONS FROM THE TRANSCRIBED DNA STRAND

As mentioned, the cell preferentially repairs lesions on the transcribed strand, thus reducing the probability of fixing a mutation in the genome.[40] In XP-C, there is a difference in the proficiency of DNA repair in particular parts of the genome whereby some parts of the genome are repaired efficiently and others not at all. Indeed, transcriptionally active β actin and dihydrofolate reductase genes are between 2- and 5-fold enriched in efficiently repaired regions in XP-C cell lines.[41] In contrast to normal cells, those derived from XP-C show a different ability to repair particular gene fragments; normal cells may completely remove cyclobutane pyrimidine dimers from two target genes within 24 hours at 10 J/m^2,[42] whereas only a portion of one target gene was repaired with the same efficiency in XP-C cells. Indeed, using DNA strand specific probes it has been shown that in the target genes the transcribed strand was repaired faster than the nontranscribed strand, but that in XP-C, repair predominantly involved the transcribed strand with the untranscribed strand being largely unaffected.[43] The situation is further complicated if we consider XP-variant cells, where the mutagenized pyrimidines were evenly distributed between both transcribed and nontranscribed strands in contrast to that in normal cells where the bias is 2:1 in favor of the transcribed strand. This could reflect a disjunction between strand specific repair processes in the XP-variant cell lines even though the overall rate of repair activity does not differ from that observed in normal cell lines.

The transcribed strand of the p53 gene is repaired faster than other genes and more efficiently than on the transcribed strand[44] and as such, one expects the majority of XP-C mutations to occur on the nontranscribed strand of the p53 gene. The inefficient repair of damaged DNA in XP results in an increased mutation frequency. Accordingly, there is a two-fold increased mutation rate in the N-*ras* oncogene[45] and a positive association with mutation of the p53 gene.[46] Probably as a consequence of gene mutation and progress towards transformation, XP lymphocytes have altered production of interferon and impaired activation of natural killer cells when compared to normal cells.[47]

8. COCKAYNE'S SYNDROME

Cockayne's Syndrome (CS) is an autosomal recessive disorder which is also often classified as a chromosome breakage syndrome. It has similarity to XP, in that there appears to be a deficiency in DNA repair after exposure to UV light. Patients exhibit photosensitivity, but unlike in XP also exhibit neurological deterioration and mental retardation. CS is not associated with an increased frequency of malignancy, although for its similarity to XP, is worthy of mention. There are at least three complementation groups (A,B,C) and of these CS-C is identical to XP-B. Other CS patients have also fallen into the XP-D and XP-G complementation groups, perhaps suggesting that more categories may exist. For both XP and CS cell lines UV damage reveals a reduced ability to recover from these lesions, although whilst XP cells show a reduced level of unscheduled DNA synthesis, CS cells do not. CS cells have a defect in the repair of the transcribed strand of active genes, whereas general repair synthesis processes appear to be normal. Thus CS may be a deficiency in an enzyme involved at identifying or directing repair enzymes to lesions on actively transcribed DNA strands. This would explain its involvement in a small subset of XP complementation groups, but not why patients suffer neurological deterioration and are not cancer prone.

Two other syndromes related to XP have been identified:

a. De Sanctis-Caccione syndrome occurs in about 18% of XP patients and is characterized by excessive neurological degeneration. It is most common in XP-D, but can occur in any XP complementation group.
b. UVA-sensitivity syndrome in which there is an autosomal dominant predisposition to various malignancies. In cell lines from these patients, exposure to long wave UVA results in an increased frequency of single strand DNA chain breaks.

CS fibroblasts repair DNA lesions at normal rates but cannot recover RNA synthesis after UV irradiation. This has recently been explained by the demonstration that CS fibroblasts have lost the ability to preferentially repair actively transcribed genes but are still competent at overall genome repair. For CS-B, the most common form of the disease, it has been demonstrated that the ERCC 6 gene is capable of correcting the defect and that this gene has sequence similarity with known helicases.[22] Similarly, ERCC 3 complements the CS-C (XP-B) mutation.[12] ERCC 3 has recently been identified as homologous to the transcription factor TFIIH.[15] The clinical phenotypes displayed by XP-B and CS patients are diverse and difficult to rationalize by a deficiency in DNA repair. To some extent these phenotypes may reflect differences in transcriptional activity with different ERCC 3 mutations being responsible for the variable degrees of severity.

References

1. Andrews A. Xeroderma pigmentosum in chromosome mutation and neoplasia. German JG, ed. New York: Liss AR 1983: 63-83.
2. Kaposi M. Xeroderma pigmentosum. Wiener mediz Jahrbücher (Oct) 1882; 619-632.
3. Kraemer K, Lee M, Scotto J. Xeroderma pigmentosum. Arch Dermatol 1987; 123:241-250.
4. Robbins JH, Kraemer KH, Lutzner MA et al. Xeroderma pigmentosum: an inherited disease with sun sensitivity, multiple cutaneous neoplasms and abnormal DNA repair. Ann Int Med 1974; 80:221-248.
5. Cohen MM, Levy HP. Chromosome instability syndromes. In: Advances in Human Genetics 1989; 18: chapter 2, 43-150.
6. Hodgson, Maher. A practical guide to human cancer genetics. Cambridge University Press 1993; part 3:163-166.
7. Stefanini M,Vermeulen W, Weeda G et al. A new nucleotide excision repair gene associated with the disorder trichothiodystrophy. Am J Hum Genetics 1993; 53:817-821.

8. Weber CA, Salazar EP, Stewart SA et al. *ERCC2:* cDNA cloning and molecular characterization of a human nucleotide excision repair gene with high homology to yeast *RAD3*. EMBO J 1990; 9:1437-1447.
9. Flejter W, McDaniel L, Johns D et al. Correction of xeroderma pigmentosum complementation group D mutant cell phenotypes by chromosome and gene transfer: Involvement of the human ERCC2 DNA repair gene. Proc Natl Acad Sci USA 1992; 89:261-265.
10. Naegeli H, Bardwell L, Friedberg EC. The DNA helicase an ATPase activities of yeast rad3 protein are inhibited by DNA damage. J Biol Chem 1992; 267:392-398.
11. Sung P, Baily V, Weber C et al. Human xeroderma pigmentosum group D gene encodes a DNA helicase. Nature 1993; 365: 852-855.
12. Weeda G, van Ham RCA, Vermeulen W. A Presumed DNA helicase encoded by ERCC-3 is involved in the human repair disorders Xeroderma pigmentosum and Cockayne's syndrome. Cell 1990; 62: 777-791.
13. Mounkes LC, Jones RS, Liang B-C. A Drosophila model for Xeroderma pigmentosum and Cockayne's syndrome: *haywire* encodes the fly homolog of *ERCC3*, a human excision repair gene. Cell 1992; 71:925-937.
14. Hughes E, Engelsberg BN, Billings PC. Purification of nuclear proteins that bind to cisplatin damaged DNA. J Biol Chem 1992; 267: 13520-13527.
15. Schaeffer L, Roy R, Humbert S et al. DNA repair helicase: A component of BTF2 (TFIIH) basic transcription factor. Science 1993; 260:58-63.
16. van Vuuren AJ, Vermeulen W, Ma L et al. Correction of xeroderma pigmentosum repair defect by basal transcription factor BTF2 (TFIIH). EMBO J 1994; 13: 1645-1653.
17. Biggerstaff M, Szymkowski DE, Wood RD. Co-correction of the ERCC1, ERCC4 and xeroderma pigmentosum group F DNA repair defects in vitro. EMBO J 1993; 12:3685-3692.
18. van Vuuren AJ, Appeldoorn E, Odijk H et al. Evidence for a repair enzyme complex involving ERCC1 and complementing activities of ERCC4, ERCC11 and xeroderma pigmentosum group F. EMBO J 1993; 12: 3693-3701.
19. Moriwaki S, Nishigori C, Imamura S. A case of xeroderma pigmentosum complementation group F with neurological abnormalities. Br J Dermat 1993; 128:91-94.
20. O'Donovan A, Wood RD. Identical defects in DNA repair in xeroderma pigmentosum group G and rodent ERCC group 5. Nature 1993; 363:185-188.
21. Scherly D, Nouspikel T, Corlet J et al. Complementation of the DNA repair defect in xeroderma pigmentosum group G cells by a human cDNA related to yeast RAD2. Nature 1993; 363:182-184.
22. Trolestra C, van Gool A, de Wit J et al. *ERCC6,* a member of a subfamily of putative helicases, is involved in Cockanye's syndrome and preferential repair of active genes. Cell 1992; 71:939-953.
23. Bankmann M, Prakash L, Prakash S. Yeast *RAD14* and human xeroderma pigmentosum group A DNA-repair genes encode homologous proteins. Nature 1992; Vol. 355:555-558.
24. Satoh MS, Jones CJ, Wood RD et al. DNA excision-repair defect of xeroderma pigmentosum prevents removal of a class of oxygen free radical-induced base lesions. Proc Natl Acad Sci USA 1993; 90:6335-6339.
25. Wang Y-C, Maher VM, McCormick JJ. Xeroderma pigmentosum variant cells are less likely than normal cells to incorporate dAMP opposite photoproducts during replication of UV-irradiated plasmids. Proc Natl Acad Sci USA 1991; 88:7810-7814.
26. Wang Y-C, Maher VM, Mitchell DL et al. Evidence from mutation spectra that the UV hypermutability of Xeroderma pigmentosum variant cells reflects abnormal, error-prone replication on a template. Molec Cell Biol 1993; 13:4276-4293.
27. Tanaka K, Satokata I, Ogita Z. Molecular cloning of a mouse DNA repair gene that complements the defect of group-A xeroderma pigmentosum. Proc Natl Acad Sci USA 1989; 86:5512-5516.
28. Tanaka K, Miura N, Satokata I et al. Analysis of a human DNA excision repair gene

involved in group A xeroderma pigmentosum and containing a zinc-finger domain. Nature 1990; 348:73-76.

29. Satokata H, Tanaka K, Okada Y. Molecular basis of group A xeroderma pigmentosum: missense mutation and two deletions located in a zinc finger consensus sequence of the XPAC gene. Human Genet 1992; 88: 603-607.
30. Sugano T, Uchida T, Yamaizumi M. Identification of a specific protein factor defective in group A xeroderma pigmentosum cells. J Biochem 1991; 110:667-674.
31. Robins P, Jones CJ, Biggerstaff M. Complementation of DNA repair in xeroderma pigmentosum group A cell extracts by a protein with affinity for damaged DNA. EMBO J 1991; 10:3913-3921.
32. Miura N, Miyamoto I, Asahina H et al. Identification and characterization of xpac protein, the gene product of the human XPAC (xeroderma pigmentosum group A complementing gene). J Biol Chem 1991; 266:19786-19789.
33. Jones C, Wood R. Preferential binding of the xeroderma pigmentosum group A complementing protein to damaged DNA. Biochemostry 1993; 32:12096-12104.
34. Legerski R, Peterson C. Expression cloning of a human DNA repair gene involved in xeroderma pigmentosum group C. Nature 1992; 359:70-73.
35. vanOostrom C, deVries A, Verbeek S et al. Cloning and characterisation of the mouse XPAC gene. Nucleic Acids Research 1994; 22:132-136.
36. Masutani C, Sugasawa K, Yanagisawa J et al. Purification and cloning of a nucleotide excision repair complex involving the xeroderma pigmentosum group C protein and a human homologue of yeast RAD23. EMBO J 1994; 13:1831-1843.
37. Hwang BJ, Chu G. Purification and characterization of a human protein that binds to damaged DNA. Biochemistry 1993; 32:1657-1666.
38. Keeney S, Chang G, Linn S. Characterisation of a human DNA damage binding protein implicated in xeroderma pigmentosum group E. J Biol Chem 1993; 268: 21293-21300.
39. Keeney S, Eker APM, Brody T et al. Correction of the DNA repair defect in xeroderma pigmentosum group E by injection of a DNA damage-binding protein. Proc Natl Acad Sci USA 1994; 91:4053-4056.
40. Dumaz N, Drougard C, Sarasin A, Daya-Grosjean L. Specific UV induced mutation spectrum in the p53 gene of skin tumours from DNA repair deficient xeroderma pigmentosum patients. Proc Natl Acad Sci USA 1993; 90:10529-10533.
41. Kantor GJ, Barsalou LS, Hanawalt PC. Selective repair of specific chromatin domains in UV-irradiated cells from xeroderma pigmentosum complementation group C. Mutat Res 1990; 243:171-180.
42. Venema J, van Hoffen A, Karcagi V et al. Xeroderma pigmentosum complementation group C cells remove pyrimidine dimers selectively from the transcribed strand of active genes. Molec Cell Biol 1991; 11:4128-4134.
43. Venema J, van Hoffen A, Natarajan T, et al. The residual repair capacity of xeroderma pigmentosum complementation group C fibroblasts is highly specific for transcriptionally active DNA. Mol Cell Biol 1989; 9:1277-1283
44. Evans MK, Taffe B, Harris C, Bohr V. DNA strand bias in the repair of the p53 gene in normal human and xeroderma pigmentosum group C fibroblasts. Cancer Research 1993; 53:5377-5381.
45. Daya-Grosjean L, Robert C, Drougard C et al. High mutation frequency in ras genes of skin tumours isolated from DNA repair deficient xeroderma pigmentosum patients. Cancer Research 1993; 53:1625-1629.
46. Sato M, Nishigori C, Zghal M et al. Ultraviolet specific mutations in p53 gene in skin tumours in xeroderma pigmentosum patients. Cancer Research 1993; 53: 2944-2946.
47. Gaspari A, Fleisher T, Kraemer K. Impaired interferon production and natural killer cell activation in patients with the skin cancer prone disorder, xeroderma pigmentosum. J Clin Invest 1993; 92:1135-1142.

CHAPTER 16

Nonchromosome Breakage Cancer Predisposing Syndromes

1. LI-FRAUMENI SYNDROME: INHERITANCE OF A TUMOR SUPPRESSOR GENE MUTATION

This dominantly acting syndrome confers susceptibility to a wide range of tumors[1,2] (Table 16.1) at an early age. There are often multiple primary tumors together with a high incidence of recurrence after radiotherapy, which perhaps suggests a susceptibility to X irradiation akin to that observed for ataxia telangiectasia. This apparently contrasts with a study showing Li-Fraumeni fibroblasts to be radioresistant in vitro.[3] The latter phenotype was paralleled by an increase in the expression of both c-*myc* and c-*raf*-1 in these cell lines. Similarly, γ irradiated fibroblasts derived from Li-Fraumeni patients and at-risk family members show resistance to cell killing when compared to either spouses or other controls.[4] Epidemiological studies have proved important in measuring the significance of Li-Fraumeni syndrome, where in a study of several members of nine kindreds there was a small but significant excess cancer risk in first degree relatives, which was consistent with an incompletely penetrant autosomal dominant gene.[5] In a second study, siblings were shown to be at a high risk of glioma, rhabdomyosarcoma and soft tissue sarcoma at a very early age.[6] Indeed, the cancer frequency in Li-Fraumeni syndrome is almost 50% in at risk patients by the age of 30, when the comparable figure in the general population is only 1%. These studies consolidated the initial retrospective 1969 epidemiological review of 600 patients by Li and Fraumeni, but the gene which was responsible was not revealed until 1990 when germ line abnormalities in the p53 tumor suppressor gene was identified as a candidate for the familial patterns of inheritance.[7] This hypothesis derived from similarities in the spectrum of cancer predisposition associated with: (a) sporadic inactivating mutations in the p53 gene (soft tissue sarcomas, brain tumors, leukemias, lung and breast carcinoma and osteosarcoma), (b) transgenic mice carrying a mutant p53 gene (soft tissue sarcomas, lung adenocarcinoma,

Table 16.1. Tumors found in Li-Fraumeni syndrome

Tumor type	Frequency in Li Fraumeni syndrome
Breast	50% (~80% diagnosed before 49 years)
Soft tissue sarcoma	29%
Brain	13%
Leukemia	8%
Pancreatic carcinomata	Elevated frequency
Lung carcinomata	" "
Laryngial carcinomata	" "
Malignant melanoma	" "

osteosarcoma, adrenal and lymphoid tumors) and (c) Li-Fraumeni syndrome itself (Table 16.1). However, the classic approaches of gene identification used for other familial syndromes such as retinoblastoma have not been possible for Li-Fraumeni syndrome for practical reasons, which includes: (a) the high mortality of affected individuals, (b) ambiguity in diagnosis of the syndrome, hence (c) a rarity of applicable tissue specimens and finally (d) the broad spectrum of tumor types means it is often difficult to distinguish cancers in those with and without the syndrome. In addition, Li-Fraumeni patients do not appear to have a readily identifiable precancerous condition to aid identification (aniridia was helpful in assignment of the Wilms' tumor locus) and it was not possible to identify a consistent karyotypic abnormality or to define linked loci. Hence, using the reverse approach, candidate genes were screened for an association with the syndrome and the p53 gene was subsequently identified to be mutated in five out of five Li-Fraumeni families.[7]

2. THE MOLECULAR BIOLOGY OF THE p53 GENE IN LI-FRAUMENI SYNDROME

A number of studies have now been carried out on affected families but not all exhibit mutations in the p53 gene. In a study of eight families, two had p53 mutations, notably at the mutational hot spot of the codon 248 CpG dinucleotide.[8] In a second study of 21 families, seven demonstrated germ line p53 mutations, one of which was an insertive/deletive in exon 4 and the remainder point mutations, three of which affected codon 248.[9] Similarly, there are a series of point mutations which have been identified in Li-Fraumeni syndrome[10,11] together with a splicing mutation.[12]

A number of studies have examined the functional effects of the mutant p53 proteins in the syndrome, particularly with regard to the ability of the mutant to act in a transdominant fashion to inhibit the activity of the wild protein.[13-16] In one of these studies,[13] six out of seven missense mutations disrupted the ability of the wild type protein to inhibit cell growth, but the other behaved as per the wild type protein. When the family was studied in greater detail, it was found that this particular germ line mutation did not form part of the mechanism of predisposition to, in this case, breast cancer. This important exception of a functionally silent germ line mutation should be considered when cancer risk is assessed. However, in the majority of the remaining cases, the germ line p53 mutants are unable to halt cell cycle progression, which is probably a step towards malignancy.

3. THE EFFECT OF p53 MUTATION UPON PREDISPOSITION TO CANCER IN LI-FRAUMENI SYNDROME

That p53 mutations are prevalent in many diverse forms of human tumor suggests that this tumor suppressor gene plays an important role in the development of tumors and may indeed be an important cancer predisposing factor in a diversity of tissues and cell types. In particular, many of the Li-Fraumeni derived cell types are heterozygous with respect to the inactivating mutation and it must therefore be supposed that conversion to the homozygous mutant cell type is a rate limiting cancer predisposing step in any of several tissues. It should be noted, however, that although showing an equivalently wide spectrum of tumor types, Li-Fraumeni syndrome cancers do not follow the same frequencies as are observed in the general population, e.g., the relative occurrence of breast and colon cancer[7] is biased in the direction of breast cancer in Li-Fraumeni syndrome, giving an additional clue as to differences in tissue specific growth control.

The role of sporadic p53 mutations in the development of neoplasia cannot be deduced from a study of Li-Fraumeni syndrome since not only is the frequency of non-Li-Fraumeni germ line p53 mutations not defined in the population, but the syndrome itself may only be manifest in an extreme set of cancer predisposed families where the p53 mutations are more penetrant in a variety of tissues. In addition, the different p53 mutations that have been observed in the syndrome would be expected to exhibit variability in the dominant effects exerted upon the wild type protein, thus manifesting in a variable phenotype.[15]

4. WILL KNOWLEDGE OF p53 MUTATION HELP DIAGNOSIS OF LI-FRAUMENI SYNDROME AND SCREENING FOR PREMALIGNANT CONDITIONS?

This brings us to the rather difficult subject of diagnosis of p53 associated familial cancers. In the first instance, it might be supposed that a polymerase chain reaction analysis for p53 mutation would allow presymptomatic testing for at risk members of known Li-Fraumeni syndrome families. However, for many of the tumor types associated with the syndrome, effective screening programs are not yet available and furthermore: (a) p53 mutations may not occur in all Li-Fraumeni families[8] and so, risk assessment on the basis of p53 mutations may be inaccurate and (b) there are cases of functionally silent germ line mutations[13] making it impossible to assign accurately cancer risk.

5. THE MOLECULAR BASIS OF RADIOACTIVE RESISTANCE IN LI-FRAUMENI SYNDROME

Cells derived from Li-Fraumeni syndrome patients are consistently more resistant to X-irradiation induced cytotoxicity than those from unaffected patients. These data have been derived from two independent studies[3,4] which represent several different affected families. What then, could be the molecular basis of this response? A consequence of mutation in the p53 gene would be an abrogation of the G1/S cell cycle check point and intuitively this should lead to radiosensitivity, as is observed in ataxia telangiectasia. The radioresistance in Li-Fraumeni syndrome indicates that there is probably selective pressure for cell survival which could either be reversion of the p53 mutation or activation of another genetic system which protects against the damaging effects of X-irradiation. This hypothesis is not likely to apply to the G2/M cell cycle checkpoint since G2 arrested (colcemid) and X-irradiated Li-Fraumeni cells accumulate chromatid aberrations (breaks and gaps) to a far greater extent than do normal cells.[17] In this particular study, six members of the family showed a radioresistant phenotype, but of these, only four were shown to have an inherited mutation in the p53 gene, showing that this phenotype may be of a more general nature than that of p53 mutation. Additionally, the differences in chromatid damage were only manifest 0.5 hours postirradiation, implicating a deficiency in the repair process, rather than a direct effect on the events at the G2/M boundary. Thus the cancer predisposing features of Li-Fraumeni syndrome are not likely to be solely manifest by a mutation in p53. There is no doubt that this plays a major role in many Li-Fraumeni cases, but we cannot discount the circumstantial evidence for a more general effect upon either repair of radiation associated damage or ability to replicate damaged DNA. Indeed, his may in part contribute to the acquisition of mutations in genes such as p53. As such, we would expect the DNA replication/perturbation repair (radioresistance) to be manifested in all Li-Fraumeni cases and p53 mutation in a smaller subset, which still allows for the observed pattern in inheritance.

6. CONVERGENCE OF TUMOR PREDISPOSITION IN AT AND LI-FRAUMENI SYNDROME

Lymphoid malignancies and especially those of T cells, are by far the most common form of neoplasia observed in AT patients and constitute approximately 80% of those observed. Similarly, in transgenic mice in which both copies of the p53 gene have been knocked out by gene targeting, there is also a high frequency of lymphoid tumors in postgestational animals. This link may well be related to an inability to correctly process DNA chain breakage, which after all, is part of the normal function of lymphocytes undergoing immunoglobulin gene rearrangements; it may well be that these cells are normally in a highly controlled recombinogenic state. Delay to or disruption of this process could result in a greater error frequency.

The similarities between AT heterozygotes and Li-Fraumeni heterozygotes (heterozygous for p53) is also worthy of note, since both have a higher frequency of both breast and other nonlymphoid cancers. In Li-Fraumeni syndrome, multiple primary cancers are frequent, as is the incidence of recurrence after radiotherapy, which may indicate susceptibility to radiation associated carcinogenesis. This, of course, is a key feature of AT. Furthermore, the increased incidence of breast cancer in AT heterozygotes may be related to low doses of radiation, which could perhaps be acquired during conventional X-ray screening.

7. ANOTHER SYNDROME WHICH PREDISPOSES TO MULTIPLE TUMOR TYPES; von HIPPEL-LINDAU SYNDROME

A number of cancer predisposing conditions are noteworthy for the wide variety of tumors to which they predispose. Of the chromosome breakage syndromes, Bloom's predisposes to leukemia, lymphoma and a number of sarcoma types. As indicated, the cause of BS is likely to be due to a deficiency in the activity of DNA ligase I, and as such, we may consider that this would have a profound effect upon a number of different cell types, particularly those undergoing regeneration. Thus it is not surprising that there is a preponderance of tumors of the hematopoietic system, followed by those in epithelial tissues, which are both usually undergoing a period of self renewal. The second syndrome we have discussed which is expressed by predisposition to a wide variety of tumors is that of Li-Fraumeni syndrome whereby the p53 tumor suppressor gene has profound effects upon the cell cycle. Again, the central role of this protein suggests it may be involved in growth control in a number of different cell types. Another syndrome, that of von Hippel-Lindau disease is also noteworthy in this regard. This disease is autosomal dominant, occurring at a frequency of 1:35,000 with the average age at diagnosis being 26.[18] Gene penetrance increases rapidly up to the age of approximately 45 and thereafter levels out in the 90% to 100% range. Sporadic incidents of von Hippel-Lindau disease may be more frequent than is realized currently, since diagnosis requires a combination of hemangioblastomas to be identified. However, given the familial incidence, the frequencies and diagnosis of inherited von Hippel-Lindau disease should be fairly accurate. This has been greatly facilitated by the availability of closely linked DNA probes to chromosome region 3p which can be used for prenatal and presymptomatic diagnosis of at risk family members.

As indicated the most common tumor types are angioblastomas, although renal cell carcinoma is the leading cause of death in von Hippel-Lindau disease, which is in part probably due to the high risk of metastasis in this condition. The majority of patients will eventually develop renal cell carcinoma if they survive and to date, the importance of this tumor type has probably been underestimated due to the later mean age of diagnosis (at 44) when compared to the hemangioblastomas.

Markers either side of the chromosome 3p region thought to be responsible for von Hippel-Lindau disease have been identified[19-21] and to date there does not appear to be significant locus heterogeneity. It is likely that the von Hippel-Lindau gene functions as a tumor suppressor gene and the genetics are similar to that observed for retinoblastoma.[18,20] Indeed, the mutation frequency (4.4 x 10^6 mutations/gene/generation) is similar to what might be expected for retinoblastoma. It is expected that the identification of the von Hippel-Lindau gene will reveal a significant tumor suppressor gene locus, not only providing a useful diagnostic tool but giving further insight into the cellular processes which contribute to loss of growth control. As with p53 and Rb, the von Hippel-Lindau gene product is expected to be a central protein in the regulation of growth and of a variety of cell types; following previous precedents, this is likely to be central to the preponderance of multiple tumor types. These syndromes (BS, von Hippel-Lindau and Li-Fraumeni) contrast with several of the other cancer predisposing syndromes (AT, FA) which are generally associated with only one or a few tumor types, with XP being somewhere in the middle, since its effect is most prevalent after mutagen exposure. It is expected that the defect in these latter syndromes will be of a more cell or tissue specific nature.

Table 16.2. Tumor frequency in von Hippel-Lindau disease

Tumor type	Frequency
Retinal hemangioblastoma	60%
Cerebellar hemangioblastoma	60%
Renal cell carcinoma	28%
Brain stem hemangioblastoma	18%
Spinal hemangioblastoma	13-44%
Pheochromocytoma	7%

(References 20,23)

8. INHERITANCE OF DEFECTS IN GENOMIC IMPRINTING; BECKWITH-WIEDEMANN SYNDROME

The characteristics of Beckwith-Wiedemann syndrome are particularly interesting with regard to possible mechanisms of cancer predisposition. Patients with this syndrome are predisposed to intra-abdominal tumors (Wilms' tumor, adrenal carcinoma and hepatoblastoma) at an early age (< 5 years). Indeed, Wilms' tumor is 700 times more frequent in Beckwith-Wiedemann syndrome when compared to the normal population. The mode of inheritance appears to be autosomal dominant but there is considerable diversity in disease expression, which is associated with incomplete gene penetrance. Familial cases indicate siblings with full penetrance (a 50% probability of being affected), but unaffected carriers show incomplete penetrance, which is increased in degree if the mother is the transmitting parent. Together with the detection of paternal disomy for chromosome 11p15, in nonfamilial cases this indicates that genomic imprinting may be involved. It is thus of interest that a loss of heterozygosity at the 11p15 location has been associated with a number of tumor types. In the mouse, two genes (H19 and IGF-II) located on the distal region of chromosome 7 undergo maternal and paternal imprinting respectively, which has now also been observed in humans.[24,25] Many Wilms' kidney tumors show biallelic expression which may be the result of either a loss or a relaxation of imprinting. If proven this could represent a new mechanism for predisposition to cancer. However, imprinting effects must be distinguished from the possibility of a Wilms' tumor arising from expansion of small population of embryonic cells which for some reason already exhibit biallelic expression at a particular locus. One candidate is the IGF-II gene which is normally expressed from the parental allele, but is expressed biallelically in Wilms' tumor. This locus has been associated with both Wilms' tumors and with Beckwith-Wiedemann syndrome. The preferred maternal transmission and variable penetrance of the Beckwith-Wiedemann syndrome 'gene' could be explained via altered imprinting of the IGF-II gene. The extent of this defect may be related to the risk of cancer development in patients with this syndrome.

References

1. Li FP, Fraumeni JF. Soft tissue sarcomas, breast cancer and other neoplasm: a familial syndrome? Ann Int Med 1969; 71:747-52.
2. Hartley AL, Birch JM, Marsden HB et al. Malignant melanoma in families of children with osteosarcoma, chondrosarcoma and adrenocortical carcinoma. J Med Genet 1987; 24:664-8.
3. Chang EH, Pirollo KF, Zou ZQ et al. Oncogenes from a cancer prone family. Science 1987; 237:1036-1039.
4. Bech-Hansen NT, Blattner WA, Sell BM et al. Transmission of in vitro radioresistance in a cancer prone family. Lancet 1987; 1:1335-37.
5. Strong LC, Williams WR, Tainsky MA. The Li-Fraumeni syndrome: from clinical epidemiology to molecular genetics. (Review). Am J Epidemiol 1992; 135(2):190-9.
6. Birch JM, Hartley AL, Blair V et al. The Li-Fraumeni cancer family syndrome. J Path 1990; 161:1-2.
7. Malkin D, Li F, Strong L et al. Geron line p53 mutations in a familial syndrome of breast cancer, sarcomas and other neoplasms. Science 1990; 250:1233-38.
8. Antibanez-Koref MF, Birch JM, Hartley et al. p53 germline mutations in Li-Fraumeni syndrome. Lancet 1991; 338:1490-1.
9. Birch JM, Hartley AL, Tricker KJ et al. Prevalence and diversity of constitutional mutations in the p53 gene among 21 Li-Fraumeni families. Cancer Res 1994; 54:1298-304.
10. Law JC, Strong LC, Chidambaram A et al. A germ line mutation in exon 5 of the p53 gene in an extended cancer family. Cancer Res 1991; 51:6385-7.
11. Srivastava S, Tong YA, Devadas K et al. Detection of both mutant and wild-type p53 protein in normal skin fibroblasts and demonstration of a shared 'second hit' on p53 in diverse tumors from a cancer-prone family with Li-Fraumeni syndrome. Oncogene 1992; 7:987-91.
12. Warneford SG, Witton LJ, Townsend ML et al. Germ-line splicing mutation of the p53 gene in a cancer-prone family. Cell Growth Different 1992; 3:839-46.
13. Frebourg T, Kassel J, Lam KT. Germ-line mutations of the p53 tumor suppressor gene in patients with high risk for cancer inactivate the p53 protein. Proc Natl Acad Sci USA 1992; 89:6413-7.
14. Hao M, Finlay, Lozano G. A functionally inactive p53 Li-Fraumeni syndrome mutant. Oncogene 1993; 8:299-306.
15. Srivastava S, Wang S, Tong YA et al. Dominant negative effect of a germ-line mutant p53: a step fostering tumorigenesis. Cancer Res 1993a; 53:4452-5.
16. Srivastava S, Wang S, Tong YA et al. Several mutant p53 proteins detected in cancer-prone families with Li-Fraumeni syndrome exhibit transdominant effects on the biochemical properties of the wild-type p53. Oncogene 1993b; 8:2449-56.
17. Parshad R, Price FM, Pirollo KF et al. Cytogenic response to G2-phase X irradiation in relation to DNA repair and radiosensitivity in a cancer-prone family with Li-Fraumeni syndrome. Radiation Res 1993; 136(2):236-40.
18. Maher ER, Iselius L, Yates JRW et al. von Hippel-Lindau disease: a genetic study. J Med Genet 1991a; 28:443-447.
19. Hosoe S, Brauch H, Latif F. Localisation of the von Hippel-Lindau disease gene to a small region of chromosome 3. Genomics 1990; 8:634-640.
20. Maher ER, Bentley E, Yates JRW et al. Mapping of the von Hippel-Lindau disease locus to a small region of chromosome 3p by genetic linkage analysis. Genomics

1991b; 10:957-960.

21. Seizinger B, Smith D, Fitting-Katz et al. Genetic flanking markers refine the diagnostic criteria and provide new insights into the genetics of von Hippel-Lindau disease. Proc Natl Acad Sci USA 1991; 88: 2864-2868.
22. Tory K, Brauch M, Linehamm et al. Specific genetic change in tumours associated with von Hippel-Lindau disease. J. Natl. Cancer Institute 1989; 81:1097-1101.
23. Fittig-Katz MR, Choyke P, Patronas N et al. Central nervous involvement in von Hippel-Lindau disease. Neurology 1991; 41:41-46.
24. Rainier S, Johnson L, Dobry C et al. Relaxation of imprinted genes in human cancer. Nature 362:747-749.
25. Ogawa O, Eccles M, Szeto J et al. Relaxation of insulin like growth factor II gene imprinting implicated in Wilm's tumour. Nature 362:749-751.

SECTION 4

Pathways to Cancer

From reading the contents of this book, one lesson should be clear: that understanding cancer as a disease is as ephemeral as the disease itself. No sooner that an interesting 'breakthrough' is discovered, than new avenues of stunning complexity are opened, always asking more questions than they answer. In this section we will attempt to draw the threads of this complex web together. Given the current state of the art, there is no panacea or universal model, yet many of the necessary tools have now been made and the scene is set for some very exciting developments.

CHAPTER 17

THE MOLECULAR MECHANISMS OF TRANSFORMATION

1. FAMILIAL INHERITANCE

Within the population, there are some obvious examples of families which are predisposed to particular types of cancer and the identification of the cause of this predisposition is of crucial importance, as is the identification of factors which may contribute to or enhance the progress of the disease. It is our treatise that we are all genetically predisposed to cancer, to a greater or lesser degree, whether this be in an obvious high gene penetrance family or more subtle effects due to inheritance of genes of low penetrance. If we are to accept the continuum of transformation hypotheses, then this must indeed be so. However, the effects of external influences throughout life and indeed, upon the preceding generations make the identification of familial clustering of such mutations extremely difficult. We have described both the molecular steps which lead to a particular colorectal carcinoma and the hormonal changes which may lead to breast cancer. Both tumor types show evidence of familial clustering, with the search for the relevant gene relying upon the application of reverse genetics, i.e., the use of genetic linkage to empirically determined markers. An additional approach is to use the pre-existing examples of the cancer predisposing syndromes to identify the responsible genes via biochemical analysis and complementation assays. It is here that defects in DNA repair, cell cycle control, tumor suppressor genes or other mechanisms may be operative and the task becomes one of extracting the valuable lessons from inherited cancer in order to apply them to the more frequently occurring forms of sporadic cancer.

A spectrum of inherited cancer predisposition can be identified within the human population and ranges from a strong family history of an uncommon cancer (e.g. retinoblastoma, multiple endocrine neoplasia) to those where the familial clustering can be identified, but due to other genetic and environmental factors, individuals may or may not be affected (e.g. breast cancer or HNPCC). In some cases, familial clusters may be either rare or very difficult to discern, e.g., differences in the ability to metabolize carcinogens. The corollary of course, is that some families may be genetically resistant to cancer and exhibit protective rather than predisposing factors. We know the benefits of caloric restriction and a high intake of fresh fruits and vegetables, both of which may be related to free radical metabolism. But these are environmental influences; are there genetic factors which remain to be discovered? Do these exhibit familial clustering?

Clearly then, the study of familial inheritance and the cancer prone syndromes affords the opportunity to elucidate the molecular changes which lead to cancer in both sporadic and inherited forms of cancer. Before discussing an integrated model for the transformation process, we will summarize those effects which may influence the choice between cell proliferation, differentiation and apoptosis.

2. INTEGRATION OF THE TRANSFORMATION RELATED PATHWAYS

The cells of a given lineage originate from a stem cell population and generally reduce in proliferative potential as they differentiate. Upon receipt of suitable signals they also retain the option to self-destruct, or apoptose. The primary source of such signals is the extracellular environment, whereby the action of cytokines impinge upon the cell surface receptors and hence transduce signals across the plasma membrane, into the cytoplasm and thus to the nucleus where they affect the transcription of relevant genes. We have discussed at length the critical role of the signal transduction pathway in control of the cell's fate and it should be obvious that there is a complex balance between interacting proteins which have both positive and negative effects. Accordingly, these have been given operational classifications as oncogenes, tumor suppressor genes, anti-oncogenes etc. There are of course many other gene products which impinge upon these processes, which have not been labeled and which are of equally profound effect upon the transformation process. Indeed, the ostensibly smaller and more subtle effects are arguably the initiating events and although they are more difficult to identify, it is these which should receive attention. Such steps include: (a) the effect of proteins which protect against deleterious effects of exogenous chemicals and toxic by products of metabolism (e.g. the phase I and II detoxification systems, those involved in destroying oxygen free radicals), (b) the effects of 'mutator genes', (c) DNA repair enzymes, (d) the intercellular interactions via adhesion molecules and the effects of local proteolysis and (e) changes in immunoresponsiveness. Intermeshed with these factors are, of course, the effects of exogenous influences such as mutagenic chemicals from the diet and environment, the effects of viral (e.g. HPV, EBV, Hepatitis B) and bacterial (*H. pylori*) infection and the effects of changes in hormone levels associated with, for example, aging and pregnancy.

3. THE IMPACT OF THE CANCER PRONE INHERITED SYNDROMES

The chromosome breakage syndromes (AT, BS, FA), together with XP, demonstrate some important principles in the development of cancer. Firstly, they emphasize the importance of DNA repair pathways at an early stage in the genesis of the tumor and secondly, they provide a general mechanism for the accumulation of mutation in human cells. To some extent the recent enthusiasm for oncogene biology has been misplaced and it is now obvious that oncogene activation is usually only a consequence of more profound changes that have gone before, notably changes in tumor suppressor gene biology and mutator phenotype. In AT the sensitivity to γ radiation has revealed a cascade which leads towards the p53 tumor suppressor gene. In the absence of one of the AT gene products, of which there must be at least five to match the number of complementation groups, the product of the GADD45 gene is not induced and in turn, neither is p53. The cell, whilst maybe still carrying out its proofreading role, cannot adequately arrest at the G1-S boundary and so attempts to replicate damaged

DNA, ultimately leading to cell death. The radioresistance phenotype which is observed in Li-Fraumeni syndrome is more difficult to reconcile, especially as some, but not all families inherit a p53 mutation. Perhaps the most likely explanation is that the p53 mutation cosegregates with a locus which confers radioresistance. In any event, acquisition of a mutant p53 will be associated with an inability to halt at the G1/S checkpoint which in both cases could increase the probability of acquiring a transforming mutation subsequent to exposure to low concentrations of oxygen free radicals. Mechanisms for radioresistance are likely to be quite complex and could involve proteins such as quinoline reductase, the cytochrome p450 complex and glutathione-*S*-transferase.

The necessity for the repair of DNA damage as a means to avoid transforming mutations is exemplified by XP, where several of the complementation groups now have proteins assigned to them. Remarkably, these cluster around the DNA nucleotide excision repair function and in particular, two of these groups encode DNA helicases which appear to act in opposite directions, presumably to aid in opening the helix to allow access to single strand binding protein and the repair complexes. Some of these proteins (e.g. the transcription factor TFIIH) are shared between the repair and replication functions, again providing a rationalization for some of the clinical characteristics of XP. The skin tumors which are prevalent in XP are likely to result from an inability to correctly repair UV associated DNA damage, particularly the highly mutagenic 6-4 pyrimidine-pyrimidones. The increased frequency of internal cancers in XP patients may be explained by the spontaneous occurrence of the 6-4 photoproducts and their inefficient repair, although this cannot be directly associated with UV light. The prevalence of neurological defects in XP is again difficult to reconcile by consideration of a DNA repair defect, but may be associated with altered transcription of relevant gene families.

The BS example is another where a pathway towards a cancer predisposing step can be identified as having origins in a DNA repair process. The inherited 'BS' mutation probably codes for a protein which has a central role in the modulation of DNA repair and DNA replication enzymes, not the least of which is DNA ligase I. Indeed, the reduced activity of DNA ligase I in BS can be used to rationalize many of the clinical and cellular characteristics of the syndrome, such as the high frequency of SCE's and the sensitivity to a wide range of mutagens. The deficiency in DNA ligase I is likely to increase the intracellular level of DNA strand breakage, which in itself is an inducing signal for the c-*myc* oncogene protein. Higher constitutive levels of c-*myc* protein may then contribute towards the transformation pathway.

Other cancer prone syndromes exemplify alternative mechanisms of cancer predisposition via inheritance, such as the maternal imprinting observed in Beckwith-Wiedemann syndrome and the inheritance of a putative tumor suppressor gene locus in van Hippel-Lindau syndrome. The latter is of course similar to the inheritance of p53 mutations in Li-Fraumeni syndrome.

Although not classified as syndromes, there are several examples of familial clustering and inheritance of cancer predisposing factors, as is observed in FAP. Similarly, several cancers may have identifiable precancerous stages which contribute towards the neoplasia, such as is observed in myelodysplastic syndrome and Barrett's esophagus.

4. THE PATHWAY TO MALIGNANCY

From the discussions herein, it should be apparent that there are a plethora of distinct stages through which a cell must transgress in order to attain a malignant phenotype. It is both the interdependence and independence of these stages which holds the key to the understanding of the transformation pathway. There are five main stages on the pathway to malignancy which can be identified as critical events, i.e., when the cell crosses each of these boundaries it reaches a 'point of no return' and different mechanisms must be used to elicit rescue, e.g., immune surveillance and apoptosis. These stages are: (a) the preinitiation step, a step above and beyond the 'background' level of cancer predisposition, (b) a tumor initiating event, expansion of the initiated population, (c) progression towards the transformed phenotype, i.e., the several steps towards malignant conversion, (d) clonal expansion and finally, (e) metastasis.

i. The Preinitiating Event

Those proteins which alter the levels of both exogenous and endogenous DNA damaging agents will affect individual tumor predisposition. For example, a reduction in the concentration of oxygen free radicals or an increase in the ability to detoxicate mutagens will all tend to be protective factors. Any change which increases the local concentration of oxygen free radical species will increase the probability of a mutagenic event. Since the cancer process requires an average of one mutation every 10 years, then even small perturbations in oxygen free radical concentration may have significant effect. Such enzymes will include the cytochrome P450 system although it should be noted that besides detoxication, these enzymes are involved in making particular compounds more mutagenic by increasing their water solubility. This is of course essential to the activation of particular chemotherapeutic agents.

In assuming a preinitiation event(s) we must also assume a background level of cancer predisposition, being the set of factors that are likely to contribute towards this process in any given individual. As we move down the pathway, the 'background ' level at any particular point in time will probably increase, being balanced by the protective factors which contrive to maintain growth control. Thus individuals with a cancer prone syndrome could have an intrinsically higher 'background' level of cancer predisposition at an equivalent point in their life cycle.

Preinitiating events may also include systemic effects such as inflammatory responses, whereby local production of cytokines (IL-1 etc.) or wounding (PDGF, EGF) may affect cell proliferation, and under certain rare circumstances, trigger a transforming change via clonal selection. Similarly, changes in the local concentration of hormones may alter the cellular growth environment.

ii. The Initiating Event

The initiating event occurs when a mutation becomes fixed within the DNA and could occur, for example, as a result of a mutator phenotype or inadequacy of the DNA repair system.

A mutator phenotype can occur with slippage of the DNA polymerase during replication, as is observed with HNPCC, where the extent of genomic instability can range from a minor addition to a substantial change in repeat length which can in itself be heterogeneous. Such mutations will defy repair since there is no departure from expected DNA structures. Overloading or reduction in DNA repair activity will also lead to mutation and this can be mediated by changes at any of the three stages of DNA repair: (a) temporary cessation of the cell cycle, (b) recognition and removal of damaged bases and (c) the activities of the DNA polymerases, DNA ligases and poly ADP-ribose polymerase. Cancer predisposition examples occur for all three stages being: (a) AT, (b) XP, CS and probably FA, and (c) BS respectively.

iii. Expansion of the Initiated Cell

The initiated cell will now have the ammunition for a selective growth advantage, depending upon which genes have been mutated. These changes must be related to a loss of cellular growth control and to some extent must participate in progression of the cell cycle. Such genes could include: extracellular signaling molecules, changes in cell surface receptors, changes in membrane associated signal transduction molecules, changes in cytoplasmic and nuclear signal transduction molecules and alterations in cell-cell communication. The clonal selection process will allow a particular cell type to expand at the expense of its neighbors and assuming that mutation is a stochastic process, the chances of acquiring a second mutation in the clone will be correspondingly higher. A particularly clear example is seen in Barrett's esophagus where the expansion of a progressively transformed cell population can be observed throughout the lifetime of the individual. However, one might argue that in the worst case, any given mutation might increase the probability of a second given mutation, further increasing the clonal selective advantage. Viral and bacterial infections may augment tumor formation by accelerating the clonal selection process and helping to select for transforming changes. There is a spectrum of potency with regard to the tumorigenicity associated with viral agents and one should not discount the contribution of apparently benign viruses; they all replicate by utilizing the cell's own DNA replication machinery and thus require a cell which is actively engaged in the cell cycle.

iv. Malignant Conversion

The final steps in the genesis of a tumor are associated firstly with the inactivation of tumor suppressor genes (loss of heterozygosity etc. in retinoblastoma, Wilms' tumor and Li-Fraumeni associated tumors) and secondly, with the activation of oncogenes. Freshly isolated tumor types often show a spectrum of different gene inactivation/activations and indeed, this may even vary within examples of the same tumor. Therefore, as a guide to tumorigenesis, these genes are often of poor diagnostic value. In addition, activated oncogenes are often of such profound effect to the cell that they are not inherited. The inheritance of tumor suppressor genes is of course permitted, because the heterozygote will have one normal copy of the relevant gene.

v. Metastasis

Usually at the end of the transformation pathway, genetic changes in metastatic potential per se cannot be said to contribute towards cancer predisposition and the two processes are probably under the control of a separate set of genes. However, it is expected that the cell adhesion molecules will prove to be critical to this process and could contribute towards clonal selection at an early stage by reducing intracellular communication and facilitating freedom from the normal local environmental growth constraints. The efficiency and effectiveness of the immune system will be of profound importance to this stage of the cancer process since this is the primary mechanism for removal of expatriated cells.

5. A Pathway to Cancer Predisposition

The cumulative effects of the protective and predisposing factors outlined in this text are indicated (Fig. 17.1). The processes of initiation and clonal selection implied therein are often of a reiterative nature with a series of mutations being acquired throughout the lifetime of the organism. In the cases of the inherited syndromes and of familial inheritance, this pathway will be accelerated by either: (a) bypassing certain steps or (b) accelerating progression through them. In the normal population, one in four will develop cancer and the probability of so doing increases with age. This is in part due to decreased efficiency of the DNA repair and immune surveillance systems, but must also reflect the cumulative acquisition of mutations, some of which may no longer be expressed. The spectrum of cancer predisposition in individuals of a given age, identical diet and exposure to environmental agents will by definition, have a normal distribution. Thus the likelihood of a given individual succumbing to cancer will be a balance between predisposing and protective factors, this being a complex combination of both interacting and noninteracting genetic influences. Shifting the balance will determine the extent of cancer proneness and cancer resistance.

The pathway to cancer is indeed complex; the myriad of relevant interacting factors has to date defied elucidation and we believe that the key to understanding the transformation process lies therein; the problem is not now one of identification of 'cancer genes' by molecular biology, but one of satisfactory dissection of the biology of the cell, of the biochemical functions of the relevant proteins and above all, how they interact to cause transformation.

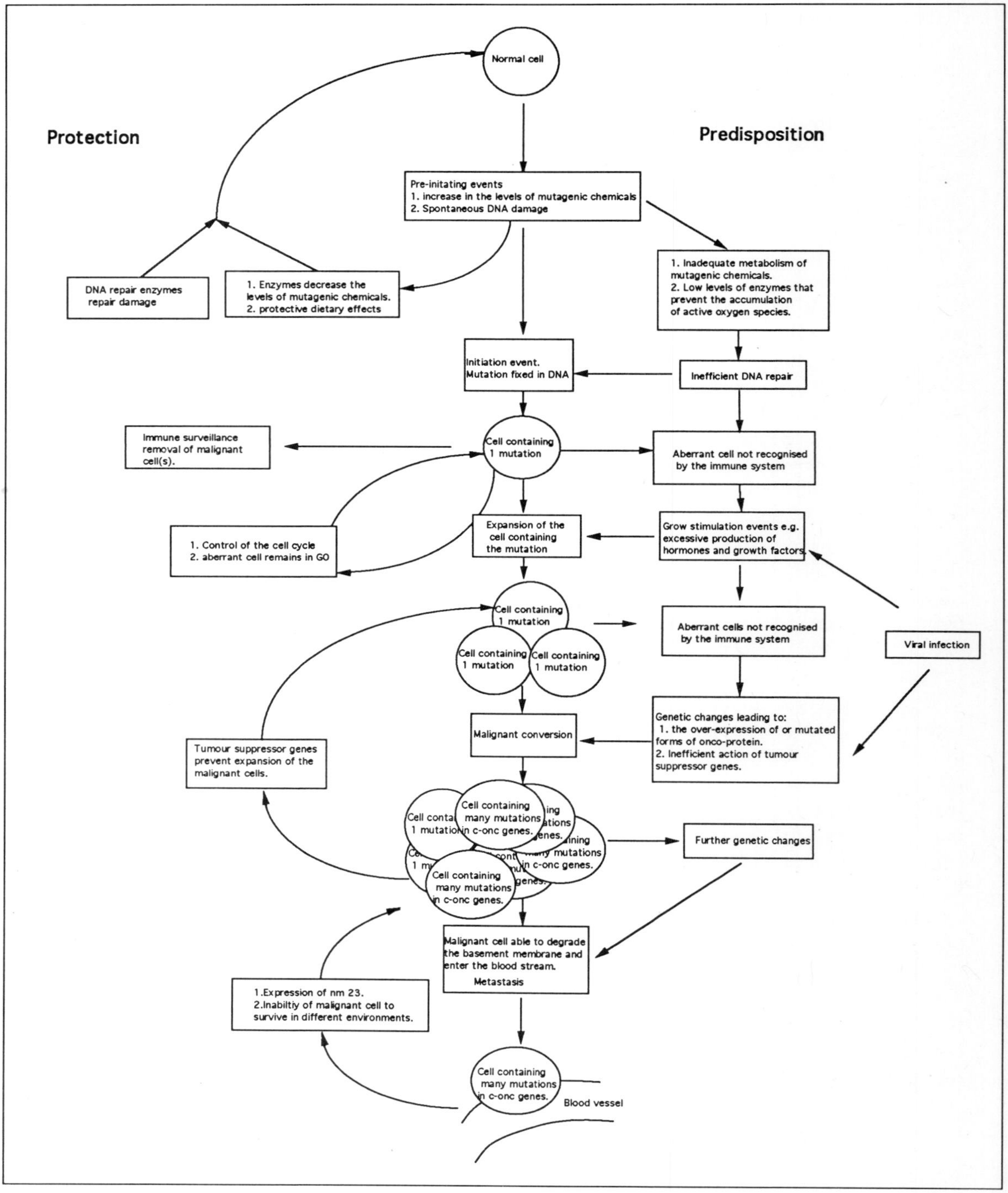

Fig. 17.1. The cancer predisposition pathway.

INDEX

Page numbers in italics denote figures (f) and tables (t).